APPRAISING RESEARCH INTO CHILDBIRTH

An Interactive Workbook

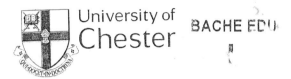

University of Chester   BACHE EDU

For Elsevier:

Commissioning Editor: Mary Seager
Development Editor: Rebecca Nelemans
Project Manager: Elouise Ball
Designer: Andy Chapman

APPRAISING RESEARCH INTO CHILDBIRTH

An Interactive Workbook

Edited by

Sara Wickham RM MA BA(Hons) PGCert

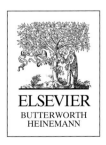

ELSEVIER
BUTTERWORTH
HEINEMANN

EDINBURGH   LONDON   NEW YORK   OXFORD   PHILADELPHIA   ST LOUIS   SYDNEY   TORONTO   2006

ELSEVIER
BUTTERWORTH
HEINEMANN

First published 2006
  Reprinted 2009

ISBN: 13: 978 07506 8849 9

British Library Cataloguing in Publication Data
A catalogue record for this book is available from the British Library

Library of Congress Cataloging in Publication Data
A catalog record for this book is available from the Library of Congress

Printed in China

ELSEVIER   your source for books,
            journals and multimedia
            in the health sciences
www.elsevierhealth.com

The
publisher's
policy is to use
**paper manufactured
from sustainable forests**

Contents

Acknowledgements

Thanks to all of the people who have helped make this book: Mary Seager, who came up with the idea; Rebecca Nelemans, who was always helpful and cheerful in the face of a million questions; Carol Hagino, whose book inspired this one; each of the chapter authors, who bravely ventured into this very different kind of writing; Trish Anderson and Nadine Edwards, who deserve special thanks for all the time they have spent on the phone helping me work out how everything could fit together; Lorna Davies, Penny Champion and Lucyann Ashdown, who read parts of Sections 1 and 6, provided really useful suggestions and excellent respite care when I needed a break; Jan Tritten, who asked me to teach research critiquing to a couple of hundred midwives first thing on a Sunday morning and thus prompted me to create some of the alternative approaches to teaching research which are in this book; Ishvar Sheran, who not only shared his professional expertise in writing a chapter with me but brought about a million cups of tea to me while I wrote; and, by no means least, all of the students, midwives and others who have allowed me to think and teach about research in different ways.

Introduction

Welcome to this book, which has been lovingly compiled for you by myself and a team of midwives and therapists who have expertise in research and who, like the authors of the original papers re-published here, have put their thoughts and theories on the line for you, the reader! As well as some information, tools, resources and discussion from me, this book contains eight chapters by different authors, and it is designed to be fun to use and read! Each of these chapters contains a full-length original research study, which is sandwiched between an introduction and a discussion written by the chapter author. The research studies themselves look very different from when they were first published in journals, as they now have little notes and questions surrounding them, which are designed to help you think more deeply about the research, and appraise its value for your practice. (I'll come back to what we mean by appraisal in a few pages, if I may, where I'll say a little bit more about how research can be fun as well!)

This book sets out to do a number of things. It aims to help people who have read a research textbook or undertaken a research module to practise what they have learned in relation to real, 'live' research. If you are reading this book without having done any study about research, and you are the kind of person who likes to have some theory before you try things out in practice, then you might want to get hold of a 'theoretical' research book as well. However, this book also aims to be a tool for the kind of people who prefer to 'do' things straight away in order to learn them, and who find they don't learn as well when they have to sit through a lot of lectures or read a load of theory before trying something out for themselves. If you are one of those people, or you are feeling particularly brave, then you might like to pile into this book without prior study, and we have provided some basic information and a few tools, tips and checklists in this introductory section to help you. However, you may find you also need to look up some of the terminology in a book or on the internet as you go along.

We have also aimed to make this book work as a revision tool for people who have studied research in the past but who feel more comfortable with one kind of research design than others, or who want to expand their skills and thinking in this area. Because it is important to make as many little neural pathways in your brain as possible, and to be able to think in different ways, we have tried hard to be creative in the way we talk about research, and we have tried to ensure that there is something new in this book for everyone, whatever your level of experience.

Getting the most out of this book...

You can use this book in a number of ways, and I have some suggestions about how you can do this, although the most important thing is that you feel free to use it in whatever way best suits your style of learning. You can, of course, start at the beginning and work through it to the end, and it has been laid out so that this will take you through research in a logical and relatively orderly manner. However, we all know that lots of people don't like to read books that way, so we have tried to cross-reference things backwards and forwards, in case you want to start somewhere in the middle! Regardless of the order in which you decide to read the book, there are also a number of ways in which you can use the individual chapters. One way is to read an article, temporarily ignoring the introductory text, boxes and questions at first, and see what you think of it. You could make a few notes and then check your thoughts against what the chapter author has said about the research. Of course, you and they might have picked up different things, and that doesn't make anybody right or wrong, but more about that in a minute... Hopefully, your confidence will get a boost when you realise that you have managed to highlight some of the same key points as someone who is experienced at critiquing. Another option is to read the whole of one section, including the introduction, and answer the questions which are in the boxes beside the article as you go along. This will help you to check your knowledge: you might find, for instance, that you know all the answers to the questions about data collection, but sometimes get stuck on questions about analysis, and this will help you find out where your learning needs are in relation to research.

If it's been a while since you studied research, or if you are returning to practice after a break, you might, again, want to use the book to test your knowledge, and see where your learning needs lie. Also, don't forget that you could include notes, reflection, etc. on the work you have done with this book in your portfolio as evidence of continuing professional development.

A word about 'right' and 'wrong'

Although we live in a society that tends to be fairly quick to judge things as 'right' or 'wrong', and to label scientific ways of knowing as superior to the knowledge we gather through our own personal experiences, this is only one way of seeing the world, and it is not the way that most of the people involved in this book see the world. As they were working on these research articles, and the questions that went alongside them, some of the chapter authors would phone me up and say things like, 'It's so difficult to ask "yes or no" questions, because there is no easy yes/no answer!'. They are absolutely right: the world we live in is often more about shades of grey than about black and white. Objective, concrete statements are, in real life, often not appropriate. In other words, our world is a very subjective one, and people have many different perspectives and ideas about it.

However, if we took the stance that there is no right or wrong to the extreme, it would be very difficult to write a research study or a book about anything! The people who do – and write up – research are exhibiting a good deal of bravery, as are the people who critique the research and share their thoughts on it. Many people are understandably afraid to publish their thoughts or their findings because they know they will be subject to criticism, which might not feel good.

There is, in my opinion, never a perfect way of doing research to find something out. Because our world is messy, complex and bursting with our humanity, there will always be things that get in the way of the goal of objectivity. Even with the kind of research that is deemed to be the most objective, the experimental randomised controlled trial, there are many things that can influence the results. For instance, many of the outcomes that are measured in research are not objective because they are based on individual interpretation. An example of a fairly objective outcome measure would be something like 'Is the baby a boy or a girl?' or 'Is this person alive or dead?'. Although there is a small area of greyness in each of these areas (the baby who is of indeterminate sex, or the person who is alive but only because he or she is on medical, mechanical life support), in most cases, there would be a high degree of agreement on the answer to these questions between different observers. However, many quantitative birth-related studies measure things like the Apgar score, or cervical dilation, or whether the woman needs to have her placenta manually removed, and different people will assess these things differently. (Are there any midwives who have not experienced the situation where someone else did a vaginal examination just after they did one and had a different opinion?!)

Researchers also have to work within a number of constraints, which might include limited resources (e.g. money, time, available expertise, assistance), ethical considerations and practical limitations. When they come to publish their findings, they might be limited by other things, including the word limit on articles in the journal in which they publish, conventions about the order in which you write up your work (something which Ruth Deery has written more about in Chapter 7) and which parts of their research the peer reviewers, journal editors and publishers want them to focus on. Journal editors and publishers, in turn, are constrained by other things that, again, serve to demonstrate just how complex all of this is in reality!

So by the time the research gets to you – the consumer – the authors of research studies have had to make lots of compromises and this inevitably leads to apparent limitations in their work. I have never read a research study that could not be criticised for something or other, and I trust that the authors, editors and publishers of the articles in this book know that we selected their work not because we felt that it was poor (in fact, we deliberately avoided research that we felt was poor because we wanted to be able to show examples of good practice as well as pointing out how hard it is to do unbiased research) and feel that the inclusion of their work in this book is a compliment because their work is interesting and useful. For all of these reasons, I would like to honour both the authors of the original studies in this book and the chapter authors who have critiqued the original articles for having the courage to share their thoughts and findings.

As you read this book, you will discover that there is an 'Answers' section after each research paper, which gives the chapter authors' answers to the questions they have posed. For all of the reasons discussed in this section, you (or whoever is teaching your research course) might disagree with some of the answers given. This might be because we have made an error, although hopefully not, as we have checked the book very carefully! It is more likely that this is because research appraisal is no more exact than actually designing and doing research. It is not uncommon for people to have subjective differences of opinion on these things. If your answer disagrees with one of those given, and you still feel that yours is correct, you might like to use this as an opportunity to reflect more on the area in question and consider why opinions might differ.

So what do we mean by appraisal?

Given everything I've said above about there being no perfect way to do research, we need to make decisions about how useful a research study is for us in practice, or in providing information upon which we can base a decision. It often comes as a surprise to the first-year student midwives that I teach when they realise that not everything published in a midwifery or medical journal is 'good' research! Appraisal, then, simply means evaluation: giving something a value, or deciding whether it is going to be useful for us. At a very basic level, for something to be useful it needs to have set out to answer a question which is relevant to our needs, and to have done that in a way which we feel will get us as close to an answer as is possible in our messy, complex, human world.

Just a couple more things!

This book is divided into six sections. The first section offers some more information about appraisal and those tools, tips and checklists I mentioned above that might help you to appraise research for use in your practice or decision making. Each of the next four sections includes a short introduction on a theme and then two chapters where you can read and work through an original research study with the help of the chapter author(s). The themes have been chosen for their relevance and importance to women and midwives and I will pop up again at the beginning of each section to talk a little bit more about each. The final section offers some further resources which might be useful if you want to look further into specific areas.

Finally, I'd like to go back to the idea of research being fun! A number of people seem to feel that things like research, science, statistics, qualitative analysis and so on are both hard to understand and boring to spend a lot of time on! This isn't helped by the ways in which these subjects are sometimes taught, especially when teachers project lots of words onto the classroom wall (one of my teaching friends calls this 'death by acetate'!) and try to get you to learn the theory, terminology and/or definitions without giving examples or otherwise 'making it real'. About 8 years ago, Trish Anderson and I were asked to teach a session on critiquing research at an international midwifery conference first thing on a Sunday morning – I couldn't imagine a worse combination of topic and timing, and it was clear that drastic action was called for! In the hope of keeping everyone up and awake rather than sending them back to bed, I came up with an idea that involved us offering sweets to the audience and planning a study to see which kind of sweet made midwives happier, simultaneously talking about all of the potential problems and sources of bias that might arise (for instance, that there is no way of making a placebo sweet, so the study cannot be 'blind'). Because the session worked better than anything else I had previously tried, I took it back into my work as a midwife teacher and began to teach research by using what became known as 'the jelly baby study'. Some of the student midwives I have taught actually told me they looked forward to learning about research because they heard from their colleagues that it would be fun, that they got to eat sweets and that they would learn through their own experiences (of being participants in a research study) rather than by looking at words on the wall.

For all these reasons I have become convinced that, if you can make research friendly and fun, if you can talk about it in real-life (rather than purely theoretical) ways, and if you can involve people by helping them think about how they might react to different things if they were participating in the study, you end up with a situation where people realise that research is not actually as difficult to get to grips with as they thought. Many of the ideas and examples that I have developed over the last few years (including a fair few references to jelly babies!) are shared in this book, and each of the people involved in this book has been invited to write in a more informal style than they might otherwise do. So if it feels at times like we are having a little chat with you rather than giving a lecture or a lesson, then we will have achieved our aim! (By the way, if you don't like the idea of us chatting to you in a book, then you will find lots of research books out there that will gladly lecture you!)

So we invite you to gather jelly babies or chocolate along with your pens and pencils, and sit back and enjoy the book!

Sara Wickham

A few tools, tips and checklists

APPRAISAL AND BIAS

As I've already said in the introduction, appraising a piece of research is simply about deciding how much value we will assign to it. There is no such thing as the 'perfect' research study and it can be helpful to think about this as a simple statement:

All research is potentially biased, and your job is simply to look for those potential sources of bias.

Once you have found the potential sources of bias, it is then a relatively simple job to decide whether the research is of use to you.

I often offer research students the idea that there are two main sources of bias to look for in studies relating to childbirth. These are:

1. bias in methods
2. bias in philosophy.

Looking for bias in the research methods includes thinking about all of the decisions made during the research and whether any of them might have led to biased results. For instance, if the authors claim that their sample is representative but you can clearly see that some groups of women were left out, you might note this as a source of potential bias. Or if, as in some of the trials that have compared an actively managed and physiological third stage, midwives were more used to offering one kind of care or intervention than another, you might think about whether this might have affected the outcomes.

Bias in philosophy can occur when it is clear that the researchers have a very different perspective to your own. For instance, if the authors of a study continually refer to women as 'patients' or 'parturients' you might suppose them to be very medical in their approach and perhaps more likely to be looking to reach conclusions that support their viewpoint. This can, of course, occur the other way around, when people who are very woman centred might be more keen to draw conclusions that favour their perspective!

My colleague Trudy Stevens calls research 'structured noseyness' (personal correspondence 2005), because you have to really want to know about things and about people's lives to carry out a good research study. Equally, the job of the person appraising research might be said to be about 'structured sniffing around', because you basically need to be a detective and sniff around for clues to potential bias.

One word of warning though – when you start sniffing around, it is very easy to find lots of sources of potential bias in a study, and end up with 50 points of criticism and no positive comments! It is also important to remember that research is hard to get perfect, and once you have sniffed out the sources of bias you might then want to think about the positive features of the study so that your critique is balanced.

If we knew what it was that we were doing, it would not be called research, would it?

ALBERT EINSTEIN

The outcome of any serious research can only be to make two questions grow where only one grew before.

THORSTEIN VEBLEN

USING RESEARCH ANALOGIES

This book uses a lot of analogies to help you relate to research in different ways and, for the people who like this kind of thing, there follows a way of thinking about research that relates to baking a cake!

Research and cakes

When you want to bake a cake (or do research), you first of all need to decide what kind of cake you want to bake; this is similar to deciding the overall aim or approach to your research. Will it be a simple chocolate cake that is quick to make and bake, or a fruit cake, which you will tend with brandy for several weeks, or maybe an extravagant wedding cake with tiers and layers and little figures on top? Although the last cake would be much more complex than the others to create, you might get more compliments at the end of your efforts if it came out well! Similarly, will the research study be a quick and simple quantitative questionnaire, perhaps to audit the demographic characteristics (age, gender, etc.) and opinions of the student midwives in one class, or a longitudinal study of women's experiences of birth, or a study that uses both quantitative and qualitative approaches to look at different aspects of an area or question?

If you are relatively new to making cakes (or, come to that, doing research), you might have to gather a bit more information before you start. You might look through some recipe books (or what, in research, is sometimes called 'the literature') to see what other people have done. You might also want to get advice from other people (who, in the world of research might be advisors, supervisors or subject specialists, like statisticians). There are obvious advantages in staying with a tried-and-tested cake; you know what the pitfalls are, you can always vary the kind of fruit or nuts that you are using to make it a bit different, and you can be fairly confident that you will get a reasonable result. However, you can also choose to be a bit more adventurous with both cakes and research! One of my friends, who often bakes cakes for things like school fetes, tries hard to make cakes that will be a bit different. Just as her cakes always stand out from the inevitable 10 plates of packet-bought fairy cakes on the cake stall, some researchers try hard to break new ground and tackle areas that have not been explored before.

When baking, some people follow recipes religiously, using exactly the right amount of everything, whereas other people put things into the bowl in a way that might look quite random to the untrained observer. The cake/research analogy falls down a bit at this point, because there are no hard-and-fast recipe books for research and *all* researchers have to use the second way! It is certainly possible to get ideas from reading other people's studies, although sometimes that can feel a bit like tasting a really good cake and wondering what on earth went into it to make it so good! With research, the exact recipe is determined by the researcher(s).

Once you've decided on the type of cake and the basic recipe, you need to gather the ingredients, the utensils and the pan that it will be baked in. Let's have a brief look at each of these things separately, before bringing them all together again.

- You could think of the cake tin as being the overall approach to the method; whether it is quantitative or qualitative, the tin (overall design) will provide the final shape of the cake (or research).
- In research, the main 'ingredient' of the study is the participants; you could think of them being like the flour – the cake wouldn't work without them. But it wouldn't be a cake if you didn't mix the flour with other things. You need to think about what kind of flour you need, because you get different cakes (results) with different kinds of flour. It is, of course, always a good idea to sift flour and, in research, you could

think of the sieve as being the ethical framework for the study – a way of making sure that the only people (flour) who make it into the study (bowl) are those that are happy to be involved.

- We need to add some kind of butter or margarine, which you could think of as the research question. (As with real butter or margarine, you sometimes need to chop the question into smaller pieces before it goes in.)
- We also need to add other ingredients and do different things to the cake, depending on the kind of cake/study we want to make. For instance, in experimental quantitative research, we might divide the mixture into two, and add a different kind of colouring (intervention) to each, so that we ended up with one of those cakes that, when you cut it, has squares of alternating colours.

If this analogy is working for you, you might already be thinking of how you could relate other cakes to other kinds of studies – if not, then you might want to skip to the next section, which takes a more logical approach!

By adding more ingredients to the bowl and mixing them all together, you are making choices about what you will put in to your study and how you will blend it to generate your data (the cake mixture). If you think about it, the order in which things go in to the cake bowl can have a profound impact on how the cake comes out, and exactly the same is true with research. If a researcher is not careful, all of the assumptions that she made can rise to the top – like raisins sometimes do!

You will then need to choose a way to bake (or analyse) the data you have generated. Will it be baked for a long time at a slow temperature, will you have to attend to it several times and turn the pan around, or, once you've put it all in the pan, will it bake quite quickly with little interference? Sometimes, you need to leave a cake alone and let it rise without interference, and, in certain kinds of quantitative studies, researchers do the same thing – they don't analyse their data until the end, in case they somehow influence the results. It is also important to think about how you will know when it's done, and how you will present it to your guests, or readers. If you are going to publish your study, you might want to add a layer of jam in the middle (discussion) and some icing sugar on the top (conclusions). If you have large amounts of data and discussion, you might want to cut slices to present in different journals or at different conferences…

This analogy is by no means perfect but, with this kind of thinking, the lack of perfection can sometimes help increase understanding – as you find the flaws, you will find that you are thinking about the area in different ways, which might help you to make further connections.

A MORE LOGICAL GUIDE TO THE RESEARCH PROCESS

If the cake analogy was a bit much for you, or you like to think in a more logical manner, the following outline of the research process might be more up your street: this outline forms the basis of 'A practical guide to critiquing 1', which appears on pages 8–10.

This outline is probably better suited to quantitative research than qualitative research, which we will talk more about in a bit. Also, researchers often move stages around, or add or delete things to suit their particular needs, so this is a fairly broad framework even for quantitative research:

1. define/formulate the research problem or broad question
2. review the relevant literature
3. begin to develop a broad framework for the research
4. formulate a specific question or hypothesis
5. develop the overall design for your research
6. specify the population you want to study

APPRAISING A RESEARCH CAKE

Now comes the really fun part! If you think about how you might analyse and evaluate a research cake, you can see that there are a number of possible approaches. You could appraise the cake as a whole to see how it works together, or you could appraise each part of the cake separately. Some of the important questions include:

- Does the cake work as a whole?
- Do the ingredients work well together?
- Was enough attention given to each individual ingredient?
- Was the sample appropriately sieved through the ethical framework?
- Was enough time allowed for the data to rise?
- Is the cake well presented in terms of the information it contains?
- Do you agree that the cake is what the creator says it is?

RESEARCH CAKES AND OTHER ALTERNATIVES

If the research cake analogy doesn't work for you, you perhaps want to give some thought to other analogies that might. May be you would be more comfortable with the idea of a research trifle, or of growing a research flower, or of a research playground – it doesn't really matter what metaphor you use, what matters is that, if you are one of the people who finds it hard to think in the very logical ways that are often used to teach the research process, you find a way of 'getting your head around' research that works for you!

7. select methods to measure the variables/outcomes
8. consider whether you need to conduct a pilot study
9. select your sample
10. collect your data
11. prepare the data for analysis
12. analyse the data
13. interpret and discuss the results
14. write up or otherwise communicate your research and findings.

APPRAISING RESEARCH: WHERE DO YOU START?!

It is possible to use a number of different approaches to critiquing research, and a few are briefly described here. The reason for offering several options is that, as I have previously mentioned, different people think and learn in different ways, and it always seems more helpful to me to present a number of options so that you can see which suits you best. Although many research books will only present one way – often, the step-by-step logical approach – this won't suit everybody as a way of thinking. Some of the following suggestions overlap each other, i.e. they are not mutually exclusive, and you can often mix and match them even more to find something which suits you.

The methodical approach

With this approach, you literally start at the beginning of the paper and read/work through to the end. As you read each part of the paper, you can make notes and write questions in the margin as you go and, by the time you reach the end, you should have a list of questions and thoughts that you can then look at more closely. The advantage of this approach is that it is unlikely that you will miss anything out. However, you will often find that some of your questions are answered by later sections of the paper and, if you are trying to read or critique a number of papers (for instance, if you are writing a dissertation), you might find that you are reading more than you need to.

The step-by-step approach

This is similar to the methodical approach but you also have a list of questions beside you as you read (such as those in the guides to critiquing below), and you set out to look for answers to them as you go along. By the time you have finished, you will have extensive amounts of notes but, again, it is labour intensive and not always the best approach if you are short of time or if you have a lot of papers to critique.

Topping and tailing

With this approach, you read the abstract and then the conclusions to the study before making a decision about whether you will read and/or critique further. This can save a lot of time if you are trying to 'weed out' the studies that are relevant to a particular question, and it can help you spot what might turn out to be the significant points right away, although it does also have a couple of significant disadvantages. Sometimes, the abstract and conclusions are not well written and so you can miss really key aspects of the study. It is also sometimes the case that the abstract and/or conclusions are a bit misleading (whether intentionally or accidentally) and so you might dismiss something that could be useful or focus too much on something that is not really significant.

The global approach

With this approach, which works well for people who like to 'meander' around what they are reading rather than starting at the beginning and finishing at the end, you start at whichever bit of the paper looks the most interesting and then follow your nose around the paper until you feel you have got what you need from it. This might mean, for instance, that you move from the title to the results section, then decide to have a look at the basic design of the study. Once you have a feeling for the study in its entirety, you might decide to look more closely at certain parts of it, or you might decide to move on to something else.

Note: in Section 6 you will also find a brief discussion on how you can draw together points from different studies into a coherent essay or dissertation. The discussion draws on some of the material discussed in the intervening chapters, which is why it comes later.

A FEW DO'S AND DON'T'S OF CRITIQUING

Do get the most out of the abstract!

Whatever your approach to reading and working through the paper, most people read the title and the abstract first. As you do this, you might find some of the following questions helpful.

- What are your first impressions?
- How do the conclusions relate to what you already know or believe? (It is important to acknowledge your preconceptions, and also to look for the preconceptions of the researchers, as in the next point).
- Who are the researchers? Might they have a personal bias? What is their experience, qualifications, role?
- Was the research funded and, if so, could the sponsors have an interest in the outcome?
- Where is the research published, and could this tell us anything about the study, or about any limitations the researchers might have faced when writing it up?

Do think about ethics!

It is important to think about ethical issues.

- Was the research fair to participants?
- Were participants able to remain anonymous? Or, if this wasn't possible (and often it isn't – with interviews, for instance, the researcher generally knows who the participant is and sometimes where they live!), were they assured of confidentiality?
- Could any perceived limitations in the research design be down to ethical issues? (For example, it is very hard to do a randomised controlled trial (or RCT) on some topics because women would not want to be randomised into one or other option. Think about the place of birth; no matter whether they plan home or hospital birth, most women would not want this decision made at the last minute by chance (randomisation) alone...)
- Was the research taken to an ethical committee for approval, and was this approval given?
- If the research was not taken to an ethical committee, are there good reasons for this? Also, don't forget that many of the people who sit on ethical committees are themselves involved in the same kinds of research as they are approving, so they might also have a vested interest in the kinds of research that are approved...

Do keep notes!

Although it is sometimes tempting to read most of the paper before you write anything down, bear in mind that it can be very helpful to make a note of your early thoughts, or first impressions, because it is easy to forget these as you read more and more of the paper, especially if you come to a point where you have to look something up, or run into something you don't understand (and more about that in the next paragraph!). Making notes from the first time you read a piece of research will enable you to remember your first impressions, even when you have read the study a number of times. If you are writing an evaluation or précis of the research, you will then have these notes to help form the framework for organising what you write.

Don't give up at the power calculation!

The vast majority of people can read and understand the title of any research paper published in a midwifery or medical journal. (They might sometimes think it sounds a bit weird or wordy, but they can generally understand what it is about!) Most will also happily make it through the abstract, although there might be a couple of unfamiliar terms that they realise they will have to ask about or look up in a dictionary. As they continue through the introduction, the background and the literature review, they are still fairly happy, because these sections tend to be written in plain English.

Then they get to the methods section. The first couple of paragraphs are OK because they talk about the basic design of the study and which kind(s) of women participated, but then the research goes on to talk about how many women were included and you see a paragraph that looks something like the one in Box 1, below.

Section 1 Box 1

We calculated that we needed to recruit 200 midwifery students in order to achieve an 80% power to detect a treatment effect of a 50% increase in happiness in the number of students feeling happy from 40 to 75%. The prevalence of happiness above 5 on a scale of 1 to 10 is reported at 40% (So and So et al 2005) and to detect a significant increase in happiness from 40 to 75% ($p = 0.05$, beta = 0.2) a sample size of 180 student midwives was required, which allowed for a 10% loss to follow-up.

Note: I have made up most of these numbers, so they do not represent a correct example, but, for our purposes, it doesn't matter at all!

As soon as people see this paragraph, three things tend to happen in quick succession.

1. Their pulse and blood pressure increase when they realise that they do not have a clue what the paragraph is talking about and wonder if they have either not paid enough attention in their classes or if they are not going to be able to understand research after all.
2. Now that they have become uncertain that they can carry on reading and understanding the rest of the research, they then decide to have a quick flick through the rest of the paper to see if there is anything else that looks a bit complicated. Because the way humans think tends to lead us towards conclusions that support our existing fears, they do, indeed, find a few tables and graphs that also look like gobbledegook, and this supports the growing idea that they are not going to be good at understanding research.
3. At this point, they often do one or more of the following things:
   i. throw the paper across the room in disgust
   ii. pour a large glass of wine
   iii. call a friend to see if s/he can empathise
   iv. cry/swear/shout at the paper/curse the researchers and/or their research lecturers

v. have a little think about alternative careers should they not manage to pass their research module

vi. go to the pub.

Many of the things in the list above can, in their place, be very therapeutic and may well make you feel a bit better, although from my perspective it would be great if you could refrain from placing too many curses on researchers and lecturers, especially if you are experienced in the magical arts! An alternative approach to doing all or any the things in the list above is to not give up at the power calculation (that is, the kind of stuff in the box above). This is because *the power calculation is only a very small part of the research as a whole*. If you don't understand it, then temporarily ignore it and assume that it is OK unless or until you can check it out with someone who does understand it. Often, researchers will note themselves (usually towards the end of the paper) whether they thought their numbers had enough 'power' to detect significant differences (e.g. in the paper in Chapter 1). Don't give up, because the chances are – if you can prevent yourself getting into the downward spiral as described above – you will be able to carry on and make sense of the majority of what follows it.

We all know that some people in the world are better at maths, statistics and all that science stuff than others, whereas other people are better at other things, like languages, painting, perineal suturing or turning cartwheels, to name just a few random examples. The people who write those paragraphs about power calculations (or who present very complex tables) either happen to be among those who understand it or else they have found somebody else who understands it to work it out and write it for them. The bottom line is that, even if you are one of those people who are better at turning cartwheels than at understanding maths, you will still be able to unearth most of the key points from a research study if you focus predominantly on the text.

Of course, there are tools to help you understand all of this maths stuff, including a few in Section 6 of this book, and, hopefully, after you have worked through the studies in this book, you will become more comfortable with that kind of information. But it is entirely possible to write a competent critique without understanding the power calculation, so, again, don't give up at that stage because you will often find that the gobbledegook lasts only for a paragraph before normal service resumes.

Do get the terminology right!

Every time I mark dissertations or research critiques there are some where the person writing has, for whatever reason, decided to try and use complex research terms but has, unfortunately, managed to get them wrong. My tips in this area would be:

- if you're not sure exactly what the term means, look it up or ask rather than guessing. This will prevent you from using terms inappropriately, because you can rest assured that the person marking your work will know the correct meaning and will be able to tell if you don't!
- be very wary of spellcheckers; they will not necessarily highlight words that are spelled correctly but are in the wrong place. Among my favourite critiques was the one about the virginal breech birth study, and I have read quite a lot over the years about randomised controlled trails!

Do strike a balance

As I've mentioned above, it is very easy to get caught up in all of the pitfalls of a study and to forget to mention the positive aspects and/or acknowledge the constraints within which the researchers found themselves. It is, then, important to identify the positive as well as the negative aspects of the research to make a fair evaluation. Of course, there are a handful of studies that have very few redeeming features, and there are also a few that are truly excellent and hard to fault, but the majority of research has both strengths and weaknesses.

Do think about the wider view

It is also easy when reading research to get caught up in the details and to forget the wider picture. Some of the questions that can help you think about the bigger picture are as follows.

- How might it have felt to be a woman (or baby, or midwife, or whatever) in this study?
- How does this research fit with:
  - your own experience?
  - what you know of women's experiences?
  - current practice where you work?
  - the beliefs held by midwives and other relevant people?
  - the midwifery literature?
- What aspects of life in our society might relate to the questions being asked here, and to the way in which they were investigated?

Do use other people's critiques – but with care

Because of the current emphasis on using research evidence in practice, along with the fact that we are expected to critique that evidence, it is not that unusual to find that someone else has published a commentary on a study that you are critiquing. With the caveat that, if your critique is going to be assessed, you should check this advice out against the advice you have been given locally, by all means use other people's critiques, but use them with care.

- Do consider going through the study yourself before you read too many other critiques, so that you can formulate your own ideas.
- Do cite them if you use them in an essay; their existence and the fact that you have used them does not detract from your own ability, but using what others have said and pretending it is your own work will!
- Do remember that, as I have mentioned elsewhere, the people who write critiques also have a word limit, and so they might have talked only about what they feel are the most relevant points.
- Do also remember that people writing critiques are also biased, and your perspective might be different from theirs – this does not necessarily mean that you are wrong! The fact that someone has managed to get their critique published in a journal or on a website does not always mean that they know more than you!

A PRACTICAL GUIDE TO CRITIQUING 1

This guide was originally designed to help people read and critique quantitative research. Although many of the questions can equally be applied to qualitative research, the guide in the next section has been designed specifically for use with qualitative research. This guide is based on the 14 steps in the section above.

Define/formulate the research problem or broad question

- Does the question relate well to practice?
- Is the question relevant to your needs?

- Is it asked in an appropriate manner?
- Is other (previous) research relating to the area discussed?

Review the relevant literature

- Was an appropriate literature search carried out?
- Is the literature cited up to date? (If not, does it matter?)
- Does the author give a fair evaluation of other people's findings?
- Are both sides of any argument presented?

Begin to develop a broad framework for the research

- Is the framework (or philosophical approach) used appropriate to the study?
- Is it suggestive of the conclusions?
- Could it suggest bias?

Formulate a specific question or hypothesis

- Is the research question or hypothesis clear?
- Is the wording of this appropriate?
- Is it suggestive of bias?

Develop the overall design for your research

- Does the design fit the question and aims of the research?
- Is the design likely to get us some way towards the 'truth' of the answer?
- Are the pros and cons of the design discussed?
- Is justification given for the use of the chosen design?

Specify the population you want to study

- Are the participants suitable?
- Who was not included in the research, and why?
- Could the exclusion of any groups be a source of potential bias?

Select methods to measure the variables/outcomes

- Are these methods appropriate?
- Do they measure 'hard' or 'soft' outcomes?
- To what extent does their measurement depend on the person measuring them?
- Would other measures be better?

Consider whether you need to conduct a pilot study

- If a pilot study was used, were the results used to improve the design?
- If a pilot study was not used, could one have improved the design of the study?

Select your sample

- How did the researchers decide who would be eligible for entry?
- Was a control group used and was randomisation used appropriately?

- Were the groups studied large enough to make a fair assessment of the effectiveness/side effects of whatever is being studied?
- Was single or double blinding used?
- Did all participants make an informed choice about being in the study?

Collect your data

- Does the paper tell you how, when and where this was done?
- Do you feel this was carried out appropriately?
- Who collected data?

Prepare the data for analysis

- Does the paper explain how this was done?

Analyse the data

- Is the method of analysis explained and justified?
- Are reasons for using particular statistics or other tests given?
- Is the probability of getting the results by chance included?

Interpret and discuss the results

- Is this process intelligible and relevant?
- Are raw figures given as well as percentages?
- Are data given in graphs and tables explained?
- Could pictorial representations of data be misleading?
- Is the discussion of results appropriate and relevant?
- Are conclusions appropriate and does the research 'fit together' well?

Write up or otherwise communicate your research and findings

- Is the research 'reader friendly' and well presented?
- Is there a logical progression to the paper?
- Are there any gaps?
- Is anything 'glossed over'?
- Are the limitations and areas of potential bias discussed honestly?

A PRACTICAL GUIDE TO CRITIQUING 2

This guide has been written by Ruth Deery. Although it says some of the things that you have just read in the guide above, different people think and learn in different ways and Ruth's background in qualitative research means that she approaches critiquing in a slightly different way from the way I approach it. Her guide is included here not only because it is more relevant to qualitative research than the first guide but also because I think it can be helpful to read through a few tools and see which appeals most to the way you think. As with everything, neither of these guides is more 'right' or 'wrong' than the other, they merely reflect different approaches!

Reviewing/critiquing a research paper

When reviewing or critiquing a research paper it is important to ask questions about each stage of the research. The stages of the research should follow the stages of the research process and should contain an introduction, a statement of the situation/ problem, and the reason why it was explored. There should then be a review of the literature and a statement of the research aim. The research method should then be described, including details of how the data were analysed. The findings of the study should precede the final section containing the discussion of the findings and recommendations for practice and for further research on the topic.

The research problem/situation and purpose

- What was the problem/situation being explored or what question was the research designed to answer?
- Is the problem/situation actually worth exploring? Is it relevant to midwifery practice and will it increase midwifery knowledge?
- Is the purpose of the study clearly presented? If it is not it will be impossible to assess whether the researcher has achieved what they set out to do.

The literature review

- Is the review comprehensive? Does it include details of studies that have been conducted in other disciplines as well as midwifery? Remember, researchers should not be blinkered – for example, what do sociologists, nurses or psychologists say about this situation?
- Is the material in the review up to date? If the literature is confined to a period of time, for example the last 10 years, has the researcher stated this?
- Is the material reviewed relevant to the topic under investigation?
- Is the review well organised, following a logical sequence?
- Has the literature been reviewed critically or has the researcher merely included details of studies without evaluating them in any way?

The research question

- Is the research question clear and unambiguous?
- Does the research question derive from the problem/situation area being explored?

The research design and method

A detailed explanation should be given of how the study was carried out, including details of the research design, e.g. experimental design or descriptive survey, and the methods employed in carrying out the study.

- Is the research method appropriate to explore the research question and is it described in detail?
- What methods were employed to collect information, e.g. observation, question-naire or interview schedule, are the methods valid (i.e. they accurately measure what they are intended to measure) and reliable (i.e. they are consistent in that if used on a number of occasions, with the same participants, they would give the same findings)? There are also alternative ways of judging the reliability and validity of a piece of research, which are discussed in Chapter 7.
- Was the sample population truly representative of the group (population) being studied? What size was the sample and what criteria were used to select them? Was

it a random sample or one of convenience? Have the characteristics of the sample been identified?

- If the study involved the voluntary co-operation of human beings, what was the response rate? What influence will the response rate have on the findings?
- Was a pilot study performed, and if so, what modifications had to be made as a result?
- Had due regard been given to the ethical implications of the study?

Data analysis

In qualitative research studies the data usually consist of fieldwork observations and/or interviews. These require transcribing and then coding so that specific categories can be identified through analysis.

- Were the methods used to analyse the data appropriate to the material collected and in accordance with the purpose of the study?

Findings

The way in which the findings are presented may intentionally or unintentionally mislead the reader.

- Are the findings presented in a clear, organised and unbiased way?
- Do the findings answer/support the research question?

Concluding discussion

- What inferences does the researcher draw from the findings? Are they justified?
- Have the limitations of the study been acknowledged and discussed?
- Have the findings of the study been critically discussed in the light of other studies on the topic?
- What recommendations for action and/or further research have been made and is the evidence produced by the research sufficiently reliable to be used as a basis for action?
- Can generalisations be made from the study that can be transferred to other situations without replication?

READY FOR TAKE-OFF!

OK, if you would like to fasten your seat belt and bring your seats and tray tables to their upright and locked positions, I think we might be ready to face some studies… Don't forget that you can return to the safety information in this section at any time, and that our attendants (in the form of the chapter authors) will be nearby to help you. You will also find more information on tables and statistics in Section 6, should you need it, although I would suggest that you at least read through Section 2, Chapter 1 before turning to that section, partly because much of the information on tables and statistics in Section 6 builds upon some of the ideas in the introduction to Chapter 1. It will also help you gain an idea of where your learning needs are. In Section, 2, Chapter 2, Nadine Pilley Edwards provides further safety information regarding qualitative research.

Each chapter contains a lifejacket in the form of all the answers to the questions asked, and don't be afraid to look at them as much as you need to. Have a safe trip, I will be checking in from time to time to talk you through the different sections, and I wish you a happy and pleasant journey towards a better understanding of research!

Women, midwives and information

INTRODUCTION

Over the past few years, the changing values of Western society have meant that both those receiving health care and those offering that health care to them have become much more aware of the need for people to have information to help them make choices. In fact, the UK-based Midwives Information and Resource Service (MIDIRS) was set up to address this very issue, and one of MIDIRS' key activities over the past few years has been the development of the informed choice leaflets, which are the subject of the two articles in this section. These research studies set out to evaluate whether these leaflets actually made a difference to women's experience of informed choice – something that, I'm sure you'll agree, is important for us to know, especially when we consider the amount of verbal and written information that is offered to women during their antenatal care.

If you want to find out whether something makes a difference to women, you can do it in any one of a number of ways. One approach is to undertake an experiment to evaluate whether the 'something' makes a difference by comparing the outcomes of two (or sometimes more) groups of women, where one group gets the 'something' and the other one doesn't. Chapter 1 gives you a chance to critique a quantitative, experimental approach to this kind of question.

However, experimental research often doesn't tell us what the women in the study think themselves, and it might not give much of an insight into other factors that come into the equation. If you want to find out about these kinds of things, a qualitative approach might be better, where you can talk to the women themselves, ask them for their thoughts and views and perhaps explore the wider issues. Thanks to the insight of the researchers who designed the evaluation of the informed choice leaflets and included both quantitative and qualitative elements to their study, we are able to include a qualitative study on the same subject, which Nadine Pilley Edwards looks at in Chapter 2. Both Nadine and I will continue this commentary as you read through the chapters so that you can see how the same kind of question can be explored by using different kinds of research.

Sara Wickham

INTRODUCTION

As discussed in the introduction to this section, one of the ways of finding out if something like an information leaflet makes a difference to women is to do a randomised controlled trial (an RCT). Although the term 'randomised controlled trial' seems quite scary to some people, in fact the principle is fairly simple and there are much friendlier ways of thinking and learning about the RCT. One of the threads leading to the development of the RCT apparently involved a woman and several cups of tea (Oakley 2000). Dr Muriel Bristol 'proved' she could tell whether milk had been added to the teacup before or after the tea was poured by drinking from several randomly arranged cups of tea and identifying which was which!

To do an RCT, you first of all need to take a large number of people and divide them randomly into two groups. (Sometimes there are more than two groups, but let's not worry about that for now, we'll save it for Chapter 6!) To make sure there is no bias in the randomisation we need to check that the groups are similar enough (comparable) to each other before we carry on. Once you have checked that the groups are comparable, you can then give the 'something' that you want to evaluate (this might be a pill, a leaflet, an intervention, or perhaps some kind of support) to one of the groups, which becomes your experimental group. The other group doesn't get the 'something' and becomes the control group. The idea behind having a control group (which, remember, we already know is similar to the experimental group) is that any external factors that might affect people's outcomes will happen fairly equally in both groups, and we can then compare the outcomes of the two groups to see if the 'something' actually made a difference to the outcomes.

This is one of the kinds of research that I teach with jelly babies! In simple terms, I divide a group of student midwives in half, and one half gets a jelly baby and the other half doesn't, and then we find out how much happier the people who got a jelly baby are than the people who didn't get one! Table 1.1 provides a quick revision of some of the key issues that come up when we are looking at an RCT in relation to jelly babies; if you are happy that you understand these issues, you might want to skip this bit and move on to the article!

There are many more issues to consider. If you want to be reminded of some basic statistics, there are a few pages on this in Section 6, but hopefully Table 1.1 will have given you the general idea, and demonstrated that it is actually very difficult to design an RCT without including potential sources of bias. As you read the article in this chapter, you will be able to see other examples of some of the difficulties that can arise when you attempt to translate the theoretical basic for studies like RCTs into real-life situations and practice, along with some of the ways in which the authors of this study attempted to reduce the risk of bias.

O'Cathian, A, Walters, SJ, Nicholl JP, Thomas KJ, Kirkham M 2002 Use of evidence based leaflets to promote informed choice in maternity care: randomised controlled trial in everyday practice. British Medical Journal 324:643

Table 1.1 Issues raised in the jelly baby study

I should probably tell you at the outset that my jelly baby study is deliberately quite flawed; this is because it allows us to look at some of the problems that can arise when you are doing an RCT and some of the sources of potential bias.

Hypothesis or question	It is important to have a clear question at the outset of any experiment – in fact, this is important in most kinds of research. At the outset of the jelly baby study I write the following question on the board, 'Do jelly babies make student midwives happy?'! Immediately you can see that we are going to have to define what we mean by 'happy' and think about how we can measure happiness – more on that in a minute – and to think about whether the question is clear and specific enough. Generally, an RCT question needs to give the reader an idea of what we are going to do, who we are going to do it to (or with) and what kind of difference we think it might make to them.
Population/sample	Are the student midwives in my classes representative of the population at large? Probably not, so we cannot say that my jelly baby study could be generalised to all women, or even to all student midwives. It is important when looking at research to see if the sample was truly representative of the group that the researchers are looking at, and to ask if anyone might have been left out, either because they were not invited to participate or because they were more likely to decline. An important implication of this last part is that, often, the women who are not represented in research studies are those who already have strong preferences about their birth experiences. For instance, a woman who already has a strong preference for either a physiological or a medically managed third stage is unlikely to want to participate in a research study where the kind of third stage she has will be determined purely by chance. Another issue with sampling is to make sure you have enough people to even out the external factors which can make people happy or unhappy: sometimes people are happy because it is their birthday or because they have recently fallen in love, and sometimes people are unhappy – with a small sample you run the risk of having one group start off happier than the other.
Outcome measures	Before I even think about giving out the jelly babies we need to come back to the question of what 'happy' actually means and think about how we will measure the happiness levels of the students before and after they have (or don't have) a jelly baby. If you think about this one for a minute you will realise that happiness, like pain or depression, is a personal thing and thus very difficult to measure objectively – my idea of happiness might be very different from yours! We can construct a scale whereby we ask everyone to rate their own happiness where 1 is 'not at all happy' and 10 is 'I couldn't be happier', but you will see that this is still going to be very subjective and potentially lead to bias.
Randomisation	With the jelly baby study, I usually randomise people into two groups by giving a jelly baby to every other person as they sit in a circle. Would you consider this a good way of randomising? People often sit in groups with people they like, and they may be of similar age and backgrounds to their friends. When looking at an RCT it is important to think about what method of randomisation was used, and whether this could have introduced potential bias. When midwives have to pick envelopes out of boxes on the labour ward to see if a woman gets one kind of care or another, they have been known to put the envelope they first chose back and then take another, perhaps because they thought that one option might be better for the individual woman. This is very woman centred, but not especially helpful in reducing bias in the research study! Telephone randomisation is often used these days, as this cannot be influenced by the person giving or carrying out the intervention.
Blinding	The ideal RCT is double blind, which describes the situation where neither the participants nor their caregivers know which group they are in. This is relatively simple to achieve if your RCT is testing a new pill, as you can have the pharmacy make you some inert, placebo pills that look and taste exactly the same as the real pills, and put them in numbered bottles so that only the pharmacists know which is which. By comparison, in a single-blind study the participants don't know which group they are in but the caregiver does, such as when somebody is receiving one of two kinds of surgery where any scarring and postoperative pain will be the same and the person is asleep while it is performed. Sometimes studies cannot be 'blinded' at all, and the jelly baby study is one of these; I have never found a way to make something that looks, smells, tastes and feels like a jelly baby but that is not, in fact, another jelly baby! Likewise, women will know whether they are having a caesarean section or a vaginal breech birth, or whether their third stage is physiological or managed.
Other sources of potential bias	There are a lot of other sources of potential bias in the jelly baby study, including that: ● the student participants are not separated into two different rooms, so some of the people who don't get a jelly baby become unhappy because of this! (I do give them jelly babies afterwards, by the way!) ● some students don't like jelly babies, or don't want to eat them because they are vegetarian or vegan. Interestingly, I have known people to have a higher happy score despite not wanting to eat the jelly baby they were given, because they found the jelly baby aesthetically pleasing to look at, or because they were simply pleased that they got one rather than being in the 'deprived' group! ● some of the women who received a jelly baby but did not want to eat it ended up giving it to their neighbour who was in the control group!

**QUESTIONS
FOR CHAPTER 1**

Papers

Use of evidence based leaflets to promote informed choice in maternity care: randomised controlled trial in everyday practice

A O'Cathain, S J Walters, J P Nicholl, K J Thomas, M Kirkham

Abstract

Objective To assess the effect of leaflets on promoting informed choice in women using maternity services.
Design Cluster trial, with maternity units randomised to use leaflets (intervention units) or offer usual care (control units). Data collected through postal questionnaires.
Setting 13 maternity units in Wales.
Participants Four separate samples of women using maternity services. Antenatal samples: women reaching 28 weeks' gestation before (n=1386) and after (n=1778) the intervention. Postnatal samples: women at eight weeks after delivery before (n=1741) and after (n=1547) the intervention.
Intervention Provision of 10 pairs of *Informed Choice* leaflets for service users and midwives and a training session for staff in their use.
Main outcome measures Change in the proportion of women who reported exercising informed choice. Secondary outcomes: changes in women's knowledge; satisfaction with information, choice, and discussion; and possible consequences of informed choice.
Results There was no change in the proportion of women who reported that they exercised informed choice in the intervention units compared with the control units for either antenatal or postnatal women. There was a small increase in satisfaction with information in the antenatal samples in the intervention units compared with the control units (odds ratio 1.40, 95% confidence interval 1.05 to 1.88). Only three quarters of women in the intervention units reported being given at least one of the leaflets, indicating problems with the implementation of the intervention.
Conclusion In everyday practice, evidence based leaflets were not effective in promoting informed choice in women using maternity services.

Introduction

There is a growing consensus that people should be informed about, and able to influence, decisions about their own health care.[1][2] Decision aids, which present the options available to patients with evidence from research on their effects, can help people to participate in decisions about their care.[3] Midwives Information and Resource Service (MIDIRS) and the NHS Centre for Reviews and Dissemination have produced a set of 10 leaflets on informed choice in maternity care. The leaflets summarise evidence on 10 decisions that women face in pregnancy and childbirth to encourage their involvement in decisions about their own care. Many maternity units buy the leaflets, yet little is known about their effectiveness.

We investigated whether the leaflets promoted informed choice and led to increased levels of knowledge, satisfaction with information, satisfaction with the way choices were made, and discussion with health professionals. We also examined whether they changed the actions women took or the services they used.

Methods

We tested the hypotheses in a cluster randomised controlled trial, with maternity units as clusters, in everyday practice. Qualitative research was undertaken alongside the trial to explore the use of the leaflets in practice and is reported separately.[4]

We randomised maternity units rather than individual women because of the risk of women sharing the leaflets in an individual level trial. Units were included if they had not already purchased the leaflets and had over 1000 deliveries annually. Twelve of the 15 large maternity units in Wales had not already purchased the leaflets and agreed to participate in the study. We also included a small unit under the managerial control of one of the 12 larger units. Maternity units were grouped into 10 clusters because some shared management or clinicians. Clusters were paired on the basis of their annual numbers of deliveries to ensure balance in the two arms of the trial. Members of pairs were randomly assigned by tossing a coin to receive the set of leaflets (five intervention units) or to continue with usual care (five control units). The intervention is described in the box.

Participants

We identified two samples of women. The first sample was all women who reached 28 weeks' gestation during a six week period and were receiving antenatal care in any setting (antenatal sample). Women were identified through hospital computer systems and the records of

1 The purpose of the introduction is to:

a) Provide a context for the research
Yes/No/Maybe

b) Explain and define any terms used
Yes/No/Maybe

c) Justify the reasons for doing the study
Yes/No/Maybe

d) Provide an overview of the findings
Yes/No/Maybe

N1 We'll look at this study in Chapter 2!

2 This risk would be a problem because (True/False):

a) It might introduce a confounding variable

b) Sharing of leaflets might contaminate the study

c) The control group should not experience the intervention

d) The design of the study is intention to treat

3 True or false?

a) This is the best method of randomisation in any study because the chances are 50/50

b) This was an appropriate method of randomisation for this study because the numbers were small

c) This was an appropriate method of randomisation for this study because units were being randomised rather than women

d) This is a poor method of randomisation because researchers may bias the randomisation

4 Apart from the women the researchers have chosen to omit (e.g. because their baby had died), can you think of any other women who would not be included in the antenatal sample of this study?

The intervention

- Ten pairs of *Informed Choice* leaflets:
- Support in labour
- Listening to your baby's heartbeat during labour
- Ultrasound scans—should you have one?
- Alcohol and pregnancy
- Positions in labour and delivery
- Epidurals for pain relief in labour
- Feeding your baby—breast or bottle?
- Looking for Down's syndrome and spina bifida in pregnancy
- Breech baby: What are your choices?
- Where will you have your baby – hospital or home?
- Leaflets were in pairs—a women's leaflet, designed to be accessible and give information about the benefits and risks of options available, and a more detailed professionals' leaflet, with references for the research on which it is based, which could be accessed by women through the midwife. The leaflets were designed to be given by health professionals to women at different stages of pregnancy
- Each intervention unit received sets of leaflets in May 1998 for an eight month period. A two hour training session was provided for staff. Training material was left with managers for cascade training
- Women in the intervention arm of the trial received the leaflets relevant to early pregnancy at their first booking appointment (10-12 weeks' gestation) and the other leaflets at 34-36 weeks' gestation

midwives and clerks in hospital and community antenatal clinics. The second sample was all women who delivered during a six week period (postnatal sample). Women were identified through child health computer records and hospital and home delivery registers. Women were excluded if they lived outside the catchment area of the hospital or in areas where antenatal care was provided by midwives from other hospitals, were under 16 years old, or had miscarried or if their baby had died or was seriously ill.

We identified an antenatal sample and a postnatal sample before the introduction of the leaflets and again nine months after they were introduced. We assessed outcomes using a postal questionnaire sent to women in these four different samples (figure). Women in the antenatal samples received the questionnaire at 28 weeks' gestation, and women in the postnatal samples received the questionnaire eight weeks after delivering their babies. Up to two reminders were sent at intervals of three weeks. The second reminder for the women in the antenatal samples was a shorter questionnaire that covered only key questions.

Outcome measures

The primary outcome was the proportion of women who answered "yes" to the question "Have you had enough information and discussion with midwives or doctors to make a choice together about all the things that happened during maternity care?" with the options "yes," "partly," "no," "there was no choice," and "did not apply." As informed choice is a difficult concept to measure[2] we also asked women about the role they took when choices were made, with six options ranging from "active" to "passive."[5]

Secondary outcomes were the "components" and the "consequences" of informed choice. The components measured were women's levels of knowledge of the 10 topics covered by the leaflets; satisfaction with information and with how choices had been made; and views of whether they had had sufficient discussion with health professionals. The consequences measured were the actions taken or services used by women. We also collected data on sociodemographic factors, parity, and women's preferences for involvement in decision making.[5]

Validation and quality assurance

We developed and piloted some measures specifically for the study on the basis of interviews with women in three maternity units not involved in this trial.[6] Other measures were modified from published sources. The questionnaires were piloted by post outside the study area. Ethical approval was obtained for the study in each area.

Sample size and statistical analysis

Assuming an intraclass correlation coefficient of 0.007 and an average cluster size of 200 we calculated we would need a sample size of 925 in the intervention units and 925 in the control units for each of the antenatal and postnatal samples. This would give us an 80% chance of detecting an increase from 50% to 60% in the proportion of women reporting that they made informed choices in the intervention units compared with no change in the control units, at a two tailed significance level of 5%. We paired maternity units to ensure balance and undertook an unmatched analysis.[7] We compared sociodemographic variables of respondents in all four antenatal samples and in all four postnatal samples at the individual level using analysis of variance and χ^2 tests. We compared any changes in the intervention units with changes over the same period in the control units using multilevel modelling.[8 9] Analysis was by intention to treat. We adjusted for women's age, age at leaving full time education, parity, and preference for involvement in decision making in the analyses. Intraclass correlation coefficients were

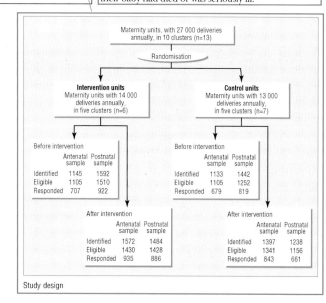

Study design

BMJ VOLUME 321   16 MARCH 2002   bmj.com

---

4 *(continued from previous page)*

5 What might be the reason(s) for excluding each of the following groups of women?
a) Women living or cared for by midwives in other areas
b) Women under 16
c) Women whose baby had died or was seriously ill

6 This table shows (True/False):
a) The number of women in each part of the trial
b) The differences in the percentage of women in the different groups
c) The response rates in each group
d) That randomisation was effective

7 List three advantages and three disadvantages of using postal questionnaires

8 Would these outcome measures best be described as:
a) 'Hard'?
b) 'Soft'?

9 Can you think of other outcome measures that might have been useful or better than the ones used in this part of the study?

10 Should ethical approval always be obtained for a study of this type? Yes/No/Maybe

N2. This kind of power calculation is discussed in Section 1.

11 Would you consider the inclusion of this kind of comparison:
a) Beneficial, but not essential?
b) Ideal, if there are more than two sample groups?
c) Essential?

12 'Intention to treat' means that:
a) The researchers had to make sure that everybody received the treatment (i.e. the leaflets) as intended
b) The researchers had to remove women from the study if they didn't receive the intended treatment
c) Even if some of the women in the leaflet group didn't receive the intended treatment, the researchers analysed the data as if they had

Table 1 Sociodemographic variables of respondents before and after introduction of intervention. Figures are numbers (percentage) of women unless stated otherwise

Variable	Before		After	
	Intervention	Control	Intervention	Control
Antenatal*				
No of women	619	622	827	743
Mean (SD) age (years)	27.4 (5.48)	27.7 (5.52)	28.0 (5.65)	27.9 (5.52)
Mean (SD) age at leaving full time education (years)	17.5 (2.15)	17.6 (2.50)	17.7 (2.43)	17.8 (2.63)
Manual occupation‡	177/518 (34)	159/516 (31)	212/696 (30)	175/617 (28)
Ethnic minority	16/616 (3)	12/606 (2)	22/822 (3)	28/739 (4)
First time mothers	280/616 (45)	292/614 (48)	350/825 (42)	352/742 (47)
Preference for active role in decisions	541/608 (89)	551/611 (90)	746/804 (93)	650/722 (90)
Postnatal				
No of women	922	819	886	661
Mean (SD) age (years)†	28.0 (5.43)	28.6 (5.62)	27.9 (5.62)	27.8 (5.98)
Mean (SD) age at leaving fulltime education (years)	17.5 (2.56)	17.8 (2.58)	17.5 (2.38)	17.6 (2.34)
Manual occupation‡	246/755 (33)	209/670 (31)	237/734 (32)	184/539 (34)
Ethnic minority	27/912 (3)	18/808 (2)	16/876 (2)	21/652 (3)
First time mothers	392/916 (43)	376/815 (46)	413/884 (47)	325/657 (49)
Preference for active role in decisions	739/880 (84)	648/786 (82)	699/851 (82)	519/639 (81)

*Sociodemographic variables collected on first and second mailings only.
†P<0.05 for analysis of variance.
‡Social class information not available for women who had never worked.

Table 3 Women's knowledge of choices in maternity services

Measure	Intervention			Control			Mean difference (95% CI)	Adjusted mean difference* (95%CI)
	Before	After	Change	Before	After	Change		
Mean (SD) antenatal knowledge score	3.74 (1.43)	3.99 (1.57)	0.25	3.79 (1.52)	3.79 (1.52)	0	0.25 (−0.05 to 0.55)	0.20 (−0.09 to 0.49)
Mean (SD) postnatal knowledge score	3.30 (1.65)	3.53 (1.64)	0.23	3.37 (1.62)	3.35 (1.61)	−0.02	0.26 (0.06 to 0.47)†	0.20 (−0.05 to 0.44)

*Adjusted for woman's age, age at leaving full time education, parity, and decision style preference.
†P<0.05.

0.01 and 0.002 for the change in informed choice in antenatal and postnatal samples respectively.

Results

Response rates—The overall response rate to the questionnaires was 64% (6452/10 070), with a rate of 65% (3164/4835) for the antenatal sample and 63% (3288/5235) for the postnatal sample. Response rates were lower in women with manual occupations and from ethnic minorities but did not differ by type of delivery, type of pain relief, parity, or age.[6]

Comparison of intervention and control groups—Sociodemographic variables of respondents in all four antenatal samples were similar (table 1). Women's age was different in the four postnatal samples, with respondents after the intervention an average of about seven months younger than respondents before.

Impact on informed choice—Before the intervention about half of women in both intervention and control units reported exercising informed choice "overall" in their maternity care. After the intervention, this proportion increased slightly in both groups (table 2) but with no significant difference in the change between groups. Results were similar for the proportion of women reporting active involvement in decision making. In the antenatal samples there were increases in knowledge, discussion, and satisfaction

Table 2 Informed choice and components of informed choice. Figures are numbers (percentage) of women unless stated otherwise

Measure	Intervention			Control			Unadjusted odds ratio (95% CI)	Adjusted* odds ratio (95% CI)
	Before	After	Change in %	Before	After	Change in %		
Antenatal								
Reporting yes to overall informed choice	357/689 (52)	532/917 (58)	6	373/663 (56)	477/820 (58)	2	1.10 (0.63 to 1.92)	1.15 (0.65 to 2.06)
Reporting "active" decision making role†	483/604 (80)	695/808 (86)	6	492/602 (82)	613/723 (85)	3	1.22 (0.59 to 2.51)	1.13 (0.47 to 2.74)
Satisfied with amount of information†	388/604 (64)	579/812 (71)	7	427/607 (70)	528/729 (72)	2	1.30 (0.96 to 1.75)	1.40 (1.05 to 1.88)‡
Satisfied with way choices were made†	416/601 (69)	612/815 (75)	6	455/608 (75)	549/722 (76)	1	1.22 (0.76 to 1.93)	1.25 (0.77 to 2.02)
Enough discussion	396/692 (57)	598/921 (65)	8	413/663 (62)	520/827 (63)	1	1.28 (0.80 to 2.07)	1.32 (0.82 to 2.14)
Postnatal								
Reporting yes to overall informed choice	499/887 (56)	500/848 (59)	3	406/788 (51)	358/637 (56)	5	0.90 (0.61 to 1.33)	0.90 (0.59 to 1.37)
Reporting "active" decision making role	664/901 (74)	638/866 (74)	0	559/797 (70)	463/647 (72)	2	0.89 (0.57 to 1.39)	0.99 (0.68 to 1.44)
Satisfied with amount of information	619/891 (70)	635/855 (74)	4	536/780 (69)	458/637 (72)	3	1.09 (0.76 to 1.57)	1.07 (0.73 to 1.57)
Satisfied with way choices were made	683/886 (77)	656/855 (77)	0	600/780 (77)	502/633 (79)	2	0.77 (0.40 to 1.48)	0.78 (0.40 to 1.54)
Enough discussion	570/883 (65)	548/847 (65)	0	481/774 (62)	414/636 (65)	3	0.86 (0.56 to 1.32)	0.82 (0.54 to 1.26)

*Adjusted for woman's age, age at leaving full time education, parity, and decision style preference.
†Not included in short questionnaire sent as second reminder to antenatal sample.
‡P<0.05.

13 Looking across this table to compare the sociodemographic variables of the women in each of the four groups will tell us that, in this study:

a) The groups were fairly well matched in all of the areas
b) The groups were fairly well matched in most of the areas
c) The groups were well matched in only a few areas
d) The groups were not well matched at all

14 What do the following abbreviations stand for?

a) CI
b) SD

15 Where $p = < 0.05$, this means that:

a) There was a 1 in 5 chance that this result came about by chance alone
b) There was a 1 in 20 chance that this result came about by chance alone
c) There was a 1 in 50 chance that this result came about by chance alone
d) There was a 1 in 200 chance that this result came about by chance alone

16 What are some of the reasons why women might answer positively to the question of whether they felt they exercised informed choice even if they did not really feel this way?

17 Could the possibility that women might not be completely honest in their answers to questions about informed choice be a significant source of potential bias in this study?

Table 5 Proportion of women who said they had received any *Informed Choice* leaflet before and after intervention. Figures are numbers (percentage) of women

	Before	After	Change in %
Antenatal			
All	580/1241 (47)	1048/1570 (67)	20
Intervention	266/619 (43)	598/827 (72)	29
Control	314/622 (50)	450/743 (61)	10
Postnatal			
All	760/1741 (44)	977/1547 (63)	19
Intervention	405/922 (44)	665/886 (75)	31
Control	355/819 (43)	312/661 (47)	4

18 Do the figures in this table give you cause for concern? Yes/No If you answered yes, then why are you concerned? If you answered no, then why are you not concerned?

19 Can you think of any ethical and fair way of removing this possible source of bias from a future randomised controlled trial which looked at the same question?

with information and with the way choices were made in intervention units (tables 2 and 3). They were not significant, however, with the exception of satisfaction with information. For this variable the difference in change was less than the minimum important difference of 10 percentage points. There was only one change in postnatal samples, with an increase of 0.24 points on a 10 point knowledge score, which was no longer significant after adjustment for covariates (table 3).

Consequences of informed choice—Given that there was no change in the proportion of women who reported that they exercised informed choice we would not expect changes in choices made. The one significant difference, which was in the proportion of women having screening tests for Down's syndrome and spina bifida, was due in part to an increase in reported uptake in the control units (table 4).

Uptake of leaflets—During the intervention period there was a significant increase in the proportion of women who reported that they had been given any of the *Informed Choice* leaflets in the intervention units compared with the control units, which showed little change (table 5). However, it was difficult to assess the uptake of the intervention leaflets with any precision. A large minority of women in the intervention units (44%) reported that they had been given at least one of the *Informed Choice* leaflets before the intervention had taken place (table 5). It is possible that a few *Informed Choice* leaflets were distributed in all the maternity units before the trial. However, most of this reported use probably relates to leaflets other than those under study because women had difficulty in distinguishing the intervention leaflets from other leaflets available in the maternity units.

Discussion

In this randomised controlled trial the use of *Informed Choice* leaflets did not change the proportion of women who reported exercising informed choice, or components or consequences of informed choice, in maternity care. This is surprising as a recent systematic review concluded that decision aids improve knowledge and increase the proportion of people who assume a more active role in decision making.[3]

Limitations in design

Possible limitations of this study are response bias, poor definition of "informed choice," and lack of power. The response rate of 64% may have introduced some bias, with under-representation of non-white women and women with manual occupations in both intervention and control groups. The pilot study of two of the leaflets suggested that women with manual occupations might benefit more from the leaflets,[10] suggesting that we may have underestimated the true effect of the leaflets. However, the main study found no relation between social class and effect of the leaflets.[6]

The question used to measure informed choice may have been insensitive. However, we used two different questions and neither showed change. Additionally, we found little change in the components of informed choice, which was consistent with a genuine lack of change in informed choice. Although we recruited fewer women than planned, the analysis for postnatal women was adequately powered due to a smaller intraclass correlation coefficient than estimated for the sample size calculation. The analysis for antenatal women had a power of about 65%. However, observed changes were small, and, although low power can explain the lack of significance, it cannot explain the size of the observed effect. Overall, it is unlikely that the study failed to detect any important change.

Everyday practice

We carried out this trial in everyday practice. We included thousands of women who might have

19 *(continued)*

20 What are your feelings about this area? Are you surprised at the results of this study? How might your existing opinion influence the way you look at the results of this study?

21 In your own words, what does lack of power mean?

22 Which of the following is most true?
a) The intervention failed and doesn't work at all
b) Women in this study did not want to make informed choices
c) The leaflets did not make a significant difference in this study, but might be shown to have an effect in future research

Table 4 Consequences of informed choice* in women using maternity services. Figures are numbers (percentage) of women

Measure	Intervention Before	Intervention After	Change in %	Control Before	Control After	Change in %	Unadjusted odds ratio (95% CI)	Adjusted† odds ratio (95% CI)
Antenatal								
More anxious	69/600 (11)	96/803 (12)	1	77/595 (13)	87/724 (12)	−1	1.16 (0.67 to 2.01)	1.28 (0.72 to 2.27)
Drank less alcohol	474/599 (79)	623/796 (78)	−1	443/592 (75)	551/696 (79)	4	0.79 (0.59 to 1.06)	0.72 (0.46 to 1.15)
Planned hospital birth	608/619 (98)	799/826 (97)	−1	604/620 (97)	725/743 (98)	1	0.50 (0.16 to 1.54)	0.52 (0.17 to 1.61)
Had screening tests	518/619 (84)	653/824 (79)	−4	437/621 (70)	589/742 (79)	9	0.48 (0.28 to 0.82)‡	0.53 (0.33 to 0.92)‡
Had ultrasound scan	619/619 (100)	826/827 (100)	0	620/622 (100)	743/743 (100)	0	NA§	NA§
Postnatal								
More anxious	99/879 (11)	86/846 (10)	−1	89/772 (12)	64/630 (10)	−2	0.97 (0.49 to 1.92)	1.13 (0.57 to 2.24)
Stayed in bed during labour	420/888 (47)	428/847 (50)	3	409/796 (51)	319/635 (50)	−1	1.19 (0.82 to 1.72)	1.26 (0.81 to 1.95)
Partner/family present during labour	867/922 (94)	836/886 (94)	0	777/819 (95)	619/661 (94)	−1	1.31 (0.79 to 2.18)	1.39 (0.66 to 2.91)
Continuous monitoring	451/922 (49)	397/886 (45)	−4	387/819 (47)	319/661 (48)	1	0.81 (0.57 to 1.16)	0.83 (0.56 to 1.22)
Had epidural	216/922 (23)	223/886 (25)	2	177/819 (22)	160/661 (24)	2	1.02 (0.59 to 1.74)	1.06 (0.57 to 1.98)
Breastfed	518/921 (56)	511/883 (58)	2	482/818 (59)	389/660 (59)	0	1.15 (0.75 to 1.77)	1.11 (0.63 to 1.97)

*Not included in short questionnaire sent as second reminder to antenatal sample.
†Adjusted for woman's age, age at leaving full time education, parity, and decision style preference.
‡P<0.05.
§Not applicable because everything was at 100%

Table 5 Proportion of women who said they had received any *Informed Choice* leaflet before and after intervention. Figures are numbers (percentage) of women

	Before	After	Change in %
Antenatal			
All	580/1241 (47)	1048/1570 (67)	20
Intervention	266/619 (43)	598/827 (72)	29
Control	314/622 (50)	450/743 (61)	10
Postnatal			
All	760/1741 (44)	977/1547 (63)	19
Intervention	405/922 (44)	665/886 (75)	31
Control	355/819 (43)	312/661 (47)	4

with information and with the way choices were made in intervention units (tables 2 and 3). They were not significant, however, with the exception of satisfaction with information. For this variable the difference in change was less than the minimum important difference of 10 percentage points. There was only one change in postnatal samples, with an increase of 0.24 points on a 10 point knowledge score, which was no longer significant after adjustment for covariates (table 3).

Consequences of informed choice—Given that there was no change in the proportion of women who reported that they exercised informed choice we would not expect changes in choices made. The one significant difference, which was in the proportion of women having screening tests for Down's syndrome and spina bifida, was due in part to an increase in reported uptake in the control units (table 4).

Uptake of leaflets—During the intervention period there was a significant increase in the proportion of women who reported that they had been given any of the *Informed Choice* leaflets in the intervention units compared with the control units, which showed little change (table 5). However, it was difficult to assess the uptake of the intervention leaflets with any precision. A large minority of women in the intervention units (44%) reported that they had been given at least one of the *Informed Choice* leaflets before the intervention had taken place (table 5). It is possible that a few *Informed Choice* leaflets were distributed in all the maternity units before the trial. However, most of this reported use probably relates to leaflets other than those under

study because women had difficulty in distinguishing the intervention leaflets from other leaflets available in the maternity units.

Discussion

In this randomised controlled trial the use of *Informed Choice* leaflets did not change the proportion of women who reported exercising informed choice, or components or consequences of informed choice, in maternity care. This is surprising as a recent systematic review concluded that decision aids improve knowledge and increase the proportion of people who assume a more active role in decision making.[3]

Limitations in design

Possible limitations of this study are response bias, poor definition of "informed choice," and lack of power. The response rate of 64% may have introduced some bias, with under-representation of non-white women and women with manual occupations in both intervention and control groups. The pilot study of two of the leaflets suggested that women with manual occupations might benefit more from the leaflets,[10] suggesting that we may have underestimated the true effect of the leaflets. However, the main study found no relation between social class and effect of the leaflets.[6]

The question used to measure informed choice may have been insensitive. However, we used two different questions and neither showed change. Additionally, we found little change in the components of informed choice, which was consistent with a genuine lack of change in informed choice. Although we recruited fewer women than planned, the analysis for postnatal women was adequately powered due to a smaller intraclass correlation coefficient than estimated for the sample size calculation. The analysis for antenatal women had a power of about 65%. However, observed changes were small, and, although low power can explain the lack of significance, it cannot explain the size of the observed effect. Overall, it is unlikely that the study failed to detect any important change.

Everyday practice

We carried out this trial in everyday practice. We included thousands of women who might have

Table 4 Consequences of informed choice* in women using maternity services. Figures are numbers (percentage) of women

	Intervention			Control			Unadjusted odds ratio (95% CI)	Adjusted† odds ratio (95% CI)
Measure	Before	After	Change in %	Before	After	Change in %		
Antenatal								
More anxious	69/600 (11)	96/803 (12)	1	77/595 (13)	87/724 (12)	−1	1.16 (0.67 to 2.01)	1.28 (0.72 to 2.27)
Drank less alcohol	474/599 (79)	623/796 (78)	−1	443/592 (75)	551/696 (79)	4	0.79 (0.59 to 1.06)	0.72 (0.46 to 1.15)
Planned hospital birth	608/619 (98)	799/826 (97)	−1	604/620 (97)	725/743 (98)	1	0.50 (0.16 to 1.54)	0.52 (0.17 to 1.61)
Had screening tests	518/619 (84)	653/824 (79)	−4	437/621 (70)	589/742 (79)	9	0.48 (0.28 to 0.82)‡	0.53 (0.33 to 0.92)‡
Had ultrasound scan	619/619 (100)	826/827 (100)	0	620/622 (100)	743/743 (100)	0	NA§	NA§
Postnatal								
More anxious	99/879 (11)	86/846 (10)	−1	89/772 (12)	64/630 (10)	−2	0.97 (0.49 to 1.92)	1.13 (0.57 to 2.24)
Stayed in bed during labour	420/888 (47)	428/847 (50)	3	409/796 (51)	319/635 (50)	−1	1.19 (0.82 to 1.72)	1.26 (0.81 to 1.95)
Partner/family present during labour	867/922 (94)	836/886 (94)	0	777/819 (95)	619/661 (94)	−1	1.31 (0.79 to 2.18)	1.39 (0.66 to 2.91)
Continuous monitoring	451/922 (49)	397/886 (45)	−4	387/819 (47)	319/661 (48)	1	0.81 (0.57 to 1.16)	0.83 (0.56 to 1.22)
Had epidural	216/922 (23)	223/886 (25)	2	177/819 (22)	160/661 (24)	2	1.02 (0.59 to 1.74)	1.06 (0.57 to 1.98)
Breastfed	518/921 (56)	511/883 (58)	2	482/818 (59)	389/660 (59)	0	1.15 (0.75 to 1.77)	1.11 (0.63 to 1.97)

*Not included in short questionnaire sent as second reminder to antenatal sample.
†Adjusted for woman's age, age at leaving full time education, parity, and decision style preference.
‡P<0.05.
§Not applicable because everything was at 100%

23 Which of the following is the most likely reason for the choice of these measures?

a) They are among the most pressing issues for women today
b) They link with important physical and psychological outcomes of birth
c) They correlated with the topics in the informed choice leaflets

24 From the raw data, are the following statements true or false?

a) Women in the antenatal sample of the intervention group drank less alcohol after the intervention than before
b) Women in the postnatal sample of the control group were less likely to have their partner present during labour than women in the postnatal sample of the intervention group
c) Every single woman who entered the study had an ultrasound scan

received the 10 leaflets, but only 70% reported receiving one of them. Studies reported in the systematic review of decision aids were explanatory trials, with the implicit assumption that all patients received the intervention.[3] One conclusion might be that the systematic review showed that decision aids can be effective under certain circumstances but that our study showed that they are not necessarily effective in the real world. The pragmatic nature of our design may have affected the outcome, but that outcome represents a true picture of the impact of introducing the leaflets into clinical practice.

Quality of implementation

There is some evidence from the trial that there were difficulties with the implementation of the intervention. The accompanying qualitative study shows that the *Informed Choice* leaflets were not introduced to women as special and different from other leaflets.[4] Additionally, not all women reported that they had been given any of the leaflets during the intervention. This limited implementation of decision aids is by no means unique to either the *Informed Choice* leaflets or maternity care.[11]

Generalisability of findings

The results are generalisable to maternity units that use *Informed Choice* leaflets to promote informed choice but not to health professionals purchasing the leaflets to guide evidence based practice or individual enthusiastic health professionals purchasing the leaflets to help meet the information needs of their clients.

We thank midwives, managers, and administrative staff in the maternity units in Wales (unnamed to ensure confidentiality of participating units), who worked so hard to help us with data collection. We thank the thousands of women who completed our questionnaires at such an important time in their lives.

Contributors: AO'C contributed to the design of the study, designed the questionnaire, coordinated data collection, contributed to data analysis, wrote the paper, and is guarantor for the paper. SJW contributed to the design of the study, undertook the data analysis, and contributed to the writing of the paper. JPN and KJT contributed to design of the study and the questionnaire, interpretation of the data, and writing of the paper. MK contributed to the design of the study and the questionnaire and writing of the paper. Helen Stapleton contributed to the design and piloting of the questionnaire. Heather Rothwell helped to establish data collection systems. Andrea Shippam and April Dagnell undertook data administration.

What is already known on this topic

Decision aids can help patients to participate in their care

Ten evidence based leaflets (*Informed Choice*) are used by maternity services in the United Kingdom to promote informed choice in women using these services

What this paper adds

The leaflets did not help to promote informed choice in maternity care

Decision aids may not be effective in the real world

Donna Mead, Laurence Moseley, Barbara Bale, Gwenan Thomas, and Sandy Kirkman were members of the research team for the wider study, of which the randomised controlled trial forms a part.

Funding: This work was commissioned by the NHS Centre of Reviews and Dissemination and funded by the Department of Health. The views expressed here are those of the authors and not necessarily those of the Department of Health.

Competing interests: None declared.

1   Charles C, Gafni A, Whelan T. International conference on treatment decision-making in the clinical encounter [editorial]. *Health Expect* 2000;3:1-5.
2   Entwistle VA. Supporting and resourcing treatment decision-making: some policy considerations. *Health Expect* 2000;3:77-85.
3   O'Connor AM, Rostom A, Fiset V, Tetroe J, Entwistle V, Llewellyn-Thomas H, et al. Decision aids for patients facing health treatment or screening decisions: systematic review. *BMJ* 1999;319:731-4.
4   Stapleton H, Kirkham M, Thomas G. Qualitative study of evidence based leaflets in maternity care. *BMJ* 2002;324:639-43.
5   Degner L, Sloan JA, Venkatesh P. The control preference scale. *Can J Nurs Res* 1997;29:21-43.
6   Kirkham M, Stapleton H, eds. *Informed choice in maternity care: an evaluation of evidence based leaflets.* York: University of York, 2001 (report 20).
7   Diehr P, Martin DC, Koepsell T, Cheadle A. Breaking the matches in a paired t-test for community interventions when the number of pairs is small. *Stat Med* 1995;14:1491-504.
8   Murray DM. *Design and analysis of group randomised trials.* Oxford: Oxford University Press, 1998.
9   SAS Institute. *SAS/STAT user's guide.* Version 6. 4th ed. Vol 2. Cary, NC: SAS Institute, 1989.
10 Oliver S, Rajan L, Turner H, Oakley A. *A pilot study of two informed choice leaflets on positions in labour and routine ultrasound.* York: Social Science Research Unit and NHS Centre for Reviews and Dissemination, 1996 (CRD report 7).
11 Holmes-Rovner M, Valade D, Orlowski C, Draus C, Nabozny-Valerio B, Keiser S. Implementing shared decision-making in routine practice: barriers and opportunities. *Health Expect* 2000;3:182-91.

(Accepted 5 October 2001)

25 Why would it have been beneficial for the informed choice leaflets to have been highlighted to the women in the study as 'special and different'?

26 Would this study change your practice in relation to your current (or future) use of informed choice leaflets? If so, then why? If not, then why not? What do you feel is the most objective conclusion for a practising midwife to draw from this study?

27 The fact that the Department of Health funded this research might lead us to assume (True/False):
a) That the Department of Health is interested in this area
b) That this is currently a key issue in midwifery practice
c) That this is an area of practice the government is keen to promote
d) That the authors wrote a good proposal for the research
e) That, because the NHS Centre for Reviews and Dissemination is involved with the informed choice leaflets, it has a particular interest in evaluating this area

28 Why does it increase the credibility of the article for authors to declare their competing interests?

ANSWERS

Q1. a) Yes, the introduction should at least begin to explain how and why this research fits with women's needs and/or current practice, although this explanation may continue into the next section(s) of the paper as well

b) Maybe: if terms need explaining or defining this should ideally happen near the beginning of the paper

c) Maybe, although some researchers may only do this briefly, especially if they feel this should be evident to the reader

d) No

Q2. a) False

b) True

c) True

d) False

Q3. a) False

b) True

c) False

d) False

Q4. Yes, women who had booked with independent midwives or who had booked later on in their pregnancies – you might be able to think of others as well

Q5. a) To prevent data contamination

b) Problems obtaining consent

c) Sensitivity/respect for the women's needs

Q6. a) True

b) False

c) False, although you could calculate this from the numbers in the table

d) False

Q7. Some possible advantages include that postal questionnaires are simple, quick, relatively cheap, easily quantified for analysis and women can remain anonymous. The disadvantages include that you may get a poor response rate, you don't know whether the respondents are misunderstanding any of the questions, you can't actually be sure that it is the woman herself who filled it out and women have no chance to elaborate if they have more to say about something than the forced choices and tick boxes on some questions allow

Q8. These outcome measures are relatively 'soft' because they measure people's opinions rather than some kind of physical parameter that is easier to measure and quantify

Q9. Well, you might have come up with other ideas here but the main issue that this question raises is the problem that arises where we want to do quantitative research on what people think and know, yet our thoughts and knowledge are far more difficult to quantify and compare than things like our height, weight or shoe size. Researchers know that this kind of data can be 'muddy', but, if we want to do quantitative studies on this kind of thing, it is all we have to work with!

Q10. Yes, because pregnant women are considered a vulnerable group

Q11. c) Essential, because it is important to show that the groups were comparable and that the randomisation was effective

Q12. c) Intention to treat analysis means that, regardless of what *actually* happened, i.e. whether all the women in the treatment groups received the leaflets and all the women in the control group didn't, the data from each of the groups are analysed as if the ideal had happened. See Wickham (2003) for further discussion on this

Q13. a) The groups were fairly well matched in all of the areas. Although there was a slight difference in age, which the authors discuss, the groups are still fairly well matched in that area

Q14. a) Confidence interval

b) Standard deviation

Both of these are discussed more fully in Section 6

Q15. b)

Q16. Women may be concerned about the impact that a negative response might have on their care, or they might want to please the midwife who had looked after them

Q17. Hopefully not; although this is the kind of thing that might bias a research study, the whole point of randomisation is that this sort of thing would occur at about the same rate in the two groups

Q18. The figures do give some cause for concern because, although they show that women in the intervention group were more likely to have said they received the leaflets than women in the control group, they also show two other things. First, not all women in the intervention group said they had received the leaflets even after the intervention; second, some of the women in the control group said they had received the leaflets. It is impossible to know whether women had actually received the leaflets; perhaps they had forgotten or had muddled the informed choice leaflets up with other leaflets that they had been given. However, it is obvious from the report of the study that the researchers were aware of these potential problems and took a pragmatic approach towards this issue

Q19. Perhaps you can think of a way, but I can't! It seems to me that it would be unfair and unethical to take other information away so that the informed choice leaflets were the only information available (although I would happily tend the bonfire of some of the other so-called 'information' leaflets (i.e. not the informed choice ones!) that are given out to women at booking!). This is one of the drawbacks of the RCT, which is why other types of study can help us gain further knowledge and understanding in this area

Q20. Everybody's answer to this will be different – mine is in the discussion that follows these answers

Q21. Hopefully, you have come up with something like, 'it means that there were not enough women in the study for any statistically significant difference between the two groups to show up'

Q22. c) More on this in the next chapter!

Q23. c) This is probably the most likely reason, but a) and b) are also important and related

Q24. a) True (but only just!)

b) False, the figure is the same for both groups

c) False. Although you might think it were true if you only looked at the percentages that were 'rounded up' – if this was the case for you, go back and look at the raw numbers in the tables!

Q25. For me, the critical thing to consider is the sheer weight of information that women receive and the chances that, if they weren't told that they were 'special and different,' they might have left the informed choice leaflets in a pile somewhere!

Q26. Well, the results certainly wouldn't make me throw away my informed choice leaflets just yet! Although it is important to acknowledge that this study didn't seem to show a significant benefit, there were a number of reasons why this might have been the case, including the fact that, as we have just discussed, the leaflets were not highlighted by the midwives as being 'special and important'. There is no evidence from this study that simply making the informed choice leaflets available to women has a significant impact on the outcomes studied. However, as the authors suggest, in the hands of individual midwives who are enthusiastic about promoting choice and basing their own practice on evidence, the informed choice leaflets might well be an effective tool – we just haven't done any research to check that out yet!

Q27. I assume that all of these are true!

Q28. It highlights whether authors have a vested interest in the result of a study, for instance whether they seek to benefit from the sales of a drug or product

DISCUSSION

To recap, this study divided maternity units into two groups, half of which gave informed choice leaflets out to women and half of which didn't. Data were collected on a number of outcomes, including whether women felt they had enough information to make informed choices, but also on things like whether their partner or another supporter was with them in labour, thus measuring the potential effect of the leaflets on some of the choices they actually made.

However, the findings suggest that the leaflets didn't make any difference to women feeling they had exercised informed choice, although they did seem to make a slight difference to women's satisfaction. The authors discuss a number of sources of potential bias; these include response bias and a poor definition of 'informed choice' and they also talk about the possibility that they didn't have enough women in the study to show an effect. Overall, though, they concluded that it was unlikely that their study failed to detect any significant change.

This RCT highlights some of the problems that can arise when we try and use this tool (i.e. the RCT) to evaluate non-physical things. Although all sorts of problems can arise even when you use RCTs to measure purely physical interventions and outcomes, when you start trying to use them to measure things like choice, thoughts and knowledge, you can end up with all sorts of areas where your study could be potentially biased. It is hard to quantify how much someone knows about a particular area, and even harder to quantify how much more or less they know than another person. One of the ways in which the authors of this study set out to reduce the potential for bias in this area was to also look at the choices women actually made: whether they had a supporter in labour, whether they had an epidural, whether they breastfed. But you don't have to think about each of these things for very long to realise that each of these choices is very complex and can be influenced of lots of factors, including the women's existing beliefs and the kind of care they experience during and after pregnancy and childbirth.

Taking both this and the results of the study into account, you might decide that the most logical conclusion to draw from this study is to say that informed choice leaflets obviously don't work. Women are influenced by lots of things, the leaflets are pretty ineffective and those of us who write them, publish them or hand them out to women might as well go home and focus our attention on something else. However, I am not prepared to draw that conclusion just yet, for a couple of reasons. One is that I have other kinds of knowledge about this area that contradict the results of the research; I have had a number of experiences in practice that have led me to believe that the leaflets are useful, and my wider knowledge about midwifery practice and women's experiences tells me that there is more to this picture than was shown in the study we have just looked at. I am not suggesting that I am planning to give these kinds of knowledge more importance than the study because I don't like its results – I have to bear in mind that I might be completely biased or wrong about this. However, I am human and therefore I do not base everything I know on research alone, so, for now, I am going to try to keep an open mind.

One of the things that really strikes me about the study is something the authors say right at the end, where they point out that the results are generalisable to maternity units but not to individual health professionals. In other words, the study shows that having the leaflets generally available in hospitals does not seem to make a difference but, in the hands of individuals who were enthusiastic about the concept of informed choice, they could have an influence.

The authors also note that the other part of this study (which we'll get to in just a minute) raised the issue that leaflets were not highlighted as 'special and different'. I can't get rid of the vision I have of women being handed great piles of stuff at booking, with the informed choice leaflets being tucked in amongst Emma's diary, the pregnancy books, the nappy adverts, the samples of creams for stretch marks and babies' bums, the pharmaceutical company leaflets discussing things like anti-D, the information on screening tests – I could go on, but you probably get the idea! How many women actually read all that stuff? More importantly, what would be the effect on women if they did read it all and found that the informed choice leaflet, based as it is on research evidence, said something entirely different to one or more of the other leaflets, which are not always based on research evidence?

It seems to me that, if we really want to look more closely at these kinds of issues, we need a qualitative study to supplement what we have learned from the RCT. Happily, the researchers involved in this study could see that there might be a need for this before they even started their research, and they ran a qualitative study alongside the RCT that you have just looked at. In the next chapter, Nadine Pilley Edwards offers an overview of qualitative research and then looks at the qualitative study of informed choice leaflets, in order to broaden and widen our knowledge on this topic.

REFERENCES

Oakley A 2000 Experiments in knowing. Gender and method in the social sciences. The New Press, New York
Wickham S 2003 Seeing women in the numbers. MIDIRS Midwifery Digest 13(4):439–44

CHAPTER 2

Nadine Pilley Edwards

INTRODUCTION

What is qualitative research all about?

Stapleton, H, Kirkham, M, Thomas G 2002
Qualitative study of evidence based leaflets in
maternity care. British Medical Journal 324:639

Doing and analysing qualitative research is neither straightforward nor easy. Researchers are continually having to develop the concepts and tools to do it. Individual readers and critical commentators have to find ways of forming an opinion about it. Collectively, we do not always know quite what to do with its findings in the context of evidence-based care. This is particularly the case when we have a long research tradition that has focused on developing strategies for carrying out and interpreting quantitative research. Nevertheless qualitative research fits well with a growing acceptance of the uncertainty and partiality of knowledge (Wickham 2004).

Unlike quantitative research, qualitative research does not strive for generalisability but tells us about the particularities of people's lives: the similarities and differences between them. It is not about truth claims, although its claims are perhaps true at that time for those people, and might ring true for others. Instead, it is an exploratory adventure designed to provide insights into the complexities of people's lives. It seeks to understand different perspectives and influences on how people live their lives. It breathes colour and vibrancy into the black and white facts and figures of quantitative research. It brings a human face to the facelessness of statistics. It demonstrates how quantitative research is a valuable, but partial, piece of the knowledge map. Above all, it shows us that knowledge comes from all sorts of places and people and is shaped by our beliefs, backgrounds and lifestyles. None of this need quench our thirst for knowledge, or prevent us from doing meaningful and useful research. It reminds us to be vigilant and humble about what we think we know, as well as open to surprises (there are endless parallels between research and midwifery!). It also reminds us that each and everyone of us contributes to knowledge and suggests that knowledge is a communal affair influenced by empirical, traditional, political, cultural and social aspects of our societies (Longino 2002).

I believe that the appearance of commentaries about qualitative research, and the appearance of research papers such as the one below in mainstream medical journals, is a positive move. It suggests that it is gaining some acceptance within science and medicine. But the emphasis is still on quantitative research, especially randomised controlled trials (RCTs), similar to the ones in Chapters 1 and 6. Because they use the language and practices of science – facts, probabilities and statistical calculation – they are often assumed to provide greatest certainty of knowledge. But, as we now know, this can be misleading. At best, the findings of RCTs suggest that the majority of people respond in particular ways to identified treatments or interventions. The RCT cannot tell us how an individual might respond to a particular treatment or intervention. Because qualitative research uses the language and practices of sociology, it is still seen by some as unscientific and therefore uncertain and untrustworthy.

Why do we need qualitative research?

Clearly, good statistical analyses can give us invaluable information about generalities and trends in populations as you have seen in the previous chapter and will see again in Chapters 3, 5 and 6. As Mary Maynard (1994) points out, quantitative research on violence against women increased our knowledge about the extent of the problem. But it was the additional qualitative research that told us about the nature of this violence. These layers of research can help us formulate plans to reduce violence against women and help those who are victims of it. In the field of birth, quantitative research tells us about the number of mothers and babies who survive, become ill and – tragically –

occasionally die, but not about the series of events that led to illness or death. It might tell us about the general effectiveness of drugs and technological procedures but it usually tells us nothing about the experiences of women and babies and their families and the quality of their lives. Yet, women are concerned about their and their families' long-term physical health, emotional and often, spiritual lives as well as their babies' short-term physical health at birth (Edwards 2005, Lewis 1990, Murphy-Lawless 1998, Noble 2001). And, as we know, women's birth experiences have a profound impact on them and their families.

Some of the most important research for women has been feminist and midwifery qualitative research that interprets women's experiences against the backdrop of cultural assumptions, expectations and practices. For example, research that showed that women desire more technology during pregnancy and birth found that this represented a desire for control rather than for technology itself (Evans 1985). Research that looked at women who do not follow medical advice and treatments (so-called 'non-compliers') showed that the constraints women face in their day-to-day lives makes it difficult for them to follow medical advice that does not take these into account (Hunt et al 1989). Research on women with chest pains assumed that if these pains did not indicate a heart problem, they must indicate a psychological problem. Qualitative, feminist research showed that chest pains can be associated with anxiety following experiences of being raped or sexually abused in other ways (Burt & Code 1995 p 32). Women who plan home births are sometimes accused of putting their own needs above their baby's safety. Qualitative research suggests that everything a woman plans in relation to home birth is to do with safety – an expanded meaning of safety (Edwards 2005).

Good qualitative research seeks to uncover the cultural, political and social themes that underpin society. For example, in maternity care, it suggests that the technocratic imperative (Davis-Floyd 1992, Davis-Floyd & St John 1998, Machin & Scamell 1997; see Chapter 8) and the power of dominant beliefs over women and midwives (Kirkham 2004) increase women's compliancy and the likelihood of them having technological births, even if they had wanted to avoid interventions.

In fact, one of the problems with quantitative research (and sometimes qualitative research) is that it tends to accept and reflect dominant values (see van Teijlingen et al 2003 and Tricia Anderson's discussion of this in Chapter 3). In childbearing these are usually obstetric values. It also risks simplifying complex ethical decisions into decisions based on statistics or evidence-based care alone. Not only can we never be sure about the accuracy of evidence-based care (Bastian 2004) but there is a further risk that those apparently advocating the exclusive use of evidence-based care to make complex decisions are making ethical judgements of their own. Attitudes towards women planning home births, water births, vaginal breech births and vaginal births after caesarean section are examples of this (see, for example, Anderson 2004).

Qualitative research is not without its problems

Of course, all research – quantitative or qualitative – has its strengths and limitations (Longino 2002, Oakley 2000, Shipman 1988). Any research depends on the skills and integrity of the researcher. Qualitative research depends on finding the people with the experiences the researcher wants to study, their willingness to share their thoughts and experiences, and the rapport between them and the researcher. All research is also political. It is always carried out by people who have backgrounds, views, assumptions, feelings and thoughts in a culture that also has many assumptions. So whereas qualitative research attempts to uncover silences and dispel unhelpful stereotyping (Burt & Code 1995, Clair 1997, Edwards & Ribbens 1998, Fine & Gordon 1992, Maynard & Purvis 1994, Morgan & Coombes 2001), it may or may not achieve this; it might even create its own silences and oppressions.

The format for reporting research is historically based on quantitative methods. This often means that complex qualitative research methodology and assumptions are only briefly reported in research findings, so it is difficult to know just how the research has been carried out and analysed and therefore how reliable it is. It tends not to be replicable. It often engages with complex social questions and requires the reader to engage with these in order to think through its meanings and implications. The reader needs to ask herself or himself about the author's stance, what assumptions have been made, whether the researcher has described what he or she found or has given some kind of context for the research and thus provided a deeper analysis of the findings.

The value of working together

Attempts to dichotomise quantitative and qualitative methods of research are unhelpful and problematic. Not least because, as Ann Oakley (2000) points out, issues of judgement cannot be erased from quantitative methods any more than a numerical base can be erased from qualitative methods. Indeed, as has been suggested above, moving across the quantitative/qualitative divide can provide detail in quantitative research that would otherwise have remained hidden, and can highlight the extent of issues in qualitative research that may equally well have remained hidden. In other words, quantitative research tells us about trends in populations and qualitative research tells us about the detail and the inconsistencies within these overall trends. Each approach both contributes to the other and demonstrates its shortcomings.

The research findings in the paper below are, I believe, particularly exciting because they provide a more sophisticated insight into the shortcomings of using only quantitative research for a social intervention (giving information leaflets to women) and demonstrate how quantitative and qualitative methods can work effectively together. The findings uncovered not only practical problems with the RCT arm of the trial, which would not otherwise have been detected and which limited its findings, but also dominant cultural beliefs that question the meaning of the RCT trial findings. The qualitative work raises questions about what can usefully be the subject of RCTs and what (if anything) a RCT *alone* can tell us.

The findings (about giving women information leaflets) help us to 'see' into the numbers of the previous paper. They uncover important background themes that explain what the numbers really mean – this is what is so important about them. Instead of telling us to abandon leaflets that inform women about their options with a sigh of relief – so that the business of 'steering' (Levy 2004) or even coercing women (see examples in Kirkham 2004) can continue as usual – it challenges us to think about how we could structure maternity services and engage with women in ways that might encourage autonomy among women and midwives (see Edwards & Leap 2006).

Qualitative research projects can be carried out in many different ways. They might involve one researcher carrying out interviews with a small number of people or, like the one in this chapter, they might involve a number of researchers in different hospitals and community settings. For example, researchers might interview people individually or in groups, observe them, and/or ask them to write diaries. The research examined here relied on four researchers carrying out a large number of interviews with women, midwives and doctors and spending many hours observing and recording interactions between them. These methods generally come under the heading of ethnographic research, a method that is further explored in Chapter 8. This kind of research is increasingly being used in childbirth studies to look at women's experiences, relationships between women and health practitioners and relationships between different kinds of health practitioners.

Qualitative research focuses on qualitative aspects of our lives. Although it is important to ask ourselves about social and cultural assumptions when critically analysing quantitative research, qualitative research particularly lends itself to these kinds of questions. Thus many of the questions that relate to this article reflect this focus and, as was suggested in the introduction, many questions have no right or wrong answers, but are designed to help us think about our own and others' assumptions and how these impact on how we read and interpret research.

QUESTIONS FOR CHAPTER 2

1   Which of the following statements are true? Non-participant observation involves:

a) Sitting quietly in a corner
b) Watching people through binoculars
c) Videoing people
d) Observing people through a unidirectional glass panel

2   Which of these statements are most true? In-depth interviews are:

a) Interviews that last at least an hour
b) Interviews during which the researcher asks a long list of questions
c) Interviews where the researcher has some prepared questions but also asks other questions that he or she thinks of as the person is talking
d) Conversations between the researcher and the person being interviewed
e) Interviews where the researcher asks only open questions

3   What might you hope to find out by observing people, asking them questions and listening to them in different settings, such as their own homes, clinics and hospitals?

4   Does including 13 maternity units sound:

a) Too few on which to base meaningful findings?
b) Too many for a qualitative study?
c) An odd number to pick?
d) A typical number for this type of research?

5   Do you think that time pressure on practitioners impacts on choice for women? Is this something you have come across in your work situation, or expect to encounter in the workplace?

6   Can you give some examples of what might generally be considered 'right' and 'wrong' choices for women to make? Why do you think these are classified as right and wrong?

7   Which of these statements are true? A hierarchical power structure means that those near the bottom of the hierarchy:

a) Have less power than others
b) Have less authority than others
c) Have less knowledge than others
d) Are more oppressed than others

8   Are the following statements true or false?

a) People are always aware of the power they have over others
b) People are always aware when they are being oppressed
c) People are always aware of their place in the hierarchy
d) People must always eventually come to accept their place in a hierarchy

9   Can you name some other hierarchical power structures in our society?

10 Why do most women trust health professionals? Is it because:

a) Professionals usually know best?
b) Professionals are more knowledgeable about birth than women?
c) Women have been brought up to trust experts?
d) Our society tends to trust professionals?

Papers

Qualitative study of evidence based leaflets in maternity care

Helen Stapleton, Mavis Kirkham, Gwenan Thomas

Abstract

Objective To examine the use of evidence based leaflets on informed choice in maternity services.
Design Non-participant observation of 886 antenatal consultations. 383 in depth interviews with women using maternity services and health professionals providing antenatal care.
Setting Women's homes; antenatal and ultrasound clinics in 13 maternity units in Wales.
Participants Childbearing women and health professionals who provide antenatal care.
Intervention Provision of 10 pairs of *Informed Choice* leaflets for service users and staff and a training session in their use.
Main outcome measures Participants' views and commonly observed responses during consultations and interviews.
Results Health professionals were positive about the leaflets and their potential to assist women in making informed choices, but competing demands within the clinical environment undermined their effective use. Time pressures limited discussion, and choice was often not available in practice. A widespread belief that technological intervention would be viewed positively in the event of litigation reinforced notions of "right" and "wrong" choices rather than "informed" choices. Hierarchical power structures resulted in obstetricians defining the norms of clinical practice and hence which choices were possible. Women's trust in health professionals ensured their compliance with professionally defined choices, and only rarely were they observed asking questions or making alternative requests. Midwives rarely discussed the contents of the leaflets or distinguished them from other literature related to pregnancy. The visibility and potential of the leaflets as evidence based decision aids was thus greatly reduced.
Conclusions The way in which the leaflets were disseminated affected promotion of informed choice in maternity care. The culture into which the leaflets were introduced supported existing normative patterns of care and this ensured informed compliance rather than informed choice.

Introduction

The organisation and provision of maternity care in the United Kingdom was challenged when the *Chang-*

 ing Childbirth report recommended that it become more "woman centred."[1] The 10 research based leaflets (*Informed Choice*)[2] were developed by the Midwives Information and Resource Service to support consumer choice.[3] The effectiveness of these leaflets has been studied in a randomised controlled trial which is reported separately.[2] To understand the social context in which the leaflets were used we undertook qualitative research alongside, but independently of, the randomised trial.

Attitudes of staff are thought to influence the choices available to childbearing women[1 5] and decision making in clinical practice.[6–8] Organisational culture affects the quality of health care.[9–11] "Socially complex interventions,"[12] such as the *Informed Choice* leaflets, should be evaluated within the context in which they are used and through a prudent combination of qualitative and quantitative methods.[13 14]

Methods

In the randomised controlled trial, 13 maternity units formed 10 clusters, five of which received the intervention of the *Informed Choice* leaflets between May and December 1998.[3 15] Four female midwifery researchers, including two of the authors (HS and GT), undertook non-participant observation and in depth interviews with health professionals and women, in both intervention and control maternity units (table). All the researchers kept detailed field notes for analysis. We used a grounded theory approach to data collection and analysis[16] and the software package QSR NUD*IST[17] to organise and interrogate the datasets.

The combination of qualitative methods enabled us to examine the same issue from a range of different perspectives and to explore beyond "official" accounts

11 Which of these statements is most true? Informed compliance is:

a) When women understand what is being said to them by professionals and agree to follow their advice
b) When women are given advice that is likely to lead them to make the decisions professionals wish them to make
c) When women agree to follow professional advice because they believe professionals know best
d) Another way of saying informed choice
e) Another way of saying informed consent

Papers

Qualitative study of evidence based leaflets in maternity care

Helen Stapleton, Mavis Kirkham, Gwenan Thomas

Abstract

Objective To examine the use of evidence based leaflets on informed choice in maternity services.
Design Non-participant observation of 886 antenatal consultations. 383 in depth interviews with women using maternity services and health professionals providing antenatal care.
Setting Women's homes; antenatal and ultrasound clinics in 13 maternity units in Wales.
Participants Childbearing women and health professionals who provide antenatal care.
Intervention Provision of 10 pairs of *Informed Choice* leaflets for service users and staff and a training session in their use.
Main outcome measures Participants' views and commonly observed responses during consultations and interviews.
Results Health professionals were positive about the leaflets and their potential to assist women in making informed choices, but competing demands within the clinical environment undermined their effective use. Time pressures limited discussion, and choice was often not available in practice. A widespread belief that technological intervention would be viewed positively in the event of litigation reinforced notions of "right" and "wrong" choices rather than "informed" choices. Hierarchical power structures resulted in obstetricians defining the norms of clinical practice and hence which choices were possible. Women's trust in health professionals ensured their compliance with professionally defined choices, and only rarely were they observed asking questions or making alternative requests. Midwives rarely discussed the contents of the leaflets or distinguished them from other literature related to pregnancy. The visibility and potential of the leaflets as evidence based decision aids was thus greatly reduced.
Conclusions The way in which the leaflets were disseminated affected promotion of informed choice in maternity care. The culture into which the leaflets were introduced supported existing normative patterns of care and this ensured informed compliance rather than informed choice.

Introduction

The organisation and provision of maternity care in the United Kingdom was challenged when the *Changing Childbirth* report recommended that it become more "woman centred."[1] The 10 research based leaflets (*Informed Choice*)[2] were developed by the Midwives Information and Resource Service to support consumer choice.[3] The effectiveness of these leaflets has been studied in a randomised controlled trial which is reported separately.[2] To understand the social context in which the leaflets were used we undertook qualitative research alongside, but independently of, the randomised trial.

Attitudes of staff are thought to influence the choices available to childbearing women[4 5] and decision making in clinical practice.[6–8] Organisational culture affects the quality of health care.[9–11] "Socially complex interventions,"[12] such as the *Informed Choice* leaflets, should be evaluated within the context in which they are used and through a prudent combination of qualitative and quantitative methods.[13 14]

Methods

In the randomised controlled trial, 13 maternity units formed 10 clusters, five of which received the intervention of the *Informed Choice* leaflets between May and December 1998.[3 15] Four female midwifery researchers, including two of the authors (HS and GT), undertook non-participant observation and in depth interviews with health professionals and women, in both intervention and control maternity units (table). All the researchers kept detailed field notes for analysis. We used a grounded theory approach to data collection and analysis[16] and the software package QSR NUD*IST[17] to organise and interrogate the datasets.

The combination of qualitative methods enabled us to examine the same issue from a range of different perspectives and to explore beyond "official" accounts

Summary of qualitative methods in study of informed choice in maternity services

Respondents	Episodes of observation	Interviews
Childbearing women	886	163 (85 antenatal, 78 postnatal)
Midwives	653	177
Obstetricians	167	28
Obstetric ultrasonographers	66	12
Obstetric anaesthetists	NA*	3
Total	886	383 (17 conducted in Welsh)

*NA=not applicable as observation of women in labour was not undertaken.

---

12 When doing qualitative research, do we need to know anything about the topic we are researching?
a) Yes, so as not to waste time and resources duplicating research
b) Yes, because it might help us decide what research should be done and how to do it
c) No, it's best not to know too much about the topic we want to research in case we become less objective and more biased
d) No, because the research that has been done is probably flawed and we do not want to be influenced by it

13 Which of the following would you describe as a socially complex intervention?
a) Reducing the number of antenatal visits for women from 14 to 6 or 7
b) Comparing continuous electronic fetal monitoring with intermittent monitoring
c) Comparing mortality outcomes for women and babies following vaginal or caesarean birth for healthy breech term babies
d) Measuring the effectiveness of using birth pools for pain relief
e) Introducing counselling before antenatal testing

14 Specify in your own words why combining qualitative and quantitative research methods was useful in this research

15 What do you think about the time scale in this study? Does it seem:
a) Too short to get good results?
b) About right for this kind of qualitative research?
c) Unnecessarily long?
d) It is difficult to know how long qualitative research should be?

16 Why would qualitative researchers keep fieldnotes?
a) For legal reasons
b) To prove that the research was accurate
c) To improve the reliability of the research
d) To improve their powers of observation and interpretation

17 Which of these statements are true? Grounded theory:
a) Is one of a number of different approaches to qualitative research
b) Cannot be used on its own
c) Always includes interviews
d) Works by looking at the deeper themes and connections in the data
e) Means that the researcher builds on the data as he or she collects them. For example, if a research subject raises an issue that the researcher had not thought of, she or he then adds this into the next interviews with new subjects

N1. NUD*IST stands for Non-numerical Unstructured Data Indexing Searching and Theorising. It is a computer software program designed to assist with the management and analysis of qualitative data. Although it is unclear what impact this has on the analysis, it provides a tool for examining large amounts of data thoroughly and systematically. NUD*IST is constantly updated and has a sister program QSR NUD*IST Vivo (NVivo). An internet search on 'NUD*IST' provides further information.

18 Why might having a range of different perspectives be useful?

19 What kind of research needs to have ethical approval?

a) All research
b) Medical research
c) Social research
d) Researchers decide

20 Which of these statements is most true? A semi-structured format means that the researcher:

a) Has a set list of questions
b) Has no preconceived ideas about what might come up in the interview
c) Has planned some questions but is open to asking unplanned questions if it seems appropriate at the time
d) Asks a mixture of open and closed questions

21 Why are openness and discussion so important in qualitative research?

N2. This links with the concept of 'rapport', which is a somewhat controversial term. Some researchers believe that, in order not to bias research, they must remain distant and impassive when interviewing subjects. Feminists and others, however, argue that a level of connection and appropriate disclosure enables women to feel more at ease and encourages them to talk more easily about their views and experiences (see Oakley 1993).

N3. Researchers rely on 'opportunistic' moments to further their research, especially in the initial phases. This means that they take any opportunity to talk with anyone who might be able to contribute to the research. As it progresses, they might want to make sure that they have included the views of certain individuals or groups of people and deliberately seek out or 'select' these people to maximise the relevance and breadth of the research data.

---

of choice and decision making from health professionals and childbearing women.

We obtained approval for the study from the local ethics committee.

Observations

We used observations of antenatal consultations (table) to identify how the leaflets were used and how informed choice and decision making occurred in practice. We made detailed field notes concerning setting, actions, words, and non-verbal cues of all present.

Interviews

We undertook face to face interviews using a semistructured format. We developed interview guides that were specific to the different participant groups, but all participants were invited to discuss the availability and quality of information, including the *Informed Choice* leaflets, receiving and conveying information, the meaning of informed choice, and the role of childbearing women in decision making. We also discussed inferences made by the researchers about behaviours and interactions during consultations. More than half of the interviews followed on from observation sessions, and this enabled us to explore issues, especially those of a sensitive nature, within the context of a previously established relationship.

Sampling

Our initial observation sample was "opportunistic," being determined by the staff on duty and whether they and their clients were willing to accommodate the researchers. We identified commonly observed responses, such as pregnant women expressing satisfaction with their care and complying with the choices offered to them, staff expressing concern about time pressures, and midwives describing the leaflets as useful tools. As the research progressed, we sampled more selectively to ensure that all women of childbearing age, all social classes, and various current and previous obstetric experiences were represented, together with women from minority groups. We sampled many more midwives than other health professionals because they provided most antenatal care and disseminated most of the leaflets. In an effort to observe and understand good practice we sampled a small number of midwives in all maternity units who were described by their managers as excellent in facilitating informed choice.

Towards the end of the intervention period we selected interviewees to confirm or refute emerging theory. As most staff and women tended to "go with the flow" of routine clinical practices, such sampling thus included women who questioned or declined the choices offered to them and staff who offered choices (and leaflets) withheld by colleagues. For midwives this revealed a link between practice and work setting. Midwives in community or domiciliary settings were generally more knowledgeable about women's individual needs and seemed more willing to advocate on their behalf. They also tended to make more openings for women to voice their concerns. Hence, we identified interplay between hierarchy, power, and trust and the impact on information sharing between women and different groups of midwives. We continued to explore themes with all relevant participant groups until repeated, rather than new, information was forthcoming and theoretical saturation was achieved.

We removed identifying information from selected transcripts and shared them with members of the research team and outside experts. This guided future data collection, guarded against any researcher dominating the analytical process, and helped to ensure validity and reliability.[18][19]

Results

The "invisible" leaflets

Most health professionals initially expressed positive views about the principles underpinning the *Informed Choice* leaflets (box 1). Within practice settings, however, they were seldom used to maximum effect. Pragmatic usage resulted in many leaflets being withheld from women because staff disagreed with the contents of the leaflet or were concerned because some leaflets promoted choices that were unavailable locally. Some midwives also made assumptions about the ability and willingness of women to participate in decision making. These assumptions were sometimes incorrect.

The potential of the leaflets was further diluted because they were often given out "wrapped" within advertising materials or concealed within the maternity folder. During interviews, questions about the leaflets usually failed to elicit any response from most women. They often confused them with other information related to pregnancy or indeed denied having received them. It was often only after coaxing by

---

22 What kind of attitudes, qualities and knowledge might those midwives who facilitate informed choice have?

N4. 'Theoretical saturation' is reached when the researcher(s) have interviewed and/or observed enough people to be reasonably sure that while there might be nuanced variations among the views and experiences of the people involved, no new, substantial themes that the researcher has not come across before are likely to be brought up.

N5. Researchers and ethics committees are rightly increasingly concerned about issues of 'confidentiality', in order to protect those people who take part in research projects. Protecting people involves more than just removing their names from the research reports. Other details might need to be omitted or changed if they make people potentially identifiable. Those belonging to minority groups may be particularly identifiable and in need of protection.

23 Can you think of a few reasons why sharing transcripts of interviews with other researchers might increase validity and reliability of the research?

24 What kind of women do you think midwives made assumptions about and what might these assumptions have been?

Box 2: Time pressures

" … at the end of the day we are governed by time, we haven't hours and hours to spend with each person… It's been good having the [*Informed Choice*] leaflets … it's a quick way out of it … You can give them a leaflet and tell them to have a read of it" (midwife, intervention site)

"It's strange, but I found that there were often things that I felt I needed to know. I was never sure whether I should ask the midwife or not … sometimes they are busy aren't they? … But if I did ask then they were brilliant … The information was there but you had to ask for it, you couldn't expect it to come pouring out" (service user, intervention site)

"I didn't feel happy throughout the pregnancy with the information I received … I constantly felt they [midwives] did not have any time for me. I was given plenty of leaflets but not enough discussion. I was never in the consulting room for any longer than five minutes at any of my antenatal appointments" (service user, intervention site)

25 Compare the qualitative findings of this research project with the quantitative results. Would you agree with the findings in the quantitative arm of the trial that informed choice leaflets make no difference?

26 From what you know of the research, routinely directing women towards relying on obstetric birth technologies seems:
a) Sensible
b) Misguided
c) Misinformed
d) Unethical

27 Do you agree or disagree with some/all of a) or b)? A strong hierarchy is:
a) A good thing because when roles are clearly defined it increases women's trust, they know where they are, it reduces the pressure on midwives to make decisions and be autonomous and makes birth safer
b) Not such a good thing because it reduces women's choices and their ability to exert their rights, midwives are less able to help women make informed decisions, they are less able to make clinical judgements, and are more like obstetric nurses, trust is reduced, medicalised birth is more likely, and birth is potentially riskier

the researcher or after her suggestion that women look within their maternity folder that leaflets were discovered and some comments were forthcoming.

Midwives generally distributed leaflets in routine ways and were rarely observed differentiating them from other information they offered women. Health professionals were seldom observed discussing the leaflets with women or asking them if they understood the information or found it useful. Women rarely initiated discussion about leaflet topics. A few women were complimentary about the leaflets and thought that they had influenced their intentions. Most women, however, did not find them helpful in decision making.

Health professionals under pressure

Most health professionals reported feeling pressured by time constraints (box 2). Midwives in particular were concerned about assuming the role of "information broker" without preparation or the allocation of additional time. Midwives on intervention sites sometimes viewed the leaflets as a pragmatic solution to time pressures. Women were often observed accommodating health professionals by limiting their questions, but some expressed dissatisfaction when written information was used as an alternative to discussion.

Lack of choice in practice

Health professionals noted that many leaflets suggested choices that were not available at a local level (box 3). Furthermore, some technological interventions, such as ultrasound scanning and monitoring in labour, have become so routine in maternity care that health professionals no longer perceive them as optional. Women sometimes made choices on the basis of their previous experiences of childbirth but were often met with resistance if their preferences contradicted established clinical norms. Staff sometimes expressed a strong dislike for an option covered by the leaflets to the extent that distribution of some leaflets was terminated on some sites. Women tended to comply with the suggestions of health professionals,

and, unless openings were made, they rarely instigated discussion about their own preferences.

Technology and litigation

Researchers observed health professionals driving decision making towards technological intervention by conveying information which either minimised the risk of the intervention or emphasised the potential for harm without the intervention. This seemed to make it difficult for women to hear alternative messages, even from obstetricians. Fear of litigation promoted notions of "right" choices with which clinicians felt clinically secure and which they thought would afford them protection against litigation. Midwives occasionally expressed frustration when such imperatives, rather than evidence based information or client choice, determined the options available. Some women were aware of the influence of technological imperatives on the attitudes of health professionals, and they occasionally experienced this as bullying. Some views are shown in box 4.

Hierarchy, power, and trust

We observed a strong hierarchy within the maternity services, with obstetricians at the top, midwives and health professionals other than doctors in the middle,

28 What do you think women's own words bring to the research?

29 What is your reaction to the quotations? Do you agree with the responses from professionals? Are the women's comments typical? Justified?

Box 3: Choices

"When you go for your hospital appointment they'll do a little scan just to see how far on you are … They have the portable scanners in all the rooms so it's very quick. Then at 18 weeks you'll have your big scan … the detailed anomaly scan" (observation of midwife interaction, intervention site)

Researcher: "Was monitoring in labour ever discussed with you?"
Woman: "No … not really… They gave me that leaflet [*Informed Choice* leaflet 2²] and told me to read it but they never said anything about what would happen in labour. They said they had to do a little trace when I first came in and then I think they just forgot to take it off" (service user, intervention site)

"With my first, I was monitored the whole time. I didn't realise that you could move round. Nobody explained that to me, but the second time around I knew that you didn't have to do it. I think the second time round I knew you had an option. You're stronger. You're a stronger person. You know what to expect" (service user, control site)

"When I declined the dating scan, the receptionist said: 'Oh, I'll just go and see if you're allowed.' … That did annoy me, you're not allowed this, you're not allowed that … I didn't have a dating scan and I had a hassle over it right up to the end" (service user, control site)

"Home deliveries are for pizzas and nothing else … women who choose to have home deliveries are very irresponsible … I know you can't stop them but I don't agree with them. If something does go wrong you haven't got a hope" (registrar, intervention site)

Researcher: "Was the option of having this baby at home discussed?"
Woman: "No … it did cross my mind. I thought I wouldn't mind considering a home birth but it wasn't mentioned. It was either a choice of [hospital X or hospital Y]."
Researcher: "And were you given this leaflet?" [researcher shows woman the *Informed Choice* leaflet on place of birth]
Woman: "Oh yes. I had that one but she [midwife] never discussed it with me … I thought she would ask me at the next visit if I'd read it but she never did so I just dropped it really. It wasn't that important … I'm quite happy with [hospital X]. I don't know why she bothered giving it me. I did wonder that…" (interview with women expecting her third baby; intervention site)

30 What is your reaction to these quotations? Are they all saying similar or dissimilar things? Do the quotations suggest a service that is woman centred, midwife led, doctor led or a combination of these?

Box 4: Technology

"Giving them a choice is not enough. They need to know the reality behind it [vaginal breech delivery] ... about the head getting stuck definitely. You can give them scare stories but you don't even have to do that. You just have to mention a complication. Something like the baby might die..." (registrar, intervention site)

The following excerpt, taken from field notes made during a routine antenatal consultation, describes an interaction between a female registrar and a working class woman with a breech presentation in her first pregnancy. The woman and her mother have both made it clear that they consider an elective caesarean section to be the only safe delivery option. The registrar attempts to present an alternative perspective:

"Well ... women still die from caesarean sections ... It's a big operation and not without its risks and complications ... What I want you to do, every morning, lunch time and tea time, is get on the floor on all fours for 10 minutes, with your forearms on the floor and your bum in the air. Do that for 10 minutes three times a day. It might encourage that baby to turn round."

The woman laughs; her mother looks disgusted (field notes, control site)

"You see there is a need for the legal document and I think rightly so because it's useful to have this in practice where there is a lot of litigation... A patient comes in, you think the foetus is OK because the Pinard has recorded everything as normal. Then the next moment you get sudden deceleration... You have no excuse for not having a tracing. If a tracing had been done perhaps it would have shown ... [an] increased risk in utero..." (consultant obstetrician, intervention site)

"... they will always guide a woman towards elective section for breech even if she wants to try for a vaginal delivery ... They're so geared towards an elective section ... Even when the woman comes in with an undiagnosed breech in labour, fully dilated, ready to push, they'll do an emergency section at that point rather than let her deliver vaginally. So what's the point of giving a leaflet [number 9²] ... What's the point of giving them information about choices they haven't got?" (midwife, intervention site)

"He [the obstetrician] is a real Jekyll and Hyde that one. He was fine as long as he thought I was going to the hospital but as soon as I said I wanted to have the baby at home it was all about haemorrhage and the risks to the baby. If anything went wrong it would be my own fault; it would be on my head. It was horrible. I came home and cried" (service user, intervention site)

"I do think you can be bullied into things, particularly if you're not strong minded about what you want. It's quite easy for them to bully you, they say things like 'The baby will die' if you don't do so and so. Or: 'You'll be in danger.' It's very easy for them because you don't really understand the medical stuff" (service user, intervention site)

---

and pregnant women at the bottom (box 5). This correlates with women's observations that midwives generally exercised little clinical influence compared with doctors. Midwives were concerned about the consequences of recommending options that contradicted obstetrically defined clinical norms. Most of the choices suggested in the leaflets required obstetric support, and hence the options offered tended to reflect the preferences of obstetricians rather than those of pregnant women or midwives. The practice of lower ranking doctors was similarly constrained by power differentials.

Women who experienced continuity of midwifery care were more likely to report trusting relationships in which they felt more able to ask questions. Such relationships, which were rarely encountered in this study, seemed to reduce imbalances in power and facilitate a partnership approach to maternity care.[20] Women who questioned practice norms in the absence of such support often reported feeling undermined and were sometimes mistrusted by health professionals.

Discussion

This qualitative study of evidence based leaflets for pregnant women found that they did not promote informed choice. This was related to time pressures on staff working within a culture that supported existing normative patterns of care rather than informed choice. The hierarchical power structures within the maternity services, and the framing of information in favour of particular options, ensured compliance with the "right" choice.

Health professionals' initial views of the *Informed Choice* leaflets were generally positive but the ways in which leaflets were distributed or withheld, however, severely diluted their potential benefits. Health professionals, pressured by time and concerned about litigation, rarely discussed the content of the leaflets or promoted their difference from other literature. The resulting invisibility helps to explain why only 70% of women in the intervention sites reported receiving a minimum of one leaflet.[15] Such findings are not unique to maternity care or to the use of evidence based decision aids.[21]

The way in which information is presented influences decision making[22] and competing "hierarchies of evidence"[14] are known to reduce the credibility of some healthcare choices. Passive dissemination of information is ineffective in changing the behaviour of health professionals.[23] Choices that are offered but not actively supported by staff are rarely taken up by pregnant women.[24] The absence of opportunities for discussion[25] that we observed is also likely to have hindered women in using the leaflets to make (informed) decisions.

The organisational and hierarchical structure of the maternity services worked against maximising the potential of the leaflets. The relative lack of continuity of care observed throughout the study made it difficult for women to follow up on issues raised in a previous consultation or to initiate discussion on leaflets and other topics related to pregnancy. Lack of continuity also precluded the formation of trusting relationships thought necessary to facilitate informed choice.[26] Societal and medical expectations tend to normalise technological interventions, and some choices promoted in the leaflets, such as whether to have ultrasound scanning or electronic monitoring in labour, were rarely available in practice because the technology had long been integrated into routine care. Health professionals generally felt responsible for anything that went wrong in maternity care, and a widespread fear of litigation caused many to promote technological interventions, even when they were contradicted by the evidence base of the *Informed Choice* leaflets.

Choice and decision making seemed to be heavily circumscribed by the pressures and norms of the local obstetric culture. The researchers observed little diversity in clinical practice between individual practitioners or maternity units. Inequalities in power and status were observed to be potent forces in maintaining the status quo, and this made it difficult to promote (informed) choice. As reported elsewhere[27 28] midwives were observed to "frame" information and "steer"[29] women towards making the "right" decisions to "protect" themselves and their clients from the

31 How far and why would you agree or disagree with the researchers' claims that the way in which information is presented (such as passive dissemination, lack of active support and little discussion) influences women's decisions?

32 Do you think some/all RCTs would benefit from having qualitative arms? Would qualitative research sometimes/always benefit from having RCTs attached? Are there subjects that lend themselves more to one than the other?

33 Which of these claims would you say best describes the term 'technological imperative'?

a) The inability of practitioners to avoid carrying out medical interventions

b) The inability of women to resist interventions

c) The reliance of our society on technology that makes it difficult for any of us to resist the use of technology

d) Technology is with us and should be used

34 What are normative practices? Can you think of a few in maternity services? In other areas of life?

consequences of inadvertently disrupting the status quo. Informed choice was therefore equated with making the locally defined "right" choice in accordance with the authoritative knowledge and experience of senior obstetricians. Unequal power relations resulted in bias towards the "objective" knowledge of health professionals and marginalised women's subjective knowledge.[30] Hence, power differentials served to reinforce informed compliance with the right choice rather than encourage informed choice. Hierarchical structures in the maternity services also made it difficult for lower ranking practitioners to support women in going against these right choices. There was little evidence to suggest that concepts such as partnership[20] or shared decision making[31] were understood by staff who generally were observed to seek women's compliance with the professionally defined right choices.

Childbearing women generally complied with expected norms in their encounters with staff, who they perceived as busy people with many demands on their time. Our results show that cultural barriers within the maternity services encourage informed compliance, even though staff adopted the rhetoric of informed choice.

Conclusions and implications

The results of this study are not specific to maternity units in Wales as similar issues have been identified in units that independently purchased the leaflets.[15] These leaflets are unlikely to promote informed choice in maternity care unless they are introduced as part of a coherent strategy addressing power imbalances and the ambiguities currently underpinning choice. The concept of informed choice carries great potential to resolve many of the issues faced by maternity services today, with informed choice and partnership in decision making lessening the burden of responsibility presently experienced by health professionals. From this and other research we can begin to understand the barriers facing the implementation of research based

What is already known on this topic

Informed Choice leaflets are widely used in maternity care but little is known about their ability to influence informed choice and decision making

High quality information is essential for promoting informed choice but is insufficient by itself

What this study adds

Time constraints and other pressures on health professionals resulted in a lack of discussion of the content of the leaflets

Fear of litigation, power hierarchies, and the technological imperative in maternity care limited the choices available

Health professionals promoted normative practices rather than choice, and as women valued their opinions this led to the promotion of informed compliance rather than informed choice

Box 5: Knowing your place

"In the later stage they [midwives] don't seem to have as much say in your care really. It's down to the consultant whether he chooses, or whether he recommends to you if the baby should be born [induced]" (service user, intervention site)

"... you wish your midwife was given more power than they are ... it comes to a certain question which they have to refer to a doctor and you think, but they know! They're in there ... But they still have to defer. They should be empowered to do this" (service user, control site)

"... the *Informed Choice* leaflets actually put midwives between a rock and a very hard place... It's unreal to encourage women to go against local policies and guidelines when we all know that if she takes that line, she'll be given a really hard time, especially by the medical profession ... I mean we've still got women in this area being threatened and struck off GPs' lists just for saying they are considering a home birth, for God's sake ... and they will have to live with the consequences of making a choice ... for a lot longer than I will" (community midwife, intervention site)

"So I was still thinking should I or shouldn't I have an epidural? This leaflet [leaflet number 6[2]] was guiding me whether I should or shouldn't. In the end I had no choice anyway. When I went to deliver my babies, I had no choice. They were deciding how I was going to deliver my babies and told me I needed an epidural. I didn't know whether I did or not" (service user, intervention site)

"... it's a consultant led service. You may disagree with what your consultant says but if you're working for that consultant that's what you've got to tell the patient ... Whether you like it or not that's what you do, whether you totally disagree, you've got to do it" (registrar, intervention site)

"They [midwives] become your friends don't they? It's not just about the pregnancy. They start to know what your husband does, what you did, what you worked as; and it's the trust thing. Going back to that word again, they become part of your life and you do put your trust in that person" (service user, intervention site)

"You start to doubt yourself if you think differently to the midwife or whoever is advising you, and if you don't agree, you think, 'Oh! I must be wrong.' Or at least, I did" (service user, control site)

"We let them [women] do what they want to do and then when things go wrong we get sued. We are ... afraid to go against the women's wishes ... [But] you get very skilled at smelling a rat. We know now when trouble is approaching and that woman [who had requested something with which the obstetrician disagreed] smells like trouble" (obstetrician, intervention site)

evidence and the use of decision aids for informed choice in various clinical settings.[14 21 26] The additional barriers we have identified are unlikely to be unique to maternity care. Their removal, however, will entail considerable cultural change at all levels of the maternity services.

We thank the women, health professionals and managers, representatives of consumer groups and other organisations, and non-NHS antenatal teachers who contributed to the research. We also thank the project advisory group; colleagues and friends who assisted the research team in many ways including critical reading of work in progress; the National Childbirth Trust, who kindly agreed to withhold dissemination of a range of their leaflets on pregnancy related topics until our study was complete; and MIDIRS (Midwives Information and Resource Service) for answering our many queries and for withholding sales of the *Informed Choice* leaflets to control maternity units participating in the research until the end of the intervention period.

Contributors: HS advised on the study design, coordinated the qualitative research team, assisted in the qualitative data collection, conducted most of the data analysis, and participated in writing the paper. MK designed the study, supervised the qualitative data collection, and assisted in data analysis and writing the paper. GT contributed to the qualitative data collection and analysis. Donna Mead, Barbara Bale, Laurence Moseley, Sandy

Kirkman, Heather Rothwell, David Cohen, and Penny Curtis were members of the research team for the wider study. Jane Durell was the project administrator. HS and MK are the guarantors.

Funding: Department of Health. The Welsh Office funded the translation into Welsh of the women's version of the *Informed Choice* leaflets and the transcribing of interviews conducted in Welsh.

Competing interests: None declared.

1 Department of Health. *Changing childbirth. Report of the expert maternity group.* London: HMSO, 1993.
2 O'Cathain A, Walters SJ, Nicholl JP, Thomas KJ, Kirkham M. Use of evidence based leaflets to promote informed choice in maternity care: randomised controlled trial in everyday practice. *BMJ* 2002;324:643-6.
3 Rosser J, Watt IS, Entwistle V. Informed choice initiative: an example of reaching users with evidence based information. *J Clin Effect* 1996;1:143-5.
4 Jones S, Sadler T, Low N, Blott M, Welch J. Does uptake of antenatal HIV testing depend on the individual midwife? Cross sectional study. *BMJ* 1998;316:272-3.
5 McCrea BH, Wright ME, Murphy-Black T. Differences in midwives' approaches to pain relief in labour. *Midwifery* 1998;14:174-80.
6 Elwyn G, Edwards A, Gwyn R, Grol R. Towards a feasible model for shared decision making: focus group study with general practice registrars. *BMJ* 1999;319:753-6.
7 Charles C, Redko C, Whelan T, Gafni A, Reyno L. Doing nothing is not choice: lay constructions of treatment decision-making among women with early-stage breast cancer. *Sociol Health Illn* 1998;20:71-95.
8 Roter D. The medical visit context of treatment decision-making and the therapeutic relationship. *Health Expect* 2000;3:17-25.
9 Davies HT, Nutley SM, Mannion R. Organisational culture and quality of health care. *Qual Health Care* 2000;9:111-9.
10 Davies C. *Gender and the professional predicament in nursing.* Buckingham: Open University Press, 1995.
11 Murphy-Lawless J. *Reading birth and death: a history of obstetric thinking.* Cork: Cork University Press, 1998.
12 Wolff N. Randomised trials of socially complex interventions: promise or peril? *J Health Serv Res Policy* 2001;6:123-6.
13 Barbour RS. The case for combining qualitative and quantitative approaches in health services research. *J Health Serv Res Policy* 1999;4:39-43.
14 Fitzgerald L, Ferlie E, Wood M, Hawkins C. Evidence into practice? An exploratory analysis of the interpretation of evidence In: Mark AL,

Dopson S, eds. *Organisational behaviour in health care: the research agenda.* London: Macmillan Business Press, 1999.
15 Kirkham M, Stapleton H, eds. *Informed choice in maternity care: an evaluation of evidence based leaflets.* York: NHS Centre for Reviews and Dissemination, 2001.
16 Glaser B, Strauss A. *The discovery of grounded theory.* New York: Aldine, 1967.
17 Gahan C, Hannibal M. *Doing qualitative research using QSR NUD*IST.* London: Sage, 1999.
18 Dingwall R. Accounts, interviews and observations. In: Miller G, Dingwall R, eds. *Context and method in qualitative research.* London: Sage, 1997.
19 Strauss A, Corbin J. *Basics of qualitative research: grounded theory procedures and techniques.* London: Sage, 1990.
20 Pairman S. Women-centred midwifery: partnerships or professional friendships? In: Kirkham M, ed. *The midwife-mother relationship.* London: Macmillan, 2000.
21 Holmes-Rovner M, Valade D, Orlowski C, Draus C, Nabozny-Valerio B, Keiser S. Implementing shared decision-making in routine practice: barriers and opportunities. *Health Expect* 2000;3:182-91.
22 Bekker H, Thornton JG, Airey CM, Connelly JB, Hewison J, Robinson MB, et al. Informed decision making: an annotated bibliography and systematic review. *Health Technol Assess* 1999;3:1-156.
23 NHS Centre for Reviews and Dissemination, Royal Society of Medicine. Getting evidence into practice. *Effect Health Care Bull* 1999;5:1-16.
24 Machin D, Scamell A. Using ethnographic research to examine effects of 'informed choice'. *Br J Midwifery* 1998;6:304-9.
25 Proctor S. What determines quality in maternity care? Comparing the perceptions of childbearing women and midwives. *Birth* 1998;25:85-93.
26 Entwistle V, Sheldon TA, Sowden A, Watt IS. Evidence-informed patient choice. Practical issues of involving patients in decisions about health care technologies. *Int J Technol Assess Health Care* 1998;14:212-25.
27 Marteau T. Framing of information: its influence upon decisions of doctors and patients. *Br J Soc Psychol* 1989;28:89-94.
28 Press N, Browner CH. Why women say yes to prenatal diagnosis. *Soc Sci Med* 1997;45:979-89.
29 Levy V. Protective steering: a grounded theory study of the processes by which midwives facilitate informed choice in pregnancy. *J Adv Nursing* 1999;29:104-12.
30 Edwards NP. Women planning homebirths: their own views on their relationships with midwives. In: Kirkham M, ed. *The midwife-mother relationship.* London: Macmillan, 2000.
31 Charles C, Gafni A, Whelan T. Shared decision-making in the medical encounter: what does it mean? (or it takes at least two to tango). *Soc Sci Med* 1997;44:681-92.

(Accepted 5 October 2001)

ANSWERS

Q1. All of these could be true, although watching people through binoculars and unidirectional glass would be rather unusual these days and might not gain ethical approval! Most non-participant observation involves being with people in their own surroundings or in a place where interactions take place that you want to know more about. You might talk with people but you would avoid deliberately influencing what they were doing and saying

Q2. c) and e) are probably most true. Interviews are unlike conversation because the researcher wants to know about the other person's views and experiences. Sharing his or her own thoughts is mainly unhelpful as it might inhibit the other person from saying what she or he really thinks. Interviews can vary enormously in length but are often around an hour or so. The researcher might have many questions but the experienced qualitative researcher will often have a few open-ended questions to begin with and be prepared to follow up what the interviewee tells him or her. Ann Oakley's (1993) chapter on interviews is a good example of the issues involved in interviewing women

Q3. It might be interesting for you to know how women and professionals behave and what they say in different settings, between themselves and to each other. If, for example, women and midwives seem to talk more easily to each other in less institutionalised settings, it is important to be aware of this when planning maternity services

Q4. In this research 13 were used because they formed 10 clusters. It was intended that five received the informed choices leaflets and five did not. This is quite a large number of units in which to carry out qualitative research but was partly to fit in with the RCT arm of the trial. There are no hard and fast rules on this. Research could be carried out in just one maternity unit, as it often is – or anywhere else

Q5. Time pressure must impact on choice for women, as choice comes about through women being informed about their options and having time to talk through the implications of these. Other influences may come into play. You will have your own experiences and examples of these. Check out others' experiences and views

Q6. You will probably have many examples. Home birth is sometimes seen as a 'wrong' choice whereas hospital birth is seen as a 'right' choice. Choices are sometimes defined as right and wrong depending on tradition: that is, what people usually do. Right and wrong might be to do with what professionals believe is right and wrong because they are seen to be experts. Most cultures have strict rules about birth and death. Robbie Davies-Floyd (1992) talks about this in terms of rituals and many sociologists have shown that right and wrong choices are to do with a society's beliefs. Raymond de Vries' (2004) book about birth in The Netherlands provides a good example of this

Q7. a), b) and d) are necessarily true; c) is more complicated because it is not necessarily those who hold most power that are most knowledgeable. In fact, those who are most oppressed often know most about how the hierarchy works because they are faced with its consequences most acutely. They have to learn about it in detail in order to develop alternative ways of knowing and doing things. How many times have we heard women saying that they need to be more informed than health professionals if they want to make choices that are seen by some professionals to be 'wrong'?

Q8. The first two are probably more often false than true. Unless we can find ways of dismantling oppressive hierarchies the second two are probably more often true. Observe interactions between people at work or socially carefully and see what you think

Q9. The Church, schools, law, even families and many more examples might have come to mind

Q10. This is actually a very complicated issue. The problem with assuming that professionals know best and that women know less is that it leads to the kind of coercion that this research is all about. It reduces ethical decision making to making 'right' choices. It is a more mechanical approach that fails to take people's unique circumstances into account. Above all, expert knowledge cannot predict outcomes accurately – it can only predict probable outcomes. There are a number of cases where women have given birth to healthy babies vaginally having been told that their babies would die if they did not have caesarean sections. As a society, we have a tendency to trust experts and women's knowledge has been undermined. For a debate about the nuances of choice see Kirkham (2004) and Edwards & Leap (2006)

Q11. b) is the closest definition of the term 'informed compliance' as it is used in this research. You can probably see that there are grey areas here and that there is some overlap between choice, consent, compliance and coercion

Q12. As is clear from this research, it is usually helpful to know something about the field of study and what is thought to be known and unknown. Given the variable quality of research, when looking at research that has been done it is important to use a critical eye. You could probably find reasons for agreeing or disagreeing with all of the statements here – give it a try!

Q13. Probably e) would be classified as a socially complex intervention – but it's possible to see socially complex aspects to most research

Q14. The quantitative research findings apparently provided an overview that giving information leaflets to women does not impact a great deal on the choices that women make. This is very important to know as the giving of leaflets is often thought to be the answer to providing good information in a fragmented service under pressure. The qualitative research told us why information leaflets do not work and what we might need to do to make them part of a more effective strategy to enable women to make decisions

Q15. It is difficult to know how long data need to be collected for in order to obtain good qualitative research. To some extent this is dictated by funding. But researchers have some idea about how long they expect to spend 'in the field' and as they observe and listen, they see and hear fewer new, unusual or surprising data – reaching what is called 'saturation'

Q16. Fieldnotes are confidential, but researchers use them for c) and d)

Q17. The most distinguishing feature is e). But a) and d) are also true

Q18. In this case, because the researchers observed and interviewed women, midwives, obstetricians, anaesthetists and ultrasonographers, they were able to explore a broad range of views and experiences from many of those involved in maternity services

Q19. a) Although qualitative research is seen as usually less invasive than, for example, drug treatments, some research asks women and men about sensitive, potentially distressing topics. Increasingly, researchers are being advised to seek ethics approval for any research. Some social research might not require it, but some journals will not publish research that has not obtained approval from an ethics committee

Q20. c)

Q21. Often, qualitative research is exploratory, so whereas researchers might have some ideas about what to ask interviewees, they might hear about issues they had not thought of. Having the flexibility to explore these avenues tends to enrich the research and improve its quality, depth and usefulness. If, for example, you were interviewing people about their dietary likes and dislikes but knew nothing about fruit, fish and chocolate, your research would have missing ingredients! If you asked open-ended questions, someone would probably mention these, so you could follow this up in subsequent interviews (drawing on grounded theory) and fill in your own knowledge gaps that would otherwise have impacted on your research findings

Q22. I am sure you have your own ideas but 'Birth centres: a social model of maternity care' and 'The midwife–mother relationship' both edited by Mavis Kirkham (2003, 2000) might give some additional ideas, as would the work on caring relationships by Sigridur Halldorsdottir and Sigridur Karlsdottir (1996)

Q23. If, as I have claimed, researchers are always influenced knowingly and unknowingly by who they are and where they come from, sharing transcripts might uncover different researchers' assumptions and blind spots. Some sociologists suggest that knowledge is communally produced and that women often work best collaboratively, as Mary Belenky and her colleagues (1986) describe

Q24. Assumptions are made about women because of their economic circumstances, their jobs, their race, their sexual orientation, their age and for many other reasons. These sometimes influence how much information midwives provide for women

Q25. That is what the results showed, following a well-designed RCT – but you might want to qualify these findings and question the ability of an RCT to measure the impact of a complex intervention on its own

Q26. From the research we have about the many potential side effects of routine obstetric interventions, b), c), and d) could all be true. Of course, technology and obstetric practices are necessary and hugely beneficial when used in the appropriate circumstances

Q27. If you align yourself more closely with a technocratic model of birth you may agree with a). If you hold a more holistic, social view of birth you may agree with b). For a good discussion about these different models of birth and what they mean, see Robbie Davis-Floyd (2002)

Q28. Perhaps it has struck you that women's own words have a power, authority and immediacy of their own

Q29 and Q30. Most of the quotations suggest that informed choice is problematic, support the notion of the technological imperative and suggest that doctors exert most control and authority while women exert least

Q31. The answer to this question will depend very much on your own perspective!

Q32. It seems important that when carrying out any research, the recipients' views about any intervention should be sought and included as a finding. It is likely that we will often want to know about the scale of a problem or incidence as well as the impact on people's lives. Issues that depend on relationships may be best researched using qualitative methods

Q33. c) is probably the best overall definition, although all of the others have been used

Q34. They are the practices that are 'authoritative' (Jordan 1997) and generally accepted by the culture as a whole. Alternatives to these are thought by many people to be dangerous, strange or unusual. In most industrialised countries, hospital birth might be an example of a normative practice; carrying out inductions when pregnancy has lasted a certain length of time is another. Managing the third stage of labour is a normative practice in most British hospitals, but not necessarily in community settings. Vaccinating children, sending them to school and living in nuclear families are all normative practices in some cultures

DISCUSSION

The value of listening to women and midwives and others cannot be overstated, as this research clearly shows. Their words do indeed breathe life and authenticity into the findings. The challenge for researchers is to leave ongoing decision-making trails so that the reader can understand how the research was done and how the researchers reached their findings (Edwards & Ribbens 1998, Ely et al 1991). Even when this is clear, we need to bear in mind that researchers might still misrepresent or misconstrue women's experiences and views (Stanley & Wise 1993).

From a woman-centred perspective, the purpose of research includes a desire to uncover structures that oppress women, and an attempt to protect their integrity by remaining close to their words and experiences. A further challenge is to remember that experience does not speak for itself and to find the fine line between discounting women's experiences and taking them on board without debate (Burt & Code 1995 p 36, Edwards & Ribbens 1998). Helen Stapleton (2004) and colleagues have done this by providing critical understandings about the ways in which women and midwives (and others) are oppressed. They weave women's and midwives' voices into the cultural constraints they face. The research thus also provides understandings about how we are all products of our culture and may accept and resist it in different ways.

What this research tells us is that decision making during pregnancy and birth is complex and is greatly reliant on what health professionals tell women, how they tell them and what they do not tell them. It tells us that the information given to women by health professionals is highly dependent on the culture in which they work and the structures of maternity services, e.g. they might have little time to spend with women and might also be victimised by those in authority if they support women to make decisions that fall outside local policies and traditions. This research also tells us that decisions that might increase the likelihood of women having normal births in a birth setting where practices frequently draw on technology are often difficult to make. It tells us that practitioners cannot easily provide individualised low-tech care to women in institutionalised settings that provide high-tech obstetric care. It tells us that institutions claim authority over knowledge, concentrate power in the hands of a few, and create unhealthy hierarchies where different views struggle to be heard. It shows that evidence-based care is difficult to introduce in these settings. Very importantly, it indicates that these barriers to information provision and decision making may be reduced when midwives are based in community settings (in women's homes or in midwifery-run birth centres) and that, when midwives are able to get to know women and spend time with them, they are more able to listen to them, provide information based on their individual needs and facilitate decision making.

Had this qualitative research not been done at the same time as the RCT, researchers would not have observed how information leaflets were withheld, or given to women in such a way that they were unused or had to be ignored. The research may then have concluded – erroneously – that women do not want research-based information, are unlikely to use it and rely on practitioners to direct their decisions. Instead, we learn that changing cultural attitudes and relationships among practitioners is essential if women are to be enabled to make decisions from a range of options during childbearing.

The findings confirm that different research approaches benefit from working more collaboratively together so that a more complex understanding of knowledge formation can be developed, based on the realities of all of our lives. This might increase our understanding of diversity and result in less judgement and blame towards those who make different decisions for different but nonetheless legitimate reasons and thus enable women to make the decisions that they believe are right for them and their families.

SUMMARY

Having now considered the findings of both the quantitative and qualitative arms of this trial on informed choices leaflets, we might want to consider whether questions need to be asked about the structure of maternity services, whereby the care that most women receive is so fragmented and mechanistic that we have to search for means to communicate and provide information that involve little connection, dialogue and trust between women and midwives. Informed choice leaflets, birth plans and a variety of forms with boxes to tick are perhaps useful when used by women and midwives who have developed relationships, but are poor substitutes for these relationships when used on their own.

References

Anderson T 2004 The misleading myth of choice: the continuing oppression of women in childbirth. In: Kirkham M ed Informed choice in maternity care. Palgrave Macmillan, Basingstoke, p 257–264

Bastian H 2004 Learning from evidence based mistakes. British Medical Journal 329:1053

Belenky MF, Clinchy BM, Goldberger NR, Tarule JM 1986 Women's ways of knowing: the development of self, voice and mind. Basic Books, New York

Burt S, Code L eds 1995 Changing methods: feminists transforming practice. Broadview Press, New York

Clair RP 1997 Organizing silence: silence as voice and voice as silence in the narrative exploration of the Treaty of New Echota. Western Journal of Communication 61(3):315–337

Davis-Floyd RE 1992 Birth as an American rite of passage. University of California Press, Berkeley

Davis-Floyd RE 2002 The technocratic, humanistic, and holistic paradigms of childbirth. MIDIRS Midwifery Digest 12(4):500–506

Davis-Floyd RE, St John G eds 1998 From doctor to healer: the transformative journey. Rutgers University Press, New Brunswick

de Vries R 2004 A pleasing birth: midwives and maternity care in the Netherlands. Temple University Press, Philadelphia

Edwards NP 2005 Birthing autonomy: women's experiences of planning home births. Routledge, London

Edwards NP, Leap N 2006 The politics of involving women in decision-making. Books for Midwives, Oxford

Edwards R, Ribbens J 1998 Living on the edges: public knowledge, private lives, personal experiences. In: Ribbens J, Edwards R eds Feminist dilemmas in qualitative research. Thousand Oaks/Sage Publications, London/New Delhi, p 1–23

Ely M, Anzul M, Friedman T et al 1991 Doing qualitative research: circles within circles. The Falmer Press/Teachers Library, London/New York

Evans F 1985 Managers and labourers: women's attitudes to reproductive technology. In: Faulkner W, Arnold E eds Smothered by invention: technology in women's lives. Pluto Press, London, p 109–127

Fine M, Gordon SM 1992 Feminist transformations of/despite psychology. In: Fine M ed Disruptive voices: the possibilities of feminist research. University of Michigan Press, Ann Arbor, p 1–25

Halldorsdottir S, Karlsdottir SI 1996 Journeying through labour and delivery: perceptions of women who have given birth. Midwifery 12:48–61

Hunt LM, Jordan B, Irwin, S, Browner CH 1989 Compliance and the patient's perspective. Culture, Medicine and Psychiatry 13:315–334

Jordan B 1997 Authoritative knowledge and its construction. In: Davis-Floyd RE, Sargent CF eds Childbirth and authoritative knowledge: cross-cultural perspectives. University of California Press, Berkeley, p 50–79

Kirkham M 2000 How can we relate? In: Kirkham M ed The midwife–mother relationship. Macmillan Press, Basingstoke, p 227–254

Kirkham M 2003 Birth centres: a social model for maternity care. Books for Midwives, Oxford

Kirkham M ed 2004 Informed choice in maternity care. Palgrave Macmillan, Basingstoke

Levy V 2004 How midwives used protective steering to facilitate informed choice in pregnancy. In: Kirkham M ed Informed choice in maternity care. Palgrave Macmillan, Basingstoke, p 57–70

Lewis J 1990 Mothers and maternity policies in the twentieth century. In: Garcia J, Kilpatrick R, Richards M eds The politics of maternity care: services for childbearing women in twentieth century Britain. Clarendon Press, Oxford, p 15–29

Longino HE 2002 The fate of knowledge. Princeton University Press, Princeton

Machin D, Scamell M 1997 The experience of labour using ethnography to explore the irresistible nature of the bio-medical metaphor during labour. Midwifery 13:78–84

Maynard M 1994 Methods, practice and epistemology: the debate about feminism and research. In: Maynard M, Purvis J eds Researching women's lives from a feminist perspective. Taylor and Francis, London

Maynard M, Purvis J eds 1994 Researching women's lives from a feminist perspective. Taylor and Francis, London

Morgan M, Coombes L 2001 Subjectivities and silences, mother and woman: theorizing an experience of silence as a speaking subject. Feminism and Psychology 11(3):361–375

Murphy-Lawless J 1998 Reading birth and death: a history of obstetric thinking. Cork University Press, Eire

Noble C 2001 Birth stories. Ginninderra Press, New Zealand

Oakley A 1993 Interviewing women: a contradiction in terms. In: Oakley A ed Essays on women, medicine and health. Edinburgh University Press, Edinburgh, p 221–242

Oakley A 2000 Experiments in knowing: gender and method in the social sciences. Polity Press, Cambridge

Shipman M 1988 The limitations of social research, 3rd edn. Longman, London

Stanley L, Wise S 1993 Breaking out again. Routledge, London

Stapleton H 2004 Is there a difference between a free gift and a planned purchase? The use of evidence-based leaflets in maternity care. In: Kirkham M ed Informed choice in maternity care. Palgrave Macmillan, Basingstoke, p 87–116

van Teijlingen ER, Hundley V, Rennie A-M et al 2003 Maternity satisfaction studies and their limitations: 'What is must still be best'. Birth 30(2):75–82

Wickham S 2004 Feminism and ways of knowing. In: Stewart M ed Pregnancy, birth and maternity care: feminist perspectives. Books for Midwives, Oxford, p 157–168

Further reading

Beech BAL 2003 Am I allowed: yes, yes, yes. Association for Improvements in the Maternity Services, Surbiton, Surrey. Available online at: www.aims.org.uk

Demilew J 2004 Integrating MIDIRS informed choice leaflets into a maternity service. In: Kirkham M ed Informed choice in maternity care. Palgrave Macmillan, Basingstoke, p 169–184

Flint C 1991 Continuity of care provided by a team of midwives – the 'Know Your Midwife' scheme. In: Robinson S, Thomson A-M eds Midwives, research and childbirth, vol 2. Chapman and Hall, London, p 72–103

Green JM, Coupland VA, Kitzinger JV 1998 Great expectations: a prospective study of women's expectations and experience of childbirth, 2nd edn. Books for Midwives, Oxford

Hewson B 2004 Informed choice in maternity care. In: Kirkham M ed Informed choice in maternity care. Palgrave Macmillan, Basingstoke, p 31–56

Kirkham M 1999 The culture of midwifery in the National Health Service in England. Journal of Advanced Nursing 30(3):732–739

Kirkham M, Stapleton H 2001 Informed choice in maternity care: an evaluation of evidence based leaflets. Women's Informed Childbearing and Health Research Group, School of Nursing and Midwifery, University of Sheffield/NHS Centre for Reviews and Dissemination, University of York

Kirkham M, Stapleton H 2004 The culture of the maternity services in Wales and England as a barrier to informed choice. In: Kirkham M ed Informed choice in maternity care. Palgrave Macmillan, Basingstoke, p 117–146

McCourt C, Page L 1997 One-to-one midwifery practice: report on the evaluation of one-to-one midwifery. Thames Valley University and The Hammersmith Hospital NHS Trust, London

McCourt C, Page L, Hewison J 1998 Evaluation of one-to-one midwifery: women's responses to care. Birth 25:73–80

Pairman S 2000 Women-centred midwifery: partnerships or professional friendships. In: Kirkham M ed The midwife–mother relationship. Macmillan Press, Basingstoke, p 207–226

Sandall J 1997 Midwives' burnout and continuity of care. British Journal of Midwifery 5(2):106–111

Sandall J, Davies J, Warwick C 2001 Evaluation of the Albany Midwifery Practice: final report. Nightingale School of Midwifery, King's College, London

Stevens T, McCourt C 2002 One-to-one midwifery practice: meaning for midwives. British Journal of Midwifery 10(2):111–115

van Olphen Fehr J 1999 The lived experience of being in a caring relationship with a midwife during childbirth. Unpublished PhD thesis, George Mason University, USA

Researching women's views

INTRODUCTION

The articles in the first section of this book add more to our understanding that, in practice, issues surrounding choice and information in childbirth are complex and laden with political issues. From the perspective of doing research, we can also see that it is not nearly as easy to find out and measure things as we might have grown up to believe. The RCT in Chapter 1 shows one thing and, if we read that alone, we might think that information leaflets weren't as helpful as we might hope, yet the qualitative part of this study in Chapter 2 offered a very different perspective on the issue.

This section explores research on a different but related theme: what are the views of women about their care and the options available to them, and how does this link with the issue of information? Again, it is possible to take either a quantitative or a qualitative approach to this question, and this section, like the previous one, offers one research article from each perspective. In Chapter 3, Trish Anderson looks at a survey, or cross-sectional study, which set out to look at women's views of their maternity care and, in Chapter 4, Mary Stewart considers a research study that took a qualitative approach to this question.

This section will enable you to look at surveys as a research method and to look more closely at grounded theory (which was also used in Chapter 2). Although it will probably not be any surprise to you to find out that, again, the different perspectives taken in researching these questions bring different challenges, advantages and disadvantages, your understanding of these issues from the previous section should help you to look at the papers even more critically in this section.

CHAPTER 3

Tricia Anderson

INTRODUCTION

We are all very familiar with surveys as a means of undertaking research. Who hasn't been stopped in the high street by someone with a clipboard asking us if we can spare 5 minutes to complete a questionnaire? Questionnaires and surveys are a good way of collating information from a large number of people in a way that appears, at first glance, to be straightforward to administer and analyse, and will produce results that are clear and unambiguous. Yet the simple questionnaire can be full of pitfalls and biases, as we shall see.

What could be more straightforward than to ask women their views of maternity care? It is an extremely valid and important area for research in this day and age of consumer-led health care, where the health service aims to meet the health needs of the population and service evaluation is a constant theme. It seems a simple enough prospect. But let's think about this for a moment.

If you were going to ask women their views of their maternity care, which women would you ask? You couldn't ask all of them – that would be impractical, and anyway, what does 'all of them' mean? So you are going to have to choose a smallish section of women to include in your survey. So how would you make sure that your small section was at least reasonably representative of everyone?

When would you ask them? During pregnancy, when they are still in the middle of their maternity care journey? Certainly their opinions would be fresh then, but they wouldn't have had time to reflect on their entire experience. In the early postnatal days, when they are tired, grappling with new motherhood and struggle even to remember what they had for breakfast? Far from ideal. Or perhaps several months after the birth, when they have had time to recover and reflect – but then will they be worrying about introducing solids and have forgotten some important details?

Last, of course, exactly what would you ask them? 'Were you satisfied with your maternity care: Yes or no' is hardly going to get the sort of useful data that you are after. And of course, being satisfied is closely linked with expectations, making this a tricky area. If a woman wasn't expecting very much from maternity care in the first place then she is going to say she was satisfied with what could have been quite a poor service, isn't she? You are going to have to decide on some specific areas to ask the women about in your questionnaire. But who decides what areas are important enough to be included? Some areas that professionals might think are very important, such as 'informed choice about pain relief' for example, might actually not be all that important to women. They might be more interested in whether the midwife smelled nice, the car parking facilities, and the toilets on the postnatal ward. Who knows? But if these areas are not included in the questionnaire, then no one will ever know!

It's trickier than you first think, and lots of maternity satisfaction surveys get it spectacularly wrong. All too often they are commissioned by 'tick-box' bureaucrats, ask the wrong questions and are seen as a justification for continuing with the existing level of services. NHS trusts love this kind of data, as do all big institutions: it can be presented in reports and presentations using colourful pie charts and graphs as hard-to-challenge 'evidence' to demonstrate what a good job they are doing. Heaven forbid if they actually had to alter something about the service as a result of a satisfaction survey!

Nevertheless, it is important that we do evaluate the care we are providing; we want to provide good-quality maternity care for women, and women are the only people who can tell us whether we are succeeding or not. This research study by Hundley et al is actually quite a good example of a well-thought-out survey – see what you think. But in future, when you read statements like '92% of women were satisfied with their maternity care' or '84% of women don't care if they know the midwife who looks after them in labour', just pause for a minute and think: which women did they ask, when were they asked, and exactly what were the questions?

Hundley V, Rennie A-M, Fitzmaurice A et al 2000 A national survey of women's views of their maternity care in Scotland. Midwifery 16(4):303–313

QUESTIONS FOR CHAPTER 3

1   This is a retrospective survey because:
a) It focuses on past events that have happened to women
b) It is based on a questionnaire design from the 1960s
c) It asks women for their views of maternity services

A national survey of women's views of their maternity care in Scotland

Vanora Hundley, Anne-Marie Rennie, Ann Fitzmaurice, Wendy Graham, Edwin van Teijlingen and Gillian Penney

Objective: a survey of women's views of their care was undertaken as part of a national audit of maternity services in Scotland. The overall aim of the audit was to determine the extent to which recommendations from recent national policy documents had been adopted in practice.

Design: a cross-sectional study seeking the views of all women giving birth throughout Scotland during a 10-day period in September 1998.

Participants: all women giving birth in Scotland within the survey period were eligible to participate in the study. Women unable to complete the questionnaire in English, women for whom the midwife deemed it inappropriate, and women who delivered but no longer resided in Scotland by their 10th postnatal day were excluded.

Data collection: a self-complete questionnaire given to the woman by her community midwife for completion on her 10th postnatal day.

Data analysis: analysis was carried out using the statistical package **SPSS** for **Windows**. Descriptive statistics were produced for all variables. Statistical tests of significance were not used, as this was primarily a descriptive survey.

Findings: of the 1152 questionnaires returned, 1137 were suitable for analysis. This gave a response rate of 69% of the eligible population (1639). Most women (80%) had the majority of their antenatal care in the community but only one third had a choice about this. Sixty-nine per cent of women received care from one or two people. However, only 37% had a choice about who these people were. The majority of women gave birth in hospital (99%). Sixty-one per cent felt that they had a choice about where they could have their baby. However, fewer women had a choice about having a home birth (41%) or a **DOMINO** delivery (23%). Just over half the women felt that it was important to be cared for by a midwife that they had met during pregnancy but only 12% of women achieved this.

Sixty-two per cent of women had talked to a health professional about what happened during labour and delivery but less than half had spoken with a professional who was present during her labour or birth.

Conclusions: considerable efforts have been made to improve information and choice for women. However, it is clear that further work is needed if women are to be offered informed choice in the provision of their maternity care. © 2000 Harcourt Publishers Ltd

Vanora Hundley BN, MSc, RGN, RM, Lecturer, Centre for Advanced Studies in Nursing, University of Aberdeen, Foresterhill Health Centre, Westburn Road, Aberdeen, AB24 2AY, UK.
E-mail: v.hundley@abdn.ac.uk

Anne-Marie Rennie BSc (Hons), MSc, RGN, RM, Research midwife, Dugald Baird Centre for Research in Women's Health, University of Aberdeen, UK

Ann Fitzmaurice MA (Hons), PgDip (information analysis), Medical Statistician, Dugald Baird Centre for Research on Women's Health, University of Aberdeen, UK

Wendy Graham DPhil (Oxon), Director, Dugald Baird Centre for Research in Women's Health, University of Aberdeen, UK

Edwin van Teijlingen MA (Hons), MEd, PhD, Lecturer, Department of Public Health, University of Aberdeen, UK

Gillian Penney MD, FRCOG, MFFP, Programme Co-ordinator, Scottish Programme for Clinical Effectiveness in Reproductive Health.

(Correspondence to VH)

Received 3 February 2000
Revised 9 March 2000
Accepted 31 May 2000
Published online 16 October 2000

INTRODUCTION

The way in which maternity care is provided in the UK has been influenced over the last decade by official reports recommending fundamental changes (House of Commons Health Committee 1992, Department of Health (DoH) 1993, Scottish Office Home and Health Department (SOHHD) 1993). These reports have advocated a shift from a maternity service in which government and professional priorities may have dominated to a more woman-centred service. The need for such a shift had been recognised by government (Department of Health 1993) and

Midwifery (2000) **16**, 303–313   © 2000 Harcourt Publishers Ltd
doi:10.1054/midw.2000.0231, available online at http://www.idealibrary.com on **IDEAL**

304 *Midwifery*

professional (Association of Radical Midwives 1986, Royal College of Midwives 1991) reports, as well as consumer organizations (Kitzinger 1981). The impetus for these changes was brought about by two policy documents 'Changing Childbirth' in England and Wales (DoH 1993) and *Provision of Maternity Services in Scotland. A Policy Review* in Scotland (SOHHD 1993). These policy documents required maternity service providers to increase women's access to information, to offer women greater choice and involvement in decision-making and to improve continuity of care and carer. It has been seven years since these documents were published; the question is, has maternity care in Scotland changed?

There is some evidence that maternity services in Scotland have responded to the policy recommendations through the introduction of new systems of maternity care provision (McGinley et al. 1995, Smith 1995). In order to ascertain the extent to which these recommendations were being adopted in practice, a national audit of maternity services was conducted by the Scottish Programme for Clinical Effectiveness in Reproductive Health (SPCERH) (SPCERH & Dugald Baird Centre for Research on Women's Health 1999).

Audit criteria were identified by a multidisciplinary Standard Setting Group from recommendations in two sets of Scottish Office Department of Health publications:

- *Provision of Maternity Services in Scotland: A Policy Review* (SOHHD 1993).
- The compendium of 13 reports produced by the Clinical Resource and Audit Group (CRAG)/the Scottish Health Management Efficiency Group (SCOTMEG) Working Group on Maternity Services and published between 1993 and 1996 (CRAG/SCOTMEG 1996).

These documents contained consensus statements developed by multidisciplinary working groups and endorsed as Scottish health service policy. However, the consensus statements and recommendations were not based on formal systematic reviews of the evidence in the manner that we would now expect for both policy documents and guidelines. In all, 28 audit criteria in four principal themes were identified (Box 1).

The audit involved two mechanisms of data collection:

1. Structured interviews with lead professionals in every consultant-led maternity unit in Scotland.
2. A questionnaire survey of all women giving birth in a 10-day period in 1998.

Both methods of data collection were required to assess many of the audit criteria and the findings have been presented in a separate report (SPCERH & Dugald Baird Centre for Research on Women's Health 1999). This paper presents the key findings of the survey to determine women's views of the care they received.

METHODS

Study design

This was a cross-sectional survey that sought the views of all women giving birth in Scotland during a 10-day period (14–23 September 1998). The study design was determined by a pilot study of four methods of distribution and follow-up. Considerable problems were encountered with each of these methods (this will be reported elsewhere) and it was decided that the most practical method was for midwives in the community to distribute numbered questionnaires to the women on their 10th postnatal day. Questionnaires were returned direct to the study team in pre-paid envelopes. The midwives informed the team of the women's names, addresses and corresponding study numbers to facilitate the reminder system. A reminder questionnaire was sent by post to women who had not responded after two weeks.

Prior to the launch of the survey, the co-operation and support from Heads of Midwifery was sought and received. All 15 Link supervisors of midwives in Scotland were approached, and through them all supervisors of midwives were contacted and informed of the survey. Information sheets were sent to all midwives who would be required to assist with distributing the questionnaire. Posters in the postnatal wards and leaflets given out following delivery provided information for women.

Participants

All women who gave birth in Scotland within the survey period were eligible to participate in the study. Women were identified by a midwife in the community and invited to take part. Ethical approval was sought from the Multi-Centre Research Ethics Committee but they considered this to be unnecessary because the study was part of an audit and not research. Exclusions included women who were unable to complete the questionnaire in the English language; women for whom the midwife deemed it inappropriate, each case being assessed individually; and women who no longer resided in Scotland on their 10th postnatal day. Midwives were asked to include women who were still in hospital on the 10th postnatal day, unless the midwife deemed it inappropriate for another reason.

---

2 The impetus behind the study was:
a) To see if maternity care in Scotland had changed since the publication of 'Provision of Maternity Care in Scotland' (1993)
b) To see if women in Scotland are happy with their maternity care
c) To assess women's views of their maternity care in Scotland

3 This survey took place during a 10-day period in September 1998. Does it matter which month it took place in?
a) Yes
b) No
c) Maybe

4 The questionnaires were distributed by community midwives on the tenth postnatal day. Do you think this is the best time?
a) Yes
b) No
c) Maybe

5 Were the women told the questionnaires would be anonymous?
a) Yes
b) No
c) We can't tell

6 Support and co-operation were sought from Heads of Midwifery. Was any effort made to gain support and co-operation from the community midwives themselves?
a) Yes
b) No
c) We can't tell

7 Supervisors of midwives were contacted and informed of the study. This was because:
a) They have a legal responsibility for maternity service provision
b) They are key stakeholders in maternity service provision
c) They could support the project by reminding the community midwives

8 If the community midwives were not supportive in a study of this kind, they might:
a) 'Forget' to give out the questionnaires
b) Give them out but with a very negative endorsement
c) Select only certain groups of women to give them out to

professional (Association of Radical Midwives 1986, Royal College of Midwives 1991) reports, as well as consumer organizations (Kitzinger 1981). The impetus for these changes was brought about by two policy documents 'Changing Childbirth' in England and Wales (DoH 1993) and *Provision of Maternity Services in Scotland. A Policy Review* in Scotland (SOHHD 1993). These policy documents required maternity service providers to increase women's access to information, to offer women greater choice and involvement in decision-making and to improve continuity of care and carer. It has been seven years since these documents were published; the question is, has maternity care in Scotland changed?

There is some evidence that maternity services in Scotland have responded to the policy recommendations through the introduction of new systems of maternity care provision (McGinley et al. 1995, Smith 1995). In order to ascertain the extent to which these recommendations were being adopted in practice, a national audit of maternity services was conducted by the Scottish Programme for Clinical Effectiveness in Reproductive Health (SPCERH) (SPCERH & Dugald Baird Centre for Research on Women's Health 1999).

Audit criteria were identified by a multi-disciplinary Standard Setting Group from recommendations in two sets of Scottish Office Department of Health publications:

- *Provision of Maternity Services in Scotland: A Policy Review* (SOHHD 1993).
- The compendium of 13 reports produced by the Clinical Resource and Audit Group (CRAG)/the Scottish Health Management Efficiency Group (SCOTMEG) Working Group on Maternity Services and published between 1993 and 1996 (CRAG/SCOTMEG 1996).

These documents contained consensus statements developed by multidisciplinary working groups and endorsed as Scottish health service policy. However, the consensus statements and recommendations were not based on formal systematic reviews of the evidence in the manner that we would now expect for both policy documents and guidelines. In all, 28 audit criteria in four principal themes were identified (Box 1).

The audit involved two mechanisms of data collection:

1. Structured interviews with lead professionals in every consultant-led maternity unit in Scotland.
2. A questionnaire survey of all women giving birth in a 10-day period in 1998.

Both methods of data collection were required to assess many of the audit criteria and the findings have been presented in a separate report (SPCERH & Dugald Baird Centre for Research on Women's Health 1999). This paper presents the key findings of the survey to determine women's views of the care they received.

METHODS

Study design

This was a cross-sectional survey that sought the views of all women giving birth in Scotland during a 10-day period (14–23 September 1998). The study design was determined by a pilot study of four methods of distribution and follow-up. Considerable problems were encountered with each of these methods (this will be reported elsewhere) and it was decided that the most practical method was for midwives in the community to distribute numbered questionnaires to the women on their 10th postnatal day. Questionnaires were returned direct to the study team in pre-paid envelopes. The midwives informed the team of the women's names, addresses and corresponding study numbers to facilitate the reminder system. A reminder questionnaire was sent by post to women who had not responded after two weeks.

Prior to the launch of the survey, the co-operation and support from Heads of Midwifery was sought and received. All 15 Link supervisors of midwives in Scotland were approached, and through them all supervisors of midwives were contacted and informed of the survey. Information sheets were sent to all midwives who would be required to assist with distributing the questionnaire. Posters in the postnatal wards and leaflets given out following delivery provided information for women.

Participants

All women who gave birth in Scotland within the survey period were eligible to participate in the study. Women were identified by a midwife in the community and invited to take part. Ethical approval was sought from the Multi-Centre Research Ethics Committee but they considered this to be unnecessary because the study was part of an audit and not research. Exclusions included women who were unable to complete the questionnaire in the English language; women for whom the midwife deemed it inappropriate, each case being assessed individually; and women who no longer resided in Scotland on their 10th postnatal day. Midwives were asked to include women who were still in hospital on the 10th postnatal day, unless the midwife deemed it inappropriate for another reason.

9 'All women who gave birth in Scotland within the survey period were eligible to participate in this study.' Is this:
a) True?
b) False?

10 The difference between audit and research is that:
a) Research studies a new development in health care; audit studies existing health care
b) Audit is primarily interested in the performance of the health care service
c) Research studies what things should be done; audit looks at how they should be done
d) Audit studies staff performance whereas research studies clients or patients

11 The Ethics Committee decided it was not necessary to submit this questionnaire to scrutiny of ethical considerations as it was part of audit and not research. Which of the following statements would you agree with most?
a) This is an appropriate decision; unlike research, audit does not have the potential to harm clients
b) This is an inappropriate decision: questionnaires for audit may have the potential to harm clients
c) This is an appropriate decision, as the purpose of audit is to evaluate services that have already happened

12 The questionnaire was only available in written format in English, thus all women who can't read and write English are excluded from this survey. Which of the following is true?
a) In Scotland this is only a small number of women and so is not important in the final results
b) The researchers used other methods to get the views of this group of women
c) It is too expensive and impractical to translate questionnaires into lots of different languages, but it would be good if it were possible
d) None of the above

13 Women were excluded from taking part if 'the midwife deemed it inappropriate'. What kind(s) of women might have been left out?
a) Women with very sick babies
b) Women who had a stillbirth
c) Women under 16 years of age
d) Women from very poor socio-economic backgrounds
e) Women with chaotic lifestyles
f) Women with mental illness, including post-traumatic stress disorder
g) Travelling women
h) Drug-using women
i) Homeless women

14 How were the 28 audit criteria developed?

a) From systematic analysis of the research
b) From a compilation of health service policy documents, which were not based on evidence
c) We can't tell

15 Were women involved in the selection of the 28 criteria to be studied?

a) Yes
b) No
c) We can't tell

16 Do you feel that the list of the 28 criteria is a woman-centred list that reflects women's priorities for their maternity care?

a) Yes
b) No
c) We can't tell

17 A closed question is:

a) A question that only has one answer
b) A question that allows the respondent a limited choice of answers
c) A question that is on a topic chosen by the researcher
d) A question that allows for easier analysis

18 The researchers state that the analysis of the answers from the open questions in the questionnaire has been reported in a separate paper. Which of the following is/are true?

a) It is good academic practice to keep the two types of data separate
b) This is acceptable as both papers 'stand alone'
c) Professional journals won't publish long articles
d) This skews the presentation of the results of the questionnaire

A national study of maternity care in scotland   305

Box 1:   Audit criteria

Equipping women to make informed choices about their care
1.   The Health Education Board for Scotland (HEBS) Pregnancy Book is a useful and comprehensive source of much of the information needed by women in the early stages of pregnancy. This book should be available to women from their GPs prior to the booking visit.
2.   There should be a hand-held maternity record which encourages the woman to be a partner in her care.
3.   Women should be given the opportunity to contribute to a birth plan which should form part of the case notes, with a copy being held by both the woman and her carers.
4.   Each Health Board area should have an antenatal education co-ordinator.
5.   Antenatal education should be an integral part of antenatal care. Educational content should be integrated into the visits at which clinical care is provided.
6.   The antenatal education provided should be regularly evaluated by both supervising professionals and consumers.
7.   The organisation of antenatal group classes should include provision for reunion groups and labour debriefing.
8.   Professional staff should have access to contact names and numbers for local and national support agencies, so that they can refer women to them.

The roles of different professional groups
9.   Each woman should have a maternity care co-ordinator responsible for the overall planning of her care. The co-ordinator may be the named midwife, the general practitioner or the consultant obstetrician.
10.   Each woman should perceive that she has had a choice of maternity care co-ordinator.
11.   All women should have the opportunity to be seen at least once during each pregnancy by a consultant obstetrician.
12.   The option of consultant-led care should be available throughout pregnancy for those women who wish it.
13.   There should be continued development of midwife-led and managed units within existing maternity hospitals.
14.   The average number of antenatal visits should be reduced from the 1991 average of 15 to the recommended number of nine.
15.   All women should be screened for postnatal depression at 6–8 weeks following delivery using the Edinburgh Postnatal Depression Scale (EPDS).
16.   Staff administering the EPDS should have received relevant training and should have access to appropriate services for women found to have abnormal scores.

Providing a choice of type of intrapartum care
17.   The number of beds for maternity care should be reduced.
18.   Women should be given the options of DOMINO delivery, home birth and early discharge.
19.   There should be a policy of reducing postnatal stays.
20.   The setting for births in hospital should be made as 'homely' as possible.
21.   Obstetric and paediatric flying squads (or other emergency transport facilities) should be maintained.
22.   Each major city should have a single flying squad overseen by a team of senior obstetrician, paediatrician and midwife. The flying squad should operate to a regularly reviewed, written protocol.
23.   Basic neonatal resuscitation comprises tactile stimulation, clearing of the airway, face mask inflation of the lungs and external cardiac massage. One of the professionals present at any birth must be trained and experienced in these skills.
24.   For planned home deliveries, two trained professionals should be present.
25.   All neonates should have routine immediate postnatal examination performed by the midwife. The findings of this examination should be recorded and should include: Apgar score, temperature, weight, length and head circumference.
26.   All neonates should have a routine medical examination within 72 hours of birth. The findings of this examination should be recorded on a standard, check-list style proforma.
27.   When phototherapy for neonatal jaundice is required, separation of mother and baby should be minimised and intermittent phototherapy (one hour in four) may have advantages.

Providing continuity of care and carer.
28.   Each woman should have a named midwife involved in her care.

19 There was a 60% response rate to the pilot questionnaire.

a) This is excellent
b) This is satisfactory
c) This is not satisfactory
d) This is very poor

20 The pilot questionnaire was distributed to women who delivered at five hospitals, using different methods of distribution. Was this:

a) Overcomplicated and unnecessary?
b) Commendably thorough?
c) Not thorough enough?

21 The researchers state that piloting the questionnaire showed it appeared to be 'easy to complete and acceptable to women'. On what evidence did they base that assessment?

a) They interviewed the women for their views
b) The return of 60% of the pilot questionnaires, appropriately completed
c) We can't tell

Data collection

Data were collected using a self-complete questionnaire. The questions focused on the criteria agreed by the multidisciplinary Standard Setting Group (Box 1); however only aspects of care that could be reported by postnatal women were included. That is, criteria that were likely to be outside the scope of the women's knowledge, for example criteria 21 and 22 (Box 1), were not assessed in this survey. The questionnaire was developed by the survey team, drawing on the above criteria and using existing, validated questionnaires (Mason 1989, Lamping & Rowe 1996, Audit Commission & Institute of Child Health 1996, Hundley et al. 1997, Rennie et al. 1998). The majority of the questions were closed, although a section for open comments was included at the end. The data from the open section have been reported elsewhere (SPCERH & Dugald Baird Centre for Research on Women's Health 1999).

The questionnaire was pre-tested on 10 postnatal women to assess its acceptability and reviewed by the audit committee for validity. Minor amendments were made and the questionnaire was then piloted to assess the acceptability of the revised questionnaire. The pilot involved distributing questionnaires to women who delivered at five hospitals in Scotland using different methods of distribution. Fifty-two women returned the questionnaires, giving an approximate response rate of 60%. The difficulties encountered in the pilot related to the methods of distribution and follow-up and these will be described elsewhere. The questionnaires appeared to be easy to complete and acceptable to women.

Analysis

Data were analysed using the statistical package SPSS for Windows (Norusis 1997). Due to the

22 The questionnaires were analysed using descriptive statistics. The other type of statistical analysis they could have used is called:

a) Correlational statistics
b) Inferential statistics
c) Significance statistics

23 Descriptive statistics are the most appropriate to use in this study because:

a) They are describing a large set of data from a large group of people
b) The researchers are not making any claims about these findings being representative of the whole of Scotland
c) They are using numbers to describe the key features found in the questionnaire results

24 175 completed questionnaires were sent in that the researchers had not been notified as having been given out. This means that:

a) There were at least 216 women who did not receive a 'reminder' second questionnaire
b) More babies were born in the study period than expected
c) The statistical analysis had to be redone

306 *Midwifery*

limited time available, it was necessary to close data entry at the end of October. Questionnaires returned after this date (n = 38) were not included in the analyses. Descriptive statistics were produced for all variables. Statistical tests of significance were not used as this was primarily a descriptive survey.

FINDINGS

Response rates

The number of questionnaires returned before the closing date was 1152. However, 14 questionnaires were completed by women who had delivered outside the study period and one questionnaire was returned blank. This left 1137 questionnaires that were suitable for analysis. A large proportion of these women requested a copy of the results (774/1137, 68%).

Calculating the response rate in this study is not straightforward and a number of different denominators can be used. The intention was to use figures provided by the midwives to calculate the response rate. However, it became obvious that we were not being notified of all women who received the questionnaire—175 questionnaires were returned from women for whom we had no notification. This is not surprising given the current constraints on midwifery workload (Skewes 1999). Thus to use the number of questionnaires that we know were given out as a denominator would have greatly inflated the response rate to 94% (1137/1209). Even adjust-

ing for these extra 175 questionnaires by removing them from the number returned would still have led to an overestimate, 80% (962/1209). We therefore sought another source of the number of deliveries occurring during the 10-day reference period.

The Registrar General's Office recorded a total of 1659 maternities, including 10 stillbirths, in Scotland during the study period (Fig. 1). Using this as the denominator, the response rate was 68.5% (1137/1659). However, it appeared that a number of women had been excluded from the survey because they had a stillbirth (n = 10), had moved away (n = 4) or for compassionate reasons, as notified by the midwives (n = 6). Reasons given included concealed pregnancy, medical reasons and very ill baby. Thus, 20 women were removed from the denominator, giving a conservative response rate of 69% (1137/1639).

When was the questionnaire completed?

The intention was that women would complete the questionnaire on, or as close as possible to, the 10th postnatal day. To assess this, the baby's date of birth was subtracted from the date the questionnaire was actually completed. The day on which the questionnaire was completed ranged from 0 to 44 days. The mean number of days was 12.3 (SD 6.5), whilst the median was 10. Whilst we asked that the questionnaires be given out on the 10th postnatal day, it appears that some midwives gave them out on the day of birth, both at home and in hospital.

25 The mean number of days that the questionnaire was completed on, following the birth, was 12.3 days. This means that (one or more answers may apply):

a) The majority of women completed their questionnaire between 12 and 13 days after giving birth
b) 12.3 days is the average and represents the most reasonably typical answer that the woman gave
c) One woman must have completed her questionnaire exactly 12.3 days after giving birth

26 One of the limitations of presenting the 'mean' as an average is that:

a) The mean can be interpreted in several different ways
b) The mean can be misleading if a lot of people have given the same answer
c) The mean can be misleading if there is a wide range within the answers

27 The median number of days that the questionnaire was completed on, following the birth, was 10 days. This means that:

a) 10 days was the middle answer in the set of responses, with the same number of answers below and above it
b) 10 days was the most frequently occurring answer
c) 10 days was the average answer in the set of responses

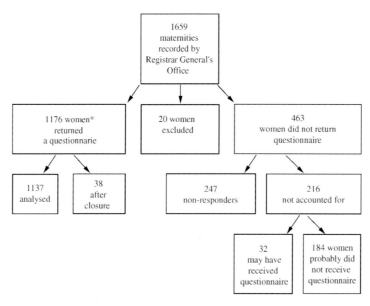

* includes one woman who returned the questionnaire blank.

Fig. I   The number of women who participated in the Scottish Births Survey and reasons for non-participation

28 Looking at the statistical description of the women who completed the survey (the demographics in Table 1), how representative is this of the women of Scotland?

a) Very representative
b) Reasonably representative
c) Not at all representative
d) We can't tell

29 The topics for the antenatal care related more to the organisation than the quality of care. Can you think of some other topic areas that could have been included?

30 A very high percentage of women felt they could ask questions (91–97%) and had the right amount of time to talk (83–89%) to midwives, GPs and hospital doctors. Does this 'ring true' with your clinical experience?

The women in the survey

Demographic data for the women in the survey are shown in Table 1. The majority of women were in the 25–35 age group with the mean age at delivery being 29.3 years (SD 5.4). Deprivation scores were calculated using postcode sectors as described by Carstairs and Morris (1991). The score is based on 1991 census data and takes into account factors such as over-crowding, male unemployment, low social class and car ownership. The higher the score (e.g. 7) the greater the level of deprivation.

Antenatal care

Nearly all women had attended both the general practitioner (GP) surgery and the hospital for antenatal check-ups (Table 2). However, the majority reported that most of their check-ups were held in the community setting. One third of women (324) said that they had a choice about where they could go for their check-ups. The number of check-ups varied considerably by geographical location, but overall almost 50% of women had between 10 and 14 check-ups. More than two thirds of women said that they had received most of their care from one or two health-care staff (midwives, GPs and/or hospital doctors) but only 37% (366) had a choice about who these staff were.

Most women felt that it was important to have one main person who was responsible for providing their antenatal care. Sixty-six per cent of women (694) reported that they did have one main person. However, half of these women said that they did not have a choice about who this person was. Women were most likely to state that the midwife was the main person responsible for providing care (Table 2). Few women (281, 29%) reported that they had a choice about whether they could have all their care, including care at delivery, from midwives.

Most women reported that they felt able to ask questions of professional staff at their antenatal check-ups. This included hospital doctors (91%),

Table I The women in the Scottish Births Survey	n	%
Age group: (n=1113)		
15–19	82	7.4
20–24	156	14.0
25–29	347	31.2
30–34	367	33.0
35–39	147	13.2
40–44	14	1.3
This birth was: (n=1136)		
One baby	1126	99.1
Twins	10	0.9
Triplets or more	0	0
Previous children: (n=1122)		
None (this was first baby)	509	45.4
One	408	36.4
Two	142	12.7
Three or more	63	5.6
Ethnic group: (n=1092)		
White	1072	98.2
Black (British, Caribbean, African, Other)	0	0
Indian	2	0.2
Pakistani	7	0.6
Bangladeshi	0	0
Chinese	4	0.4
Other	7	0.6
Who the woman lives with: (n=1120)		
Husband/partner	996	88.9
Mother and/or father	81	7.2
Other children	593	52.9
Siblings	31	2.8
Other	15	1.3
Deprivation score: (n=1006)		
1 (affluent)	64	6.4
2	126	12.5
3	242	24.1
4	263	26.1
5	155	15.4
6	102	10.1
7	54	5.4

Table 2 Antenatal care	n	%
Number of antenatal check-ups during pregnancy: (n=1050)		
0	2	0.2
1–4	31	3.0
5–9	321	30.6
10–14	496	47.2
15 or more	200	19.0
Location attended for check-ups:		
Hospital clinic (n=1033)	843	81.6
GP surgery (n=1030)	909	88.3
Community clinic (n=1031)	226	21.9
At home (n=1037)	155	14.9
Other (n=1034)	12	1.2
Location of most check-ups: (n=1028)		
Hospital clinic	149	14.5
GP surgery	675	65.7
Community clinic	108	10.5
At home	13	1.3
Equal hospital and GP	45	4.4
Equal GP and community	23	2.2
Some other combination	14	1.4
Proportion of women who had: (n=1028)		
Most care in hospital	149	14.5
Most care in the community	828	80.5
Most care combination	51	5.0
During pregnancy, women got most of their care from: (n=1046)		
One or two people	717	68.5
Different people each time	329	31.5
Importance of having one main person responsible for care? (n=1048)		
Very important	534	51.0
Quite important	394	37.6
Not important	120	11.5
If the woman had a main person responsible for providing antenatal care, who was this? (n=688)		
GP	232	33.7
Midwife	328	47.7
Hospital doctor/obstetrician	105	15.3
Combination	23	3.3

308 *Midwifery*

hospital midwives (96%), GPs (97%) and community midwives (97%). In general, women felt that the amount of time available to talk at check-ups was about right (doctor's surgery/midwife clinic 89%, hospital 83%).

Antenatal information and advice

Three quarters of the women were given the name of a midwife that they could contact during pregnancy for advice. Of these women (784), 33% had contacted the midwife, 66% did not try and 1% had tried but been unable to contact the midwife. Most women (84%, 952) reported that they had received the *New Pregnancy Book* published by the Health Education Board for Scotland and distributed free to all pregnant women. Half of the women (51%, 568) had attended antenatal classes or groups during pregnancy. Not surprisingly, women were more likely to attend classes if this was their first baby (79%) rather than a subsequent baby (27%). The type of classes and groups are shown in Table 3. Most women who attended felt that the classes or groups had prepared them reasonably well for childbirth and for looking after the baby.

Labour and delivery

The majority of women had a normal delivery and gave birth in hospital (Table 4). The mean gestation at delivery was 39.6 weeks (SD 1.6). Of the eight home births, five were planned. Sixty-one per cent of women (597) felt that they had a choice about where they could have their baby. However, fewer felt that they had a choice about having a home birth (41%) or a DOMINO

delivery (23%). Nearly half the women (46%) reported that they did not know what a DOMINO delivery was.

Just over half the women (54%) felt that it was important to be cared for by a midwife that they had met during pregnancy (Table 4). However, only 12% achieved this. Women who were cared for by a midwife that they had met during pregnancy were more likely to say that this was very important, whereas those women who had not met the midwife were more likely to say that it was not important (Fig. 2). Fifty-eight per cent of women (589) reported that they had preferences about their care during labour and delivery. Of these women, 74% (420) had recorded these preferences. In most cases preferences were written in a formal birth plan (73%), but in 23% of cases they were written directly into maternity records. The remaining women recorded their preferences on a separate sheet of paper. Only 79% of women who had a birth plan reported that they themselves were involved in its preparation. Others who were involved included the midwife (62%), husband/partner (55%), obstetrician (7%), GP (3%) and friend/relative (3%). Most women who had a written birth plan felt that it was taken into consideration (Table 4).

31 73% of the women had a formal birth plan in their notes.

a) True
b) False
c) We can't tell

Table 3   Antenatal information

	n	%
Which antenatal classes or groups did women attend: (n=568)		
Hospital antenatal classes	316	55.6
Community antenatal classes	285	50.2
National Childbirth Trust	23	4.0
Active Childbirth	7	1.2
Aquanatal classes	12	2.1
Breast-feeding classes/workshop	11	1.9
Other	22	3.9
How well did women feel that the classes prepared them for *childbirth:* **(n=552)**		
Well	244	44.2
Reasonably well	276	50.0
Not enough	26	4.7
Not at all	6	1.1
How well did women feel that the classes prepared them for *looking after the baby:* **(n=539)**		
Well	156	28.9
Reasonably well	285	52.9
Not enough	70	13.0
Not at all	28	5.2

Table 4   Intrapartum care

	%	n
Place of birth: (n=1136)		
In hospital – NHS care	1122	98.8
In hospital – private care	4	0.4
At home (total)	8	0.7
Born before arrival/in transit to hospital	2	0.2
How important did women feel it was to be cared for in labour by a midwife whom they had met during pregnancy? (n=1116)		
Very important	241	21.6
Quite important	361	32.2
Not important	514	46.1
Proportion of women who were cared for in labour by a midwife whom they had met during pregnancy: (n=1109)	134	12.1
How important did women feel it was to have a written birth plan: (n=1104)		
Very important	303	27.4
Quite important	384	34.8
Not important	417	37.8
Did women who had a written plan feel that it was taken into consideration? (n=409)		
Yes fully	226	55.3
Yes partly	144	35.2
No	36	8.8
Not applicable (had caesarean section)	3	0.7
Type of birth: (n=1135)		
A normal vaginal delivery	776	68.4
An assisted vaginal delivery	149	13.1
A planned caesarean section	94	8.3
An emergency caesarean section	116	10.2

32 Most women were happy with a 3–5 day postnatal stay in hospital.

a) True
b) False
c) We can't tell

33 Figures 2 and 3 are examples of graphic representation of the data called:

a) Pie charts
b) Histograms
c) Bar charts
d) Line graphs

34 Which of the following is correct?

a) Figure 3 is a vertical sloped bar chart
b) Figure 3 is a horizontal histogram
c) Figure 3 is a vertical line graph
d) Figure 3 is a stacked vertical bar chart

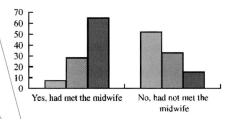

Fig. 2 How important do you think it is to be looked after during labour by a midwife that you have already met? ■ Not important; ■ Quite important; ■ Very important.

Postnatal care

Sixty-two per cent of women (700) had talked to a health professional about what happened during labour and delivery. It is not surprising that women were most likely to talk to midwives (Table 5). However, less than half had spoken with a professional who was present during the woman's labour or birth. Fifteen per cent of women (161) said that there was someone they would have liked to talk to but had not done so. In most cases this was the midwife who was present during labour and delivery.

Sixty per cent of women reported that they had or were still breast feeding their babies and the majority of these women reported that they had received enough help, encouragement, advice and privacy (Table 5). With regard to postnatal advice in general, 26% of women (279) reported that they had been confused or worried by the different advice that they had received from health professionals.

The majority of women who delivered and/or received postnatal care in hospital (77%) reported that they had a choice about how soon to go home after the birth. On average, women's stay in hospital was between 3 and 5 days and most women were happy with this.

Satisfaction with care

Women were asked a closed question about satisfaction for each time period: antenatal, intrapartum and postnatal. For example, 'Thinking about your antenatal care, how satisfied were you with the care you received?'. Figure 3 shows women's responses to these questions. In all three time periods most women reported that they were satisfied with the care they received. Satisfaction was greatest with care received in the postnatal period, while dissatisfaction was greatest with care received during labour and delivery.

DISCUSSION AND CONCLUSION

The Scottish Policy Review recommended informed choice as 'the key to giving women

Table 5	Postnatal care		
		n	%
Professionals the women *had* talked to: (*n*=681)			
Hospital doctor–present during labour/birth		115	16.9
Midwife–present during labour/birth		253	37.2
Hospital doctor–*not* present during labour/birth		80	11.7
Midwife–*not* present during labour/birth		507	74.4
GP		233	34.2
Health Visitor		42	6.2
Someone else		27	4.0
Professionals the women would have liked to talk to: (*n*=161)			
Hospital doctor–present during labour/birth		46	28.6
Midwife–present during labour/birth		104	64.6
Hospital doctor–*not* present during labour/birth		11	6.8
Midwife–*not* present during labour/birth		7	4.3
GP		19	11.8
Someone else		7	4.3
Proportion of women who breastfed their baby: (*n*=1125)		678	60.3
Of these women, the proportion who were given enough:			
Help (*n*=668)		592	88.6
Encouragement (*n*=660)		598	90.6
Advice (*n*=653)		579	88.7
Privacy (*n*=645)		604	93.6
Length of hospital stay: (*n*=1120)			
Less than 6 hours		9	0.8
7–12 hours		45	4.0
13–24 hours		102	9.1
1–2 days		320	28.6
3–5 days		542	48.4
6 days or more		102	9.1
Women thought that the length of hospital stay was: (*n*=1119)			
Too long		44	3.9
Too short		99	8.8
The right length		976	87.2

the level and quality of service which they want' (SOHHD 1993 p20). However, in common with women in England and Wales (Garcia et al. 1998), the majority of our respondents reported having no choice about whom they saw for antenatal care and where they went for that care. While most women had one main person responsible for providing care during pregnancy, only half of these women had a choice about who this person was.

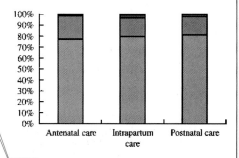

Fig. 3 How satisfied were you with the care you received? ■ Dissatisfied; ■ Satisfied in some ways; ■ Satisfied.

35 In Table 5, the percentages in each section add up to more than 100%. This is because:

a) There is an error in the calculations
b) Women could tick more than one box
c) Some women did not fill this section in correctly

310 *Midwifery*

The picture was slightly better with regard to choice about where to have their baby and is an improvement on the findings of the 1993 MORI survey, which found that the majority of women reported that they had no choice about place of birth (MORI 1993). Less than half of the women said that they had a choice about whether they could have a home birth. However, this is still considerably higher than the recent comparable national survey in England and Wales (Garcia et al. 1998).

Improved access to information is essential if women are to have real choice. Most women felt able to ask questions of professional staff during their antenatal care and, if they attended antenatal classes, they felt that the classes prepared them well for childbirth. Written information may also facilitate choice and the majority of women reported receiving the recommended pregnancy and childbirth book. However, the fact that nearly a third of women did not know that they could have all their care from midwives and almost half did not know what a DOMINO delivery was, clearly indicates that these methods of providing information do not always convey the available options for care. The interviews with maternity care staff, carried out in the first phase of the audit, highlighted the problems of providing a DOMINO service within current staffing levels (SPCERH & Dugald Baird Centre for Research on Women's Health 1999). As a result, staff may feel unable to provide women with information and choice about all available options because to do so would over-commit the midwife. This control of information as a means of self-preservation has been found in a previous study that explored midwives' views of continuity of carer (University of Glasgow & Royal College of Midwives Scottish Board 1997). Indeed, a recent Scottish study of women's choice of DOMINO delivery found that women were only offered a DOMINO birth because of dissatisfaction with a previous experience of care (Mansion & McGuire 1998).

MIDIRS Informed Choice leaflets have been suggested as a means of improving communication between women and professional staff (Rosser 1995). However, resource implications (Rosser 1996) and areas of controversy (Rosser 1997) may mean that they are not used in all hospitals. It is not possible from this survey to determine the proportion of hospitals in Scotland currently using these leaflets.

It is concerning to find that one fifth of women who had a written birth plan were not involved in its preparation. It is possible that the question might have been interpreted as relating to the actual writing of the plan, something that could have been carried out by staff if the birth plan was written directly into the maternity records. Another explanation may be that although a birth plan is traditionally thought to be an expression of the woman's preferences (Whitford & Hillan 1998), some women may see the birth plan as documentation of the health professionals' plan for their labour and delivery. This form of documentation would be most likely where complications were anticipated. However, we found no association between mode of delivery and involvement in the preparation of the birth plan. It is known that some women prefer to leave the decisions to health professionals believing that 'they know best' (Bluff & Holloway 1994) and this may be the reason for their lack of involvement. Indeed this has been found in a recent study of birth plans (Whitford & Hillan 1998). In these cases the birth plan may simply document the woman's wish to let the doctor or midwife decide the care. It is not possible in our study to determine the content of the women's birth plans. However, the proportion of women in this study who did not feel that they were involved is sufficiently high to warrant further investigation.

Postnatal discussion regarding labour and delivery, sometimes called debriefing, has been recommended both in the literature and by government reports (Alexander 1998). The Scottish Policy Review recommended that women should be given 'the opportunity to talk over the birth' during their postnatal care in hospital (SOHHD 1993 p23). Nearly two thirds of women in this study had the opportunity to do this, however, few were able to discuss their experience with a health professional who was actually present during their labour or delivery. The area of debriefing is under-researched (Alexander 1998) and the importance of having a professional who was actually present is uncertain. Further research is needed in this area.

It is evident that there is still considerable work to do to achieve the Scottish Policy Review recommendation to improve 'communications with women so that they can be more involved in decisions about the management of their own pregnancies' (SOHHD 1993 p54).

The second key feature of care highlighted by the Scottish Policy Review was continuity of carer. It is clear from qualitative research that this was something which women valued (Bostock 1993). Unlike Changing Childbirth (DoH 1993), the Scottish Policy Review did not set a target regarding the proportion of women who should know the carer at delivery but stated that 'health boards should secure a system where more women are given the options of DOMINO delivery, home births and/or early post-natal discharge where appropriate and these options should incorporate continuity of care...' (SOHHD 1993 p53). However, with only 12% of women reporting that they knew the person who cared for them during labour and delivery, this must surely be seen as a failure to meet this recommendation.

It is reassuring then to find that the majority of women were satisfied with the care that they received. However, we must exercise caution in interpreting these findings. There are numerous difficulties in measuring satisfaction (Locker & Dunt 1978, Fitzpatrick & Hopkins 1983, Fitzpatrick 1991) and in particular satisfaction with childbirth (Lumley 1985, Jacoby & Cartwright 1990, Hundley et al. 1997). Although the study team tried to overcome the problems associated with using an overall measure by asking about satisfaction antenatally, intrapartum and postnatally, it is likely that smaller areas of dissatisfaction will have been overlooked. A further problem is that respondents tend to be reluctant to criticize their carers (Fitzpatrick 1991) and this may have been compounded by our choice of study design. The timing of the survey may also have led to an overestimation of satisfaction as there is some evidence that postnatal women are more likely to express negative feelings about the birth experience some time after the event (Erb et al. 1983 Bennett 1985).

Limitations of the study

The study design relied on service providers to distribute the questionnaire. This caused two obvious problems, a logistical problem and a difficulty in interpreting the actual response. The logistical problem arose when, prior to the circulation, staff were asked to predict the number of deliveries in their area in the 10-day period. Some centres gave inflated projections and this led to a shortage of questionnaires at some locations and excess at others. Although this problem made the survey more complex to organise, the main concern is that some women may not have received the questionnaire.

The second problem relates to the large discrepancy between the number of maternities recorded by the Registrar General's Office and the number of women receiving a questionnaire according to the midwives (Fig. 1). Of the 463 maternities identified by the Registrar General's Office, for whom we did not receive a questionnaire, 247 can be considered non-responders as the midwives reported that they had been given a questionnaire. We might estimate that 15% of the other 216 women received a questionnaire but the midwives did not give us the women's details, as this would be a similar percentage to the responders. That leaves 184 women, 11% of the eligible population, who did not receive a questionnaire. It is likely that this is not a random group in terms of either their demographic and obstetric characteristics or their geographical location. However, our data show that the study participants were compar-

able to national statistics on maternal age, parity and deprivation (SPCERH & Dugald Baird Centre for Research on Women's Health 1999).

A further problem is that of health-care staff acting as gatekeepers to the research. The research team was keen that all women who wanted to participate in the research should be given the chance to do so. However, we were also aware that women who had a difficult birth or stillbirth might find the questionnaire too upsetting to complete. For this reason the midwives were asked to assess each woman individually and to inform the research team if a woman did not wish to be part of the survey. The team was informed of six women who were not given a questionnaire for compassionate reasons, but it was clear from the responses that none of the women who had a stillbirth completed a questionnaire. Although it is possible that these women did not wish to be part of the survey, we were not notified of this. It may be that the midwives automatically excluded them as these women tend to be excluded in surveys of this type. It follows that other women could also have been excluded, perhaps members of minority ethnic groups. The limited resources available for the study meant that we were unable to have the questionnaire translated and therefore our exclusion criteria included women who could not read English. We were not told of any such women and it may be that they had friends or family who could translate the questionnaire for them. However, as no Scottish maternity statistics by ethnic origin are available, we cannot be certain that all groups are adequately represented. However, these are the groups least likely to have access to information, choice and continuity of carer (Neile 1997).

The Scottish Births Study provides an overview of women's service use and satisfaction with services in one particular 10-day period and we caution against using the findings as a means of determining the needs of women. A needs assessment exercise would require more detailed demographic and epidemiological data than we have available to allow the preferences of specific sub-groups of women to be taken into account. Such subgroups might be women from ethnic minority groups or women with complications of pregnancy.

Application of these findings to clinical practice is further complicated by large geographical differences in practice. This is best demonstrated by comparing the number of antenatal check-ups in four areas with the national figures (Table 6). The national figures suggest that approximately one third of women have the recommended number of check-ups, nine or less (CRAG/SCOTMEG

36 Do you feel the researchers pulled out all the most important findings to explore in their discussion?

a) Yes
b) No
c) We can't tell

37 Now go back and re-read the abstract. Do you feel that the abstract faithfully summarises the key findings of the study?

a) Yes
b) No

---

312 *Midwifery*

Table 6 Geographical differences in the number of antenatal check-ups

	Number of antenatal check-ups			
	0–4 %	5–9 %	10–14 %	15 or more %
Grampian (*n*=108)	3.7	42.6	39.8	13.9
Tayside (*n*=87)	3.4	42.5	46.0	8.0
Forth Valley (*n*=73)	1.4	16.4	57.5	24.7
Highland (*n*=43)	2.3	4.7	53.5	39.5
Scotland (*n*=1050)	3.2	30.6	47.2	19.0

1995). However, at health board level the proportion of women who achieve this can be as low as 7% and as high as 46.3%. Such differences might call into question the value of national figures.

To conclude, there have been considerable efforts to improve information and choice for women. However, it is clear that further work is needed if women are to be offered informed choice in the provision of their maternity care.

ACKNOWLEDGEMENTS

We are extremely grateful to all the women who gave their time in completing the questionnaires and to the midwives, Supervisors of Midwives and Link Supervisors who assisted with the distribution of the questionnaires and thus made this study possible. The study was commissioned by the Scottish Programme for Clinical Effectiveness in Reproductive Health (SPCERH) which is funded by the Clinical Resource and Audit Group (CRAG) of the Scottish Executive Health Department (SEHD). However, the views expressed in the paper are those of the authors and not the funding bodies. This paper has been produced on behalf of the Scottish Births Survey Team, the members are Frances Findley, Ann Fitzmaurice , Wendy Graham, Maureen Heddle, Vanora Hundley, Fiona Preston, Anne-Marie Rennie, Pamela Smith and Edwin van Teijlingen.

REFERENCES

Alexander J 1998 Confusing debriefing and defusing postnatally: the need'for clarity of terms, purpose and value. Midwifery 14: 122–124

Association of Radical Midwives 1986 The Vision: proposals for the future of the maternity services. A.R.M., Lancashire

Audit Commission and Institute of Child Health 1996 Maternity Care Survey. Audit Commission/Institute of Child Health, Bristol

Bennett A 1985 The birth of a first child: do women's reports change over time? Birth 12: 153–158

Bluff R, Holloway I 1994 'They know best': women's perceptions of midwifery care during labour and childbirth. Midwifery 10: 157–164

Bostock Y 1993 Pregnancy, childbirth and coping with motherhood. What women want from the maternity services. Framework for Action Working Group on Maternity Services, Edinburgh

Carstairs V, Morris R 1991 Deprivation and health in Scotland. Aberdeen University Press, Aberdeen

CRAG/SCOTMEG Working Group on Maternity Services 1995 Antenatal care. (MSP 2/95) CRAG, Edinburgh

CRAG/SCOTMEG Working Group on Maternity Services 1996 Final report. CRAG, Edinburgh

Department of Health (DoH) 1993 Changing Childbirth, Report of the expert maternity group. HMSO, London

Erb L, Hill G, Houston D 1983 A survey of parents attitudes towards their caesarean births in Manitoba Hospitals. Birth 10: 85–91

Fitzpatrick R 1991 Surveys of patient satisfaction: I - important general considerations. British Medical Journal 302: 887–889

Fitzpatrick R, Hopkins A 1983 Problems in the conceptual framework of patient satisfaction research. Sociology of Health and Illness 5: 297–311

Garcia J, Redshaw M, Fitzsimons B et al. 1998 First class delivery. A national survey of women's views of maternity care. Audit Commision and National Perinatal Epidemiology Unit, Bristol

House of Commons Health Committee 1992 Second Report of the House of Commons Health Committee on Maternity Services for the session 1991–92 (HCP29). HMSO, London

Hundley V, Milne J, Glazener C et al. 1997 Satisfaction and the three Cs-continuity, choice and control-women's views from a randomised controlled trial of midwife-led care. British Journal of Obstetrics and Gynaecology 104: 1273–1280

Jacoby A, Cartwright A 1990 Finding out about the views and experiences of maternity-service users. In: Garcia J, Kilpatrick R, Richards M (eds). The politics of maternity care-services for childbearing women in twentieth-century Britain. Clarendon Press, Oxford

Kitzinger S 1981 Change in antenatal care. A report of a working party set up for the National Childbirth Trust. NCT, London

Lamping DL, Rowe P 1996 Users' manual for purchasers and providers: survey of women's experience of maternity services. (Short form). London: Health Services Research Unit, School of Hygiene and Tropical Medicine, London

Locker D, Dunt D 1978 Theoretical and methodological issues in sociological studies of consumer satisfaction with medical care. Social Science and Medicine 12: 283–292

Lumley J 1985 Assessing satisfaction with childbirth. Birth 12 (3): 141–145

Mansion EM, McGuire MM 1998 Factors which influence women in their choice of DOMINO care. British Journal of Midwifery 6 (10): 664–668

Mason V 1989 Women's experience of maternity care–a survey manual. Office of Population Censuses and Surveys. HMSO, London

McGinley M, Turnbull D, Fyvie H et al. 1995 Midwifery development unit at Glasgow Royal Maternity Hospital. British Journal of Midwifery 3 (7): 362–371

MORI (Market and Opinion Research International) 1993 Maternity services research study conducted for the Department of Health. MORI, London, SE1 0HX

Neile E 1997 Control for Black and ethnic minority women: a meaningless pursuit. In: Kirkham MJ, Perkins ER (eds) Reflections on Midwifery. Bailliere Tindall, London

Norusis MJ 1997 SPSS for Windows. 7.5. Reference Manuals. SPSS Inc., Chicago

Rennie AM, Hundley V, Gurney E et al. 1998 Women's priorities for care before and after delivery. British Journal of Midwifery 6 (7): 434–438

Rosser J 1995 Informed choice initiative. MIDIRS Midwifery Digest 5 (4): 382–384

Rosser J 1996 New series of Informed Choice leaflets. MIDIRS Midwifery Digest 6 (3): 269–270

Rosser J 1997 Informed Choice Series II. MIDIRS Midwifery Digest 7 (1): 22

Royal College of Midwives 1991 Towards a Healthy Nation, every day a birth day. RCM, London

A national study of maternity care in scotland 313

Scottish Office Home and Health Department (SOHHD) 1993 Provision of Maternity Services in Scotland. A Policy Review. HMSO, Edinburgh

Scottish Programme for Clinical Effectiveness in Reproductive Health (SPCERH) and the Dugald Baird Centre for Research on Women's Health 1999 Maternity care matters: an audit of maternity services in Scotland 1998. S.P.C.E.R.H. Publication Number 9. S.P.C.E.R.H., Aberdeen

Skewes J 1999 Message to midwives on pay. RCM Midwives Journal 2 (11): 340–341

Smith K 1995 Secret success. Nursing Standard 8(45): 18–19

University of Glasgow and the Royal College of Midwives Scottish Board 1997 Midwives and Woman Centred Care. Royal College of Midwives, Edinburgh

Whitford HM, Hillan EM 1998 Women's perceptions of birth plans. Midwifery 14: 248–253

ANSWERS

Q1. a) Like most questionnaires, this asks for views of services that have already happened. Occasionally you may come across a 'prospective' survey, in which participants are recruited and complete questionnaires at the beginning of their care

Q2. a) and c). There is an explicit, two-fold aim: as well as assessing women's views, the researchers introduce a comparative element in which they compare the outcomes of this survey with a MORI poll in 1993. However, we are given no details about this MORI poll and so it is not possible to comment on whether the researchers are comparing like with like

Q3. a) Yes, sometimes it can make a big difference to the findings. Happiness or consumer spending surveys in January, for example – think empty purses, cold, grey, damp! – will get different results from those done in sunny June! There are often peaks in birth numbers in March and September. September 1998 might have been a particularly busy month, which could have affected women's experiences and quality of care. When evaluating the questionnaire results, it is important to be aware of any events during September 1998 that might have impacted on the survey findings

Q4. c) This is a tricky area; there is no 'best' time. Ten days postnatal might not be the best time but it is probably the most practical and thus is a pragmatic compromise. If you distribute a questionnaire a few days after the birth, women are still recovering from the immediate effects. We also know that they experience the 'halo' effect, inasmuch as feelings about the birth are often overshadowed by having a healthy baby. However, if you wait until they have been discharged from community midwifery care, it is much harder to control the distribution of your questionnaire as women do not see health visitors on such a regular basis. But we do know that women change their views over time and a proportion of women who were 'satisfied' in the early days and weeks move to becoming more negative as the months pass (and vice versa). What would have been useful is if the researchers could have followed up their questionnaire with a second one, say 6 months later, as we know that the effects and memories of childbirth experiences can have lifelong consequences

Q5. c) It is not made explicit. The researchers do not say specifically that the questionnaires were anonymous, but they state that each questionnaire had a study number. With these numbers they were able to 'map' the returning questionnaires to named women, so they could send out reminder questionnaires to those who hadn't responded within 2 weeks. Clearly if women were aware that their questionnaire could be traced back to them it has the potential to inhibit their responses

Q6. b) The community midwives were sent an information sheet; this is not the same as gaining their support and understanding for the project. Gaining the support of the people 'on the ground' who are actually going to be distributing or administering your questionnaire is extremely important in any research study, as they have the power to make or break it, as we shall see in the next question

Q7. c) The researchers do not state why they felt the need to contact all the supervisors of midwives. It is often the case that senior staff are informed of these types of projects and the staff on the ground (who are expected to implement them) are left out. Having said that, it is good practice to inform all key personnel in any project you are doing, to generate good will and deter saboteurs!

Q8. a), b) and c)! This is an important part of any research study – that those people who are directly implementing it at grassroots level are 'on board' and supportive, otherwise they have the potential to sabotage the study and make any results invalid. Can you think of other ways in which midwives could sabotage research studies?

Q9. b) This is most likely to be false. How did the researchers aim to include the views of women who chose to give birth unattended (a small but increasing number), women whose partners forbade them to contact maternity services, or women who gave birth with independent midwives? This is likely to be a small number of women but they are important in this kind of survey because they are precisely the kind of women whose needs are not being met by existing maternity services. It would be very valid to try and ascertain the number and views of women who are so dissatisfied with mainstream NHS maternity care that they seek alternatives, and leaving them out altogether skews the results considerably.

Q10. b) But this is a very grey area. Primarily audit aims to map the performance of the health care service against pre-agreed targets/standards/performance indicators. Research aims to increase our body of knowledge and understanding – to find out new things or gain greater understanding of existing phenomena which can be in any area

Q11. b) The divide between audit and research is far from clear. It can be just as distressing to fill in an audit questionnaire as one for research, and there are still important ethical issues such as client exploitation, confidentiality and prejudice to consider. Principles of ethical research and audit have developed considerably over the last few years, and it is likely that in future these types of questionnaire, even if it is part of an audit programme, will have to undergo scrutiny from an ethics committee

Q12. d) This is a perennial problem with research: how do we really include and hear the voices and experiences of the women whose first language is not English and whose literacy skills may be limited? When evaluating maternity services they are an important group whose voices should not be excluded, particularly as we know that this group of women may be at increased risk of not accessing services and having poorer health outcomes. To exclude them from a survey of women's views will skew the results. But translating leaflets into lots of languages has not been shown to be the answer either (Woolridge 2004), as many women are not literate in their spoken language nor familiar with complex form-filling. The most effective way to include the views of these women is through undertaking one-to-one interviews, focus groups and so on, with interpreters if need be. This can be time-consuming and expensive and thus these women often get overlooked

Q13. a), b), c), d), e), f), g), h) and i) That is, all of the above! One of the problems of using the midwife as 'gatekeeper' to the questionnaire is that she may have her own prejudices and stereotypes of who is likely to fill in what was, after all, a long written questionnaire. Even though they were asked to give it to every woman within the study period, the midwives were given discretion to decide whether it was appropriate or not. Some midwives might have self-selected out clients who they felt could not or would not fill in the questionnaire. Others might carefully 'screen out' women who they think might give a negative response. But if you leave out all of the women in the groups above, your survey is going to be very limited – and these may well be the very women whose needs are not well met by the maternity services

Q14. b) The researchers acknowledge that these audit criteria were based on policy documents that did not meet current standards of evidence-based health care

Q15. b) No, the health service policies that were used to identify these 28 criteria were endorsed by multi-disciplinary professional committees and taken as health service policy but there is no mention of any consumer involvement. Thus a major weakness is that it is professionals who have decided the areas to study, not the women who are at the receiving end of the services

Q16. b) No, this appears to be a very service-led agenda about health care structure and organisational matters, rather than criteria that might relate to individual women's views of their care. An alternative approach might have been to carry out in-depth interviews or focus groups with women to generate a list of criteria of things that are important to them, which could then be explored through a survey

Q17. b) and d) Closed questions limit the possible range of answers, whereas open questions invite a totally free range of answers. Both types have their uses. Open questions allow people to say whatever they want and can lead to rich, interesting data. However, they are more time-consuming for people to complete and often end up being left blank. They can be complex to analyse and to make clear comparisons between people's responses. Closed questions, on the other hand, can be clear, simple and quick to complete. But the limitation of closed questions is they simplify things. A questionnaire of closed questions offers a wide range of people a limited range of pre-set options, which may not in fact represent their views. Most of us have experienced the frustration of wavering between two boxes on a questionnaire, knowing that neither of them is 'really right'!

Q18. c) and d) It is true that most professional journals won't publish articles of much more than 2000 words, which means that researchers often have to 'squeeze' their research to fit. Clearly, separating the analysis of the open and the closed questions is one way to do this. However, it then means that what we are reading in this article is only a part of what the women wanted to say – and it may or may not be a fair representation. We can't say. There are often respondents who cover questionnaires in writing, writing long detailed and deeply felt answers to open questions, and sometimes even unbidden. If you wanted to make a thorough assessment of this questionnaire you would need to get both papers and read them side by side.

Q19. b) Anything less than a 50% response rate and there is no certainty that the responses are in any way representative of the group sent the questionnaire; thus the findings cannot be generalised in any way. Postal questionnaires have a generally low response rate which limits their usefulness but interestingly in maternity research the response rate is frequently very high – 80% and more. This shows the importance that women ascribe to their maternity care

Q20. b) This was very thorough when it comes to including women who have had NHS hospital-based maternity care, but does not include tackling the issues of piloting the questionnaires with women who have given birth at home; again, a small but important group when it comes to assessing satisfaction with maternity care

Q21. b) It seems that they based this assumption on the fact that 60% of the questionnaires were returned and completed appropriately. However, did the 40% of women who did not return the pilot questionnaire do so because they found it unacceptable, too difficult to complete, or irrelevant to them? We don't know

Q22. b) Inferential statistics, as their name implies, aim to make inferences about the results to a wider population, most commonly aiming to estimate the probability that the findings in a sample reflect those that may be found in the population as a whole. They can also be used to test out hypotheses about links and causation between different factors under study

Q23. b) and c) This is acceptable for this kind of survey, but it limits the wider application and generalisability of the results. The reader must be very aware that no inferences have been made to try to generalise or apply these results to a wider population of women – but of course, that is what often happens!

Q24. a) This error in the recruitment and notification process will have introduced bias into the results. The 216 women who were not accounted for may have been given a questionnaire by community midwives which was not completed, and these women would not have received a reminder, as the midwives did not notify the researchers that they had been included

Q25. b) The average can be a useful quick calculation but it tells us nothing about the range or spread of answers. For example, there might have been some women who completed the questionnaires anything from one to hundreds of days after giving birth; these women are invisible when a simple average is presented

Q26. c) One of the problems with the mean is that, if there have been one or two people who have given answers that are very different, it will 'pull' the mean towards them. In this example, for instance, if one woman had completed her questionnaire 129 days after giving birth but the majority had completed it within 10–15 days, when you added all the answers up and divided them by the number of respondents, the mean would be 'artificially high'

Q27. a) It is the mode that is the most frequently occurring answer, and it would have been useful if the researchers had given the mode, in addition to the mean and median, both of which can be misleading. Giving all three measures of central tendency (where they differ) gives the most complete picture

Q28. d) The authors make the claim that the group they studied is comparable to the national statistics of maternal age, parity and deprivation (1999), but do not give any details of how closely comparable it is. Does it match it precisely? (Unlikely!) Is it 'roughly' comparable? If so, were there any groups where it was more, or less, comparable? We need a little more information if we are to accept that this sample of women who gave birth in the study period, and who answered the questionnaire, is representative of all new mothers in Scotland

Q29. They could have included questions on many, many other aspects of care. Just as a starter, how about whether the woman liked the caregiver, felt she could trust them, felt they were competent, knowledgeable and professional, felt they treated her as an individual, how long she had to wait to be seen, whether any enquiries or phone calls were answered promptly, the facilities at the health centre/surgery, whether test results were available promptly and sensitively. You can probably think of lots of others. This makes you realise that although at first glance this questionnaire appears very comprehensive, it is in fact quite limited in its scope

Q30. It certainly doesn't ring true with what I've heard pregnant women say! This is an example of the kind of superficial statistic thrown up by quantitative surveys, which, on first glance, seems to be extremely positive. But we have mentioned already how expectations link to satisfaction. If you only expect to see your doctor or midwife for a 5–10-minute appointment, then if you get 10 minutes you will be satisfied; if you get 15 minutes you will be extremely satisfied. If you only expect to ask your midwife questions about technical/ clinical matters, then you won't be disappointed that you can't discuss your fears about the birth or your worries about coping with four children

Q31. b) False. This is an example of how statistics can be presented in a misleading way, and the dangers of 'skim-reading'! If you read this paragraph carefully, it states that: (i) 58% (589) of women had preferences; (ii) of these women only 74% (or 420 women) had recorded these preferences; (iii) of these women, only 73% (or approximately 307 women) had recorded these preferences in a formal birth plan. That leaves us with 307 women out of a possible 1137 analysed questionnaires had a formal birth plan in their notes; approximately 27% – a very different result!

Q32. c) I don't think we know about their happiness! The researchers make an inference from a question that asked whether they thought the length of hospital stay was too long, too short or just right, with 87.2% answering that it was just right. Again, there could be many different interpretations of that fact. If you had been socially conditioned into thinking that most women stay a few days in hospital after giving birth, then that is what you think will be 'right', that is what you will expect and that is what you will be satisfied with. A lot of women don't know that they can leave as soon as they have given birth, if they want. Neither have women been offered the opportunity of staying 2 weeks in a beautiful postnatal hotel! If the hospital postnatal ward is dirty, overcrowded and has too few staff, then staying a few days until you have mostly recovered and then going home is likely to seem the best option – especially if you have never been offered any alternatives

Q33. c)

Q34. d) Bar charts can be presented either horizontally or vertically. They can be shown with each 'bar' separate, or 'stacked' where each bar equals 100%, divided into the range of possible sub-groups. One of the problems with this kind of presentation in journals is that while they work well in colour, they can be very hard to read in black and white!

Q35. b)

Q36. b) There are a number of strong findings in the data that are not mentioned in the discussion. As many people only ever read the abstract and the conclusions of a study, this is one way in which awkward findings get 'buried'. They are simply omitted from the discussion section and it is as if they never happened. One example would be that only 55% of women (who had a written birth plan) felt their birth plan was fully taken into consideration; the remainder (just under half the group) felt it had only been taken partly, or not at all into consideration. Read through and see what other findings that you think would be worthy of comment and discussion have been omitted from the final section

Q37. b) For example, there is no mention in the abstract of the findings about birth plans, postnatal care and breastfeeding. Of course, authors can't put everything into an abstract, so they have to make choices about what to highlight. Abstracts are actually very powerful things! Many people, myself included, skim-read journals, scanning the abstracts to see if any article is worth reading in full. It is always interesting to compare the full text of any results section with the results that the authors choose to highlight in the abstract; you will quite often find a difference. If controversial or politically sensitive findings are carefully not mentioned in an abstract, they may get buried for ever! Equally, and perhaps more worryingly, claims and conclusions made in an abstract may not always be supported by the research findings themselves. Never rely on an abstract! Read Henci Goer (2002) for some shocking examples of this type of manipulation of research findings

DISCUSSION

Although there has been an increase in the use of maternity care satisfaction surveys, their results are sadly often unreliable or skewed. In a key paper entitled 'What is, must still be best', van Teijlingen et al (2003) reflect on this Scottish birth survey, which sought the views of all women who gave birth in Scotland during a 10-day period in 1998. As you have just read, women were overwhelmingly satisfied with the care they received, as is typical in these types of surveys, and reports of dissatisfaction were relatively low. One variable that did emerge was that, the fewer the number of carers the women experienced, the more likely she was to be satisfied. However, the authors explain in detail how women tend to value what they have experienced, i.e. the status quo, over innovations in care of which they have no knowledge or experience. Satisfaction surveys thus have major limitations when it comes to exploring ways in which to develop or improve maternity services.

When it came to developing a relationship with a known professional, for example, two-thirds of women who had experience of one primary carer providing their antenatal care rated it as very important. However, of those women who had never experienced it, three-quarters said it was not important. It is perhaps surprising that as many as a quarter of the sample of women who had *never* experienced continuity of antenatal carer *did* rate it as important! In labour this figure went up to 54% – more than half the women rated knowing the midwife beforehand as important, even though only 12% achieved this. Given the bias already mentioned with women tending to value the status quo, this is an extraordinarily strong finding; stronger than the simple percentage implies.

Another important point when considering the research evidence around women's experiences of childbirth is that women change their opinions over time significantly (Waldenstrom 2003, 2004). Thus any research that looks at women's experiences, such as maternal satisfaction surveys and so forth, needs to be scrutinised carefully in the light of when, in relation to the birth experience, it was done. Of course, it is not possible to say which is the 'real' feeling: feelings and perceptions at 1 week after the birth are as valid as those 6 months after the birth. But inasmuch as the earlier one is transitory and the later one likely to be longer lasting, the later feelings need perhaps more consideration than they currently receive. Waldenstrom has done some helpful work here. Working with a longitudinal cohort of 2428 women who completed questionnaires in early pregnancy, and then at 2 months and 1 year after the birth, she first looked at women's memories of childbirth at 2 months and 1 year after birth; 60% made the same assessment of the birth at both time points but a quarter (24%) had become more negative as the year had passed, and 16% more positive (Waldenstrom 2003). Waldenstrom then analysed data from the 2428 women to try and tease out the reasons why some women changed their minds. She found that changing opinion from positive to less positive was associated with difficult births, such as very painful labour and caesarean section. Negative feelings about labour care – overall dissatisfaction with care in labour, the midwife not being sufficiently attentive and still having unanswered questions about the birth – were also statistically significant, as were psychosocial variables – single status, depressive symptoms and worry about the birth in early pregnancy.

Changing opinions the other way, i.e. from negative to less negative, were associated with less worry about the birth in early pregnancy and a more positive memory of support by the midwife during labour. Waldenstrom's conclusions are that 'measures of satisfaction with childbirth soon after delivery may be coloured by relief that labour is over and the happy birth of a baby. More negative aspects may take longer to integrate. Supportive care may have long-term effects and may protect some women from a long-lasting negative experience' (Waldenstrom 2004 p 102).

The real challenges thrown up by maternity satisfaction surveys are that: (i) women can only talk about what they know; (ii) for most women the 'halo' effect of having a healthy new baby tends to overshadow any dissatisfaction with what happened on the labour ward for at least the first postnatal weeks; and (iii) many women have quite low expectations of maternity services anyway. Questionnaires tend to focus on existing services with existing, unchallenged assumptions. But if you've only ever tasted lemonade, you're not going to know that champagne even exists! If women have never had the experience of a waterbirth, say, then they might be quite happy giving birth on a narrow bed and, when asked, will say it was fine. Have you ever heard a woman say 'I wish the delivery beds in hospital were softer'?! No, she puts up with them because she thinks that's how giving birth has to be. Most of us are also quite sceptical of new ideas and have an innate conservatism so when women are presented with a new idea (such as a local birth centre), their hypothetical response is likely to be less enthusiastic than it might be once the service is established. So there are major issues about using these kinds of surveys to lead service improvements and innovation – they actually tend to lead to maintaining the status quo. Consumer-led health care is another of those tricky things that sounds good in theory but is actually rather slippery in reality. It's a rare pregnant woman who says 'Yes I have studied maternity services around the world and actually what would make me the most happy is a mixture between the Dutch and New Zealand systems with a little bit of the Albany practice philosophy thrown in'.

But it doesn't mean that we throw in the towel. There are many innovative ways in which women can be directly involved in developing new maternity services that do meet their needs and wishes – through creative focus groups, discussions and interviews, exposure to new ideas and services from around the world, artwork and so on – all to help 'out-of-the-box' thinking.

Questionnaires and surveys have their place in the research cupboard; they can give us a 'snapshot' of a large number of people's views on pre-set subjects fairly easily. But hopefully this exercise has also made you aware of some of their limitations. It is important that we do ask women what they think of the maternity services they receive, but it is also important that we understand the ramifications of who we ask, how we ask them, what we ask them and when we ask them. If you are ever involved in evaluating maternity services provision, you can consider using methods other than just a simple questionnaire, and you'll be much more aware now of the importance of asking the right questions.

References

Goer H 2002 The assault on normal birth: the OB disinformation campaign. Midwifery Today 63:10–14

van Teijlingen ER, Hundley V, Rennie AM 2003 Maternity satisfaction studies and their limitations: what is, must still be best. Birth 30(2):75–82

Waldenstrom U 2003 Women's memory of childbirth at two months and at one year postpartum. Birth 30:248–254

Waldenstrom U 2004 Why do some women change their opinions about childbirth over time? Birth 31(2):102–107

Woolridge M 2004 The LIFT Project: effective interventions to promote breastfeeding. Mother and Infant Research Unit, University of Leeds. Conference presentation at UNICEF 7th Annual Conference: 'Reducing inequalities in breastfeeding: evidence and support for success', 10–11 November 2004, Glasgow

CHAPTER 4

Mary Stewart

INTRODUCTION

Madi BC, Crow R 2003 A qualitative study of information about available options for childbirth venue and pregnant women's preference for place of delivery. Midwifery 19(4):328–336

One of the key qualities of good midwifery practice is openness: openness to new ideas, to uncertainty, to complexity and to the endlessly fascinating, sometimes challenging lives that people lead. This is one of the reasons why I believe that grounded theory method lends itself to midwifery research. Grounded theory requires researchers to be open-minded and to avoid prescriptive guidelines (Sarantakos 2005). In turn, this means that researchers might have to give up their own preconceived ideas to show alternative perspectives and to acknowledge the perceptions and beliefs of the people they research (Holloway & Wheeler 1996). When used by midwives, it is essentially very woman-centred research.

However, as discussed in Chapter 2, it would be naïve to suggest that a midwife who chooses to use grounded theory method can put aside all her preconceptions and undertake the research from a neutral stance. We are all products of the social and cultural systems in which we live and work. We all have deeply held beliefs that help us to make sense of our lives, although articulating, or even acknowledging, these beliefs is not always easy. A key aspect of all qualitative research is the need for reflexivity; that is, the researcher acknowledges their own influence on data collection and analysis, as well as their own subjectivity (Silverman 2000).

Another key aspect of this research method is that the theory is generated from the data (Holloway & Wheeler 1996), whereas the reverse tends to be true in quantitative research. Sarantakos (2005) points out that the notion of theory being 'grounded in data' suggests a level of empiricism and objectivism that is incompatible with qualitative research. However, one of the main aims of this book is to demonstrate that different research paradigms are not mutually exclusive. The supposed barriers between and amongst dissimilar methods are all surmountable and the best research will use elements from both.

The study by Madi and Crow is a good example of an interesting and important research question that has been answered using grounded theory in an appropriate and relevant way. Having said that, however, the same broad question (what information do women have about place of birth and how does the midwife influence that choice?) could have been answered in different ways, for example, using a questionnaire or an ethnographic approach. One method is not better than another and each could have produced rich data. However, as Madi and Crow point out, little research has been done in this area, so there was a prime opportunity for gathering data in order to develop new theories.

I am passionate about the subject of home birth. It is the place where women have had their babies across centuries and cultures. Despite a growing re-emphasis on the importance of normal birth, led by influential thinkers in midwifery such as Soo Downe (2004), the rate of home birth in the United Kingdom remains at 2%. Madi and Crow's study helps to explain why this might be so.

A qualitative study of information about available options for childbirth venue and pregnant women's preference for a place of delivery

Banyana Cecilia Madi and Rosemary Crow

Aim: to explore the level of information about possible venues for childbirth among pregnant women, and to establish the midwives' involvement in giving information and helping women to make choices about where they want to give birth.

Design: qualitative study using tape-recorded unstructured interviews.

Setting: the South East of England.

Participants: 33 pregnant women; 20 planning a hospital birth and 13 planning a home birth recruited between 32 and 42 weeks of pregnancy.

Findings: women planning a home birth were well informed about the options available to them, while the majority of those planning a hospital birth were less informed about the availability of home birth and assumed that the hospital was the only option. Midwives did not initiate the discussion of availability of home birth but supported those who already knew and asked for it.

Conclusions: almost a decade after the adoption of *Changing Childbirth* (DoH 1993) recommendations as policy in England there is still evidence of lack of information among pregnant women regarding services available to them. In this study the midwives' reluctance to inform women about home birth as a possible venue for childbirth, has been demonstrated. © 2003 Elsevier Ltd. All rights reserved.

Banyana Cecilia Madi
PhD, MSc, RM, RGN
Wellcome Trust
Postdoctoral Fellow,
Department of Social
Statistics, University of
Southampton, Highfield,
Southampton, SO17 1BJ, UK

Rosemary Crow
PhD, MA, RM, RGN
Professor of Nursing,
University of Surrey, UK

(Correspondence to BCM,
E-mail: bcm@socsci.soton.
ac.uk)

Received 3 July 2002
Revised 15 October 2002;
30 April 2003
Accepted 20 May 2003

BACKGROUND

The publication of *Changing Childbirth* (Department of Health (DoH) 1993), and the subsequent adoption of its recommendations as policy in England in 1994 brought some hope that real choice and control would be in women's hands (Ralston 1994). Midwives were recommended as better placed to take charge of the care of all women with normal pregnancies (DoH 1993). The policy document recommended that women should be empowered by being given adequate information about all services and choices available to them to enable them to make informed decisions about their care, including the choice of where they want their babies to be born. Prior to this policy document, it was very difficult for women to have a home birth because

recommendations for a place of delivery favoured institutional deliveries (Ministry of Health 1959, Department of Health and Social Security 1970, House of Commons Social Services Committee 1980). The hospital was considered the quintessence of safety in childbirth for both mother and baby. The view that the hospital was safer than the woman's own home for childbirth, and the policy of encouraging all women to give birth in hospital became the subject of debate as others disagreed on the basis that the evidence did not support the premise (Tew 1977, 1985, 1990, Russell 1982, Campbell & Macfarlane 1987, 1994, Murphy & Fullerton 1998).

A MORI poll commissioned to inform the Changing Childbirth committee found that 72% of the respondents were not given a choice about the place of delivery (Market Opinion Research Institute (MORI) 1993). The House of Commons Health Committee pointed to widespread demand for choice, from women, about the type of maternity care, and the concomitant frustration due to the lack of choice provided by the maternity services (House of Commons Health Committee 1992). Earlier studies have suggested a desire for more information about childbirth, and problems with getting adequate information (Oakley 1979, Reid & Mcllwaine 1980, Jacoby 1988, Mander 1993, Kirkham 1999). Even more important, subsequent studies still suggest a lack of information about options for childbirth, including the place of delivery (Mckay & Smith 1993, Gready et al. 1995, Davies et al. 1996, Chamberlain et al. 1997, Garcia 1999, Hundley et al. 2000, O'Cathain et al. 2002). A recent survey using 1188 pregnant women found that 43% wanted more information about maternity care choices (Singh et al. 2002). Another study has suggested that only 5% of midwives routinely offer home birth as an option at 'booking' (Floyd 1995).

Other countries of the UK have policies that promote woman-centred care (Welsh Office 1991, Scottish Office 1993, Department of Health and Social Services Northern Ireland 1994). However, The Royal College of Midwives (RCM) has observed that since the introduction of woman-centred care the home birth rate has increased only slightly compared to the number of women who would like the service (RCM 2002). The RCM reiterates that women have a right to choose where to give birth, and that helping women to make informed choices and promoting home birth is good practice, which is congruent with government policy (RCM 2002).

Making real choices involves a process of giving and sharing of information that would assist in the decision making. Exercising choice in childbirth would involve women first getting information about the issues to be considered, and the options available to them from their midwives and/or other sources. However, in a literature review of women's views on their maternity care in the UK (Dowswell et al. 2001) some of the reviewed studies suggested that women did not perceive that they were offered choice about their care (Gready et al. 1995, Davies et al. 1996, 1997, Chamberlain et al. 1997, Garcia 1999). There is a dearth of descriptive literature on the specific topic of women's views about the information they are given about available venues for childbirth, and the midwives' involvement in helping them make choices about where to give birth. Most studies on the subject have looked at general views about preferences for home and hospital deliveries using quantitative methods (Mather 1980,

Soderstrom et al. 1990, Cunningham 1993, Waldenstrom & Nilsson 1993, Jones & Smith 1996, Davies et al. 1996, Fordham 1997, Viisainen et al. 1998, Churchill & Benbow 2000, Hundley et al. 2000) while few used qualitative methods (Kleiverda et al. 1990, Mackey 1990, Coyle et al. 2001). The main findings are that women choosing to have their babies at home are hoping to have more flexibility, choice and control during the birth process (Kleiverda et al. 1990, Mackey 1990, Soderstrom et al. 1990, Davies et al. 1996, Fordham 1997). The other suggestion from the studies is that women choosing a hospital birth are concerned about safety (Mather 1980, Mackey 1990, Soderstrom et al. 1990, Cunningham 1993, Jones & Smith 1996, Chamberlain et al. 1997).

The present study is part of a wider qualitative study that examined women's views about factors affecting their preference for place of delivery. The aim of the current study was to elucidate how much information women have about the availability of home and hospital as childbirth venues, and how their midwives are involved in helping them make their choice of where to give birth.

METHODS

Design

A grounded theory approach (Glaser & Strauss 1967) was used to elicit pregnant women's views about their knowledge of possible venues available to them for childbirth, and to elicit midwives' involvement in giving pregnant women information, and assisting them to decide where to give birth. Unstructured interviews were conducted by the researcher (BCM) at the women's own homes; each participant was interviewed only once.

Access and ethical considerations

The study was conducted in two areas in the South-East of England using one hospital in each area as a base for recruiting women. Ethical approval was obtained from one research ethics committee that served both hospitals. During the planning stages of the study, midwifery managers at the two hospitals were contacted to discuss the proposal, and possible use of their maternity units for conducting the study. The managers consulted with the relevant consultant obstetricians and general practitioners and they collectively gave permission for the study to be conducted. Once research ethics approval had been gained, meetings were held with midwives at the two maternity units to

QUESTIONS FOR CHAPTER 4

1 Grounded theory takes an *inductive approach* to research. Essential features of an inductive approach are (True/False):

a) Starts with a theory or hypothesis
b) Moves from the general to the particular
c) The researcher attempts to influence data collection
d) The researcher interprets the research from their own perspective
e) Based on a philosophy that people should be valued as individuals

2 List three advantages and three disadvantages of unstructured interviews

3 The interviewer may directly affect interviews. List some of the interviewer effects that might apply in this research

4 The venue for the research is relevant because (True/False/Maybe/Unclear):

a) Women were likely to feel more relaxed in their own home
b) Their responses were more honest
c) Partners and other family members could contribute

5 The purpose of ethics committees is (True/False):

a) To protect research participants from possible harm
b) To ensure that the research is properly supervised
c) To ensure that the confidentiality of participants is protected
d) To ensure adequate procedures for gaining informed consent from participants

6 What research term is often applied to the midwifery managers, consultant obstetricians and general practitioners in this context? Give a brief definition and explanation of that research term

7 Which of the following statements about information leaflets is *least* true?

a) They should be written in clear and unambiguous language
b) They should highlight all the risks that might be involved in taking part in the research
c) They make clear that individuals who choose not to participate in the research will not be disadvantaged
d) They give individuals the opportunity to withdraw from the research at any stage, without explanation

8 Pseudonyms are used to protect the anonymity of research participants. List three other procedures that should be followed to ensure anonymity

9 Does this statement reflect practice in your own area of work? (If you do not work in the community you might want to check with a colleague who does.) What are the implications of excluding women below 32 weeks gestation?

13 Open coding involves the following processes (Yes/No/Maybe).

a) New theories are converted to hypotheses
b) Data are broken down and new concepts are sought
c) Hypothetical relationships between data are tested
d) Data are labelled, and conceptual patterns are sought in order to create categories
e) New categories are compared to others to identify the most important
f) The central phenomenon of the data is sought

330 *Midwifery*

discuss the study and how the midwives could help. Midwives at the two hospitals were divided into two teams, those assigned to work in the community, and those who were based in the hospital. For the purpose of the study, the researcher worked with both teams. Community midwives were consulted about women who were planning a home birth, and hospital midwives about women who were planning a hospital birth. It was agreed that midwives would distribute information leaflets explaining the study to potential participants during antenatal visits and ask if they would be interested in participating. This approach was taken because it was felt that women would not feel pressured to participate if asked by their midwives rather than a stranger. As well as explaining the purpose of the study, the information leaflets explained that participation in the study would involve one interview at the woman's chosen place. The potential participants were also clearly informed that they could refuse to participate without any prejudice to their normal care, and that if they chose to participate they could still withdraw at any time. Women who showed interest in participating were asked to sign consent to be contacted by the researcher by telephone to discuss a convenient time and place to meet to discuss the study further and possibly conduct the interview.

After the study was explained by the researcher, participants were asked to sign a consent form to participate in the study and to have the interviews tape-recorded for later transcription and analysis. At the interview stage each woman was given a foreign pseudonym and was referred by it during the interview so that the transcript would identify her as such to disguise her identity.

Participants

Pregnant women were invited to participate in the study if they met the following criteria:

- 32–42 weeks of pregnancy.
- Low obstetric risk pregnancy; including singleton pregnancy, no known complications, cephalic presentation.

The criteria were chosen because women of low obstetric risk are unlikely to have restrictions on where they could give birth. Secondly, it was thought that in the second trimester women might have started thinking about where they might want their babies to be born, and that the midwives might also have started to talk to them about options for childbirth venue.

Two groups of women were selected, one comprising 20 women planning a hospital birth and another made up of 13 women planning a

home birth. The home birth group included all women who were in the home birth antenatal register at the time of the study. The hospital birth group comprised a purposefully chosen sample from the hospital birth antenatal register.

Data collection

All participants preferred to be interviewed in their homes. Prior to the interview, participants were reminded of the objectives of the study and asked if they had any questions about the study, particularly the content of the information leaflets. They were reminded that participation in the study was voluntary, and that they could stop the interview at any time if they did not wish to continue. The researcher then asked an open question about how they made the decision about where they were going to give birth; the question was asked as a continuation of the conversation that had already started at the beginning of the meeting. There was a question guide intended for use if the participant was not forthcoming with information. The question guide included areas of discussion such as, how much the woman knew about the options that were available, what the source of the information was, how the midwife was involved, when the decision was made, who was involved, and the main reason for preferring their chosen place to the alternative place. All interviews were tape-recorded with the participant's permission. Notes were also made about the interview soon afterwards. Information about the participants' demographic variables was extracted from their antenatal records.

Data analysis

The process of data analysis was iterative with data collection, after the first interview was conducted, it was immediately transcribed verbatim and the transcript checked against the recording for accuracy. The transcript and accompanying notes were read and re-read then analysed by hand using open coding (Glaser 1992) to identify emerging themes as indicated by significant words and sentences. A pictorial representation of all the categories and themes that came out of the interview was drawn. The findings of the analysis of the first interview were used to guide the subsequent interview and the process continued like that until the last interview.

The constant comparative method of analysis (Glaser & Strauss 1967, Strauss & Corbin 1990) was employed, where all data relevant to a category are identified and examined and compared to the rest of the data. The iterative process of interview–analysis–interview allowed questions to be refined, or more questions to be asked for clarification of points made earlier.

10 Pick the correct definition of purposeful sampling from the list below.

a) The researcher chooses a few respondents and asks them to recommend other people who may be willing to participate in the research
b) The researcher considers all significant aspects of the research sample and ensures that each aspect (e.g. ethnicity, education, etc.) is represented
c) The researcher identifies and chooses people who, in her opinion, are relevant to the research
d) The researcher approaches people who are available and easily accessible when collecting data

11 These are often referred to as field notes. The purpose of field notes is to (True/False):

a) Record non-verbal communication
b) Summarise the context in which interview took place
c) Start the process of data analysis
d) Record the researcher's personal thoughts

12 Select words and phrases from the following list in order to create a definition of the iterative process of data analysis.

- Literature
- Domains
- Validity
- Repetitive
- Findings
- Constant comparison
- Moves from participants' responses to researcher's synthesis
- Symbolic categories
- Data

14 Theoretical sampling can be defined as (True/False):

a) Entails an ongoing process
b) Depends on selection of typical cases
c) Sample is identified at beginning of the study
d) Is guided by emerging theory
e) Is concerned with developing and validating theory

15 Data saturation is said to occur when (True/False):

a) The sample size is representative
b) Links between categories are clearly established
c) Each category has been illustrated using the data
d) No new information on a category can be found
e) The category has been described in detail, identifying any variations

16 Auditability is important because (tick all that apply):

a) It allows the research to be replicated
b) It increases the transparency and believability of the research
c) It demonstrates that the researcher's findings are correct
d) It enables the reader to scrutinise the research process
e) It demonstrates that the research has been carried out objectively

17 Can you identify any problems with Table 1?

18 Some possible advantages of including women with differing characteristics are (True/False/Maybe):

a) The heterogeneity of the sample is increased
b) Findings are more generalisable
c) It is easier to test theories
d) The findings are more robust

Available options for childbirth venue   331

Theoretical sampling (Patton 1980, Guba & Lincoln 1985, Morse 1989, Strauss & Corbin 1990, Kuzel 1992) was used, where subsequent participants are chosen because of the possible contribution they could make to the already developing story line as suggested by the analysis. For example, the first three women interviewed from the hospital group were all unmarried and they mentioned that they had not discussed the issue of where the baby was going to be born with their partners. The researcher wanted to understand why there was such a pattern. Therefore the next participant from the hospital group was purposefully chosen as married, and a deliberate decision was made to ask her whether she had discussed the place of delivery with her partner. This helped to understand the context of the theme that was emerging from the data.

The process of data collection and analysis continued until no new findings were forthcoming, this stage was considered to be the data saturation stage (Morse 1989, 1995). Another researcher, not involved in the study repeated the analysis for a third of the transcripts and came up with similar findings.

FINDINGS AND DISCUSSION

All women who were invited to participate in the study did. All were of British, Caucasian origin except for one whose origin was Indian. The age, marital status, and parity of those who participated are presented in Table 1. Women in the home birth group had more college and university degrees than those in the hospital birth group. Other studies have also found women planning a home birth to be generally better educated (Cohen 1982, Schneider 1986, Eakins 1989, Rooks et al. 1989, Soderstrom et al. 1990).

There was only one woman in the home birth group expecting her first baby, whereas in the hospital group there was an even distribution of parity. This finding is in line with those of other studies, which found an under representation of first-time mothers in out-of-hospital births (Cohen 1982, Schneider 1986, Littlefield & Adams 1987, Howe 1988, Rooks et al. 1989, Anderson & Greener 1991, Viisainen et al. 1998).

Information was found to be one of the main themes in the findings. The women's preferences for a place of birth seemed to be influenced by what information they had about available options. Under the main theme of information, subcategories of 'presumption of a hospital birth', 'midwives' involvement', 'partners' involvement' and 'influence of others' emerged. The subcategories emerged because:

- some women assumed that they were going to give birth in hospital (*assumption of hospital delivery*);
- some had discussions with their partners about the place of delivery while some had not (*partner's involvement*);
- others referred to the discussions they had with their midwives (*midwife's involvement*);
- some had friends or neighbours who had had babies at home which encouraged them in their choices (*influence of others*).

Presumption of a hospital delivery and midwife's involvement

Most women planning a hospital birth had assumed that the hospital was the only place to go. Women seemed to have come to the assumption because no one had talked to them about what other options were available:

Well, I am having it at (name of hospital) because, basically there is nowhere else to have it, I don't think. (Tshidi, hospital)

I don't know how I came to the decision that I am going to have my baby in hospital; um (pause) I suppose I probably assumed from the start that I would. I have always presumed that it would be at the hospital. I didn't even think about having it at home, I don't know why I didn't even consider it... I have never known anybody to have a baby at home before. I just presumed that was the normal thing to do you know. (Gaboelwe, hospital)

I think you just grow up knowing you are going to have your baby in hospital. Just, you know, you immediately think that you are going to have your baby in hospital. I didn't really give home birth a thought and I

Table 1	Characteristics of women in the study	
Characteristic	Home birth $n=13$	Hospital birth $n=20$
Age		
20–25	2	4
26–31	4	6
32–37	6	8
38–43	1	2
Marital status		
Married	10	3
Single	15	5
Number of pregnancies		
First	1	6
Second	4	5
Third	6	6
Fourth	2	3
Education		
Primary	3	8
Secondary	5	7
University/college	5	5

332 *Midwifery*

just had hospital in mind really. (Segosha, hospital)

Some women specifically said that their mid-wives encouraged them to go to a particular hospital or gave them a choice between the two hospitals in the area:

Oh it's only been a choice of hospital; I can't even remember being asked the question whether I wanted a home birth. I was given the choice of two hospitals, basically [1 or 2], but again I suppose I was familiar with 1, I'd had a baby there I was more than happy with the care that I got there so I saw no reason to go and change to a different hospital. (Montlenyane, hospital)

I wouldn't say a 100%, but I think they really want you to go to hospital. I would say that they give the information that they have to give, but they would slightly, not force you, that's the wrong word, but in the way that it's presented and the rest of it would encourage you to go to [name of hospital]. Yes, you would probably be encouraged that way. (Boithatelo, hospital)

Some women mentioned that they thought one had to indicate interest in having a home birth for the option to be considered:

I think a lot of them make an assumption and think well, yes, you come under [name of hospital] or [another hospital] or whatever and say, 'you will be going along there to have the baby, won't you?' And, people, unless they have specifically thought about it and are willing to state, 'well, actually, no, I won't,' then they will not get the option at all. You do have to ask about things, and even when I said I want a home birth, I already knew the process because I had spoken to my neighbour about it, but there was nothing given to me. You have to go looking for it or ask for the information yourself definitely. (Maipelo, homebirth)

I don't really remember anybody telling me about the options of home and hospital birth. I think it is just presumed that is the decision you make and if you are not giving any other decisions you are sort of rail-roaded into that scenario and you don't think of anything else (hospital birth). (Pedzani, hospital)

The findings that women felt they were not given information about options for childbirth is in tandem with findings of other studies that looked at different aspects of satisfaction with provision of maternity services and found that women feel they are often not offered a choice about their care (MORI 1993, Gready et al. 1995, Davies et al. 1996, Chamberlain et al. 1997,

Davies 1997, Garcia 1999). These findings there-fore support the argument made by other researchers and commentators that women are being persuaded to give birth in hospital (Bathgate & Ryan 1995, Devenish 1996, Leap 1996, Pengelley 1996, Walcott 1997, Warshal 1997, Stapleton 1997, Hosein 1998, Kargar 1998). Others have argued that consumer choice is limited to the services on offer, such that those who extol choice also define the choices available (Kirkham & Perkins 1997). The view of the House of Commons Health Committee is that the available choices are 'often more illusory than real' (House of Commons Health Committee 1992, para 51).

Some women mentioned that their midwives asked them where they were going to deliver, and the response to this question was always the local hospital. The researcher wanted to know why this question was interpreted this way and therefore some of the participants were asked what choice they thought the question implied. The following is a conversation between the researcher and one participant about that question:

I was just asked where I wanted to have my baby and when I said (name of hospital) that was it, it wasn't taken any further they didn't even explain the difference between the two hospitals. (Mampenene, hospital)

Researcher: When you were asked where you wanted to have your baby, what did you understand the question to mean?

Just the literal, what (pause), I wasn't asked about wanting a home birth or anything like that. I wasn't asked if I wanted a home birth. I just took it to mean which hospital I want to go to. (Mampenene, hospital)

It appears from the interaction above that the way information was presented may have had an impact on how women understood it. The question could have meant either;

1. Was she going to have the baby at home or in hospital, or
2. Which of the two hospitals was she going to.

The woman above and others planning a hospital delivery, understood the question to mean the latter.

It was evident, particularly among women planning a home birth, that if you knew about the availability of home birth, and wanted that option then the midwives were willing to listen and sometimes even supportive of the choice:

My main midwife, she just said to me, if you want to have it at home you can have it at home, that's no problem. So she was suppor-tive, she didn't sort of try and persuade me

19 What are the possible implications of this comment (i.e. that it is 'an interesting finding')?

one way or the other, that was really her only comment on it. (Bonyana, home)

I went for my 28-week check and was very nervous about mentioning it to the midwife. I thought I can't possibly ask for a home birth for my first baby, but I did and the idea was welcomed by the midwife. (Segametsi, home)

An interesting finding was that although some women felt that they should be informed about all the options of where to have a baby, most women who were planning a hospital birth were protective of their planned place of delivery, and felt that it probably would not have made any difference to their choice if they had been informed of the availability of home as a possible venue for childbirth:

I think at the booking visit I was asked which hospital I would be going to, home birth wasn't mentioned. Now we are talking about it, I think perhaps it should have been mentioned as a matter of course. But I feel personally that I, you know, that I'm intelligent enough to decide whether I want to ask about it, and then I'd make a decision that way. But I suppose it wouldn't instill a lot of confidence in people if it wasn't mentioned at all, and they were there thinking, well, actually I think I like the idea of a home birth If you then just ask which hospital would you like to go to, I suppose it makes it difficult to say I'd rather have it at home. (Leungo, hospital)

Home birth is not something I would have wanted anyway, but it wasn't mentioned. (Mampenene, hospital)

I mean you only ever know as much as anybody ever tells you or you bother to find out. I am sure there's lots more information if I can be bothered to find out and things, you know, I can get and do. But I mean, I think you only, I personally only asked as much information as I particularly want to know and once I've got all the information I particularly need them I'm happy, so, you know, I'm happy with the package that I've got. (Boithatelo, hospital)

This finding resonates with that of an earlier study that found that women are usually happy with the care that they receive whatever it is (Porter & Macintyre 1984).

Partner's involvement

There was a distinct difference between women planning a home birth and those planning a hospital birth with regard to their partner's involvement in the decision making. All women in the home birth group had discussed the issue of place of birth with their partners or husbands. Some of the women's partners were very supportive of their home birth choice, but some were not in support of home birth initially, but after discussions with their partners they came to support them:

My husband said to me, whatever you want is fine by me. So, yes, he is quite understanding and just said well, I can't understand why you want to have it at home, but I'm with you a 100%. (Gaolape, home)

At first he was apprehensive. He is American and they are very used to birth being a very medical thing …his mother had five caesarean sections, so his attitude was initially was very negative but he came round so quickly, it was like probably took less than a day to convince him. (Senyana, home)

My husband and I had an argument about it last night (pause). He is frightened, he is very frightened. My husband is just, just hasn't got the faith that I have because he hasn't got the knowledge that I have despite what I tell him…. But it is a two-way thing, I can't do this without my husband's support and I must respect his decision and his attitude. (Nnese, home)

On the other hand, most women who were planning a hospital birth had not discussed the place of delivery with their partners:

We never really discussed it because we knew when [name of hospital] closed down, we just thought oh well, next time we have a baby it will be at [name of hospital]. So, um, yes, it wasn't something we discussed, it was just, that was where we were going to go. (Olebogeng, hospital)

We just assumed it would be in hospital, we didn't really talk about it. We didn't discuss it at all. (Gaboelwe, hospital)

The finding that women who were planning a hospital birth had not discussed where they were going to give birth with their partners may strengthen the argument that these women did not know that there was another option apart from the hospital, and therefore there was no point in discussing the obvious. Actually, some of the women were asked why they did not consider a home birth and the reaction was that it was not mentioned:

When someone plants a seed of thought in your head, like perhaps home birth, and gives you some information, you may consider it more, but because that seed was never

334 *Midwifery*

planted, I didn't even consider it (hospital). (Gaboelwe, hospital)

Influence of others

The subcategory of influence of others applies only to women who were planning a home birth. Most of them mentioned someone they knew who had a home birth and said that their positive experiences had either influenced or encouraged them to pursue their home birth:

> I suppose you are idealistic to a certain extent but the lady who is down the road who has had two babies at home just said that the experiences didn't compare. You know, having a baby in hospital or having a baby at home is, was just so different and it was just relaxed and you just had the baby and carried on. (Segametsi)

> My neighbour next door also had an influence because she had a baby six months ago and she had a home birth. (Maipelo)

Summary

In this qualitative study some insight into the specific role played by midwives in the South-East of England in pregnant women's decision making about the place of delivery has been provided. A reflective perspective by pregnant women about how they decided on where they were going to give birth has also been presented. The nature of the study implies that findings cannot be generalised to other populations. However, because data were collected and analysed until saturation, the identified issues may be relevant to other pregnant women in similar circumstances. Other researchers have identified that women are not given adequate information about services on offer. The present study adds to the existing knowledge, and goes further by allowing women to reflect on circumstances leading to their planned place of delivery. Women were encouraged to reflect on how their midwives were either stepping-stones or impediments in the decision-making.

The findings would suggest that midwives may not be comfortable with freely giving out information about home birth but it was beyond the limits of the study to ask midwives their reasons. Some studies have suggested that midwives view childbirth in a medical fashion (Olsson et al. 2000), while others feel that midwives fear being blamed (Kirkham 1999) and are therefore disempowered.

Implications for practice

The central aim of *Changing Childbirth* (DoH 1993) is for midwives to uphold the principle of informed consent and maximise opportunities for women to make choices about their care, including the choice of where to give birth, but studies are still suggesting that women are not informed. More efforts are therefore needed to tackle the problem of midwives' failure of their duty to inform women. Talking to women about their services and their rights and choices is one of the ways that could help in providing truly woman-centred care, and the principle of informed choice and consent is fundamental to good maternity care.

It is fitting to end by giving a quotation from one of the women who took part in the study who said:

> I think we need to educate our midwives and suss out why midwives are so against home births, some midwives are and some midwives aren't. .... but the midwife has to be very unbiased in giving an informed choice and I think most (pause), some midwives are biased to hospital births. (Nnese, home birth)

ACKNOWLEDGMENTS

This study was fully funded by the European Institute of Health and Medical Sciences, University of Surrey as part of a PhD study by Banyana Cecilia Madi.

REFERENCES

Anderson A, Greener D 1991 A descriptive analysis of home births attended by CNMs in two nurse-midwifery services. Journal of Nurse-Midwifery 36: 96–103

Bathgate W, Ryan MHM 1995 Divided views among health professionals on place of birth. British Journal of Midwifery 3(11): 583–587

Campbell R, Macfarlane A 1994 Where to be born? The debate and the evidence 2nd edn. National Perinatal Epidemiology Unit, Oxford

Chamberlain G, Wraight A, Crowley P 1997 Home births: the report of the 1994 confidential enquiry by the National Birthday Trust Fund. Parthenon Publishing Group, London

Churchill H, Benbow A 2000 Informed choice in maternity services. British Journal of Midwifery 8(1): 41–47

Cohen RL 1982 A comparative study of women choosing two different childbirth alternatives. Birth 9(1): 13–19

Coyle K, Hauck Y, Percival P, Kristjanson L 2001 Ongoing relationships with a personal focus: mothers' perceptions of birth centre versus hospital care. Midwifery 17: 171–181

Cunningham JD 1993 Experiences of Australian mothers who gave birth either at home, at a birth centre, or, in hospital labour wards. Social Science & Medicine 36(4): 475–483

Davies J 1997 The midwife in the Northern Region's 1993 homebirth study. British Journal of Midwifery 5(4): 219–224

Davies J, Hey E, Reid W, Young G 1996 Prospective regional study of planned home births. BMJ

20 Generalisability involves (tick all that apply):

a) Findings can be applied to the wider population
b) Results are produced consistently
c) May also be described as fittingness
d) The search for objective truths
e) Increased if study is systematic

Available options for childbirth venue

335

313(7068): 1302–1306. http://bmj.com/cgi/content/abstract/313/7068/1302

Department of Health (DoH) 1993 Changing childbirth, Part I: report of The Expert Maternity Group (chair, Lady Cumberlege) HMSO, London

Department of Health and Social Security 1970 Domiciliary midwifery and maternity bed needs: report of the sub-committee (chair, Sir John Peel) HMSO, London

Department of Health and Social Services Northern Ireland 1994 Delivering choice: the report of the Northern Ireland maternity unit study group. DHSS, Belfast

Devenish S 1996 Home birth: the midwife's dilemma. MIDIRS Midwifery Digest 6(1): 9–12

Dowswell T, Renfrew MJ, Gregson, Hewison J 2001 A review of the literature on women's views on their maternity care in the community in the UK. Midwifery 17: 194–202

Eakins P 1989 Free standing birth centers in California: program and medical outcome. Journal of Reproductive Medicine 34: 960–970

Floyd L 1995 Community midwives views and experience of home birth. Midwifery 11: 3–9

Fordham S 1997 Women's views of the place of confinement. British Journal of General Practice 47: 77–81

Garcia J 1999 Mothers views and experiences of care. In: Marsh G, Renfrew MJ (eds) Community-based maternity care. Oxford University Press, Oxford

Glaser BG 1992 Basics of grounded theory analysis: emergence vs forcing. Sociology Press, Mill Valley

Glaser BG, Strauss AL 1967 The discovery of grounded theory: strategies for qualitative research. Aldine, Chicago

Gready M, Newburn M, Dodds R, Gauge S 1995 Birth choices: women's expectations and experiences. National Childbirth Trust, London

Guba EG, Lincoln YS 1985 Effective evaluation: improving the usefulness of evaluation. Results through evaluation and naturalistic approaches. Jossey Bass, San Francisco

Hosein M 1998 Home birth: is it a real option? British Journal of Midwifery 6(6): 370–373

House of Commons Health Committee 1992 Health Committee Second Report, Session 1991–92: Maternity Services (chair Nicholas Winterton). HMSO, London

House of Commons Social Services Committee 1980 Perinatal and neonatal mortality: second report, session 1979–1980. HMSO London

Howe K 1988 Home births in South-West Australia. Medical Journal of Australia 149: 296–301

Hundley V, Rennie A-M, Fitzmaurice A, Graham W, Teijlingen E, Penney G 2000 A national survey of women's views of their maternity care in Scotland. Midwifery 16: 303–313

Jacoby A 1988 Women's views about information and advice in pregnancy and childbirth: findings from a national study. Midwifery 4: 103–110

Jones O, Smith S 1996 Choosing the place of birth. British Journal of Midwifery 4(3): 140–143

Kargar I 1998 Concerning rotten apples and barrels. Midwifery Matters (77): 4–5

Kirkham MJ 1999 The culture of midwifery in the national health service in England. Journal of Advanced Nursing 30: 732–739

Kirkham MJ, Perkins ER 1997 Reflections on midwifery. Bailliere Tindall, London

Kleiverda G, Steen A, Anderson I, Treffers P, Everaerd W 1990 Place of delivery in the Netherlands: maternal motives and background variables related to preferences for home or hospital confinement. European

Journal of Obstetrics and Gynecology and Reproductive Biology 36: 1–9

Kuzel AJ 1992 Sampling in qualitative inquiry In: Crabtree BF, Miller WL (eds) Doing qualitative research, Vol. 3. Sage, Newbury Park

Leap N 1996 Persuading women to give birth at home or offering real choice? British Journal of Midwifery 4(10): 536–538

Littlefield VM, Adams BN 1987 Patient participation in alternative perinatal care: impact on satisfaction and health locus of control. Research in Nursing and Health 10: 139–148

Mackey MC 1990 Women's choice of childbirth setting. Health Care For Women International 11: 175–189

Mander R 1993 Who chooses the choices? Modern Midwife 3(1): 23–25

Market Opinion Research Institute 1993 Maternity services report: research study conducted for the Department of Health. Department of Health, London

Mather S 1980 Women's interest in alternative maternity facilities. Journal of Nurse-Midwifery 25(3): 3–10

Mckay S, Smith SY 1993 What are they talking about? Is something wrong? Birth 203: 142–147

Ministry of Health 1959 Report of the Maternity Services Committee (Cranbrook report). HMSO, London

Morse JM 1989 Qualitative nursing research: a contemporary dialogue. Sage, Newbury Park

Morse JM 1995 The significance of saturation. Qualitative Health Research 5(2): 147–149

Murphy PA, Fullerton J. 1998 Outcomes of intended home births in nurse-midwifery practice: a prospective descriptive study. Obstetrics and Gynecology 92(3): 461–470

O'Cathain A, Thomas K, Walters SJ, Nicholl J, Kirkham M 2002 Women's perceptions of informed choice in maternity care. Midwifery 18: 136–144

Oakley A 1979 Becoming a mother. Martin Robertson, Oxford

Olsson P, Jansson L, Norberg A 2000 A qualitative study of childbirth as spoken about in midwives' ante- and postnatal consultations. Midwifery 16: 123–134

Patton MQ 1980 Qualitative evaluation and research methods, 2nd edn. Sage Publications, Newbury Park

Pengelley L 1996 GP's and home birth. New Generation Digest 16: 4–5

Porter M, Macintyre S 1984 What is must be best: a research note on conservative or deferential responses to antenatal care provision. Social Science & Medicine 19(11): 1197–1200

Ralston R 1994 How much choice do women really have in relation to their care? British Journal of Midwifery 2(9): 453–456

RCM 2002 Position paper 25: home birth. RCM Midwives Journal 5(1): 26–29

Reid ME, McIlwaine GM 1980 Consumer opinion of a hospital antenatal clinic. Social Science & Medicine 4: 363–368

Rooks J, Weatherby N, Ernst E, Stapleton S, Rosen D, Rosenfield A 1989 Outcomes of care in birth centers: the national birth center study. New England Journal of Medicine 321: 1804–1811

Russell J 1982 Perinatal mortality: the current debate. Sociology of Health and Illness 4(3): 302

Schneider D 1986 Planned out of hospital births. New Jersey 1978–1980. Social Science & Medicine 23: 1011–1015

Scottish Office 1993 Provision of maternity services: a policy review. The Scottish Office, Edinburgh

Singh D, Newburn M, Smith N, Wiggins M 2002 The information needs of first-time pregnant mothers. British Journal of Midwifery 10(1): 54–58

336 *Midwifery*

Soderstrom B, Stewart PJ, Kaitell C, Chamberlain M 1990 Interest in alternative birth places among women in Ottawa-Carleton. Canadian Medical Association Journal 142(9): 963–969

Stapleton H 1997 Choice in the face of uncertainty In: Kirkham MJ, Perkins ER (eds) Reflections on midwifery. Bailliere Tindall, London

Strauss AL, Corbin J 1990 Basics of qualitative research: grounded theory procedures and techniques. Sage, Newbury Park

Tew M 1977 Where to be born? New Society 39: 120–121

Tew M 1985 The place of birth and perinatal mortality. Journal of The Royal College of General Practitioners 35: 390–394

Tew M 1990 Safer childbirth? A critical history of maternity care, 2nd edn. Chapman & Hall, London

Viisainen K, Gissler M, Raikkonen O, Perala ML 1998 Interest in alternative birth settings in finland. Acta Obstetricia et Gynecologica Scandanavica 77: 729–735

Walcott L 1997 Achieving a home birth. Midwifery Matters 75: 10–11

Waldenstrom U, Nilsson CA 1993 Characteristics of women choosing birth center care. Acta Obstetricia et Gynecologica Scandanavica 72: 181–188

Warshal S 1997 Home birth hassles. AIMS Journal 8(4): 3–5

Welsh Office 1991 Protocol for investment in health gain: maternal and early child health. DHSS, Cardiff

ANSWERS

Q1. a) False – this is a *deductive approach*
b) True
c) False
d) False – they try to interpret from the perspective of the participants
e) True

Q2. Advantages: information is not 'forced' from participants; responses may be more open, spontaneous and honest; participants more active/researcher more passive
Disadvantages: analysis likely to be more time-consuming; may be difficult to draw conclusions as interviews may cover very different issues; may not go in the direction the interviewer wanted or hoped

Q3. Possible answers include the interviewer's age, gender, ethnicity, social class, accent, and demeanour. All of these characteristics may have an inadvertent effect, e.g. they may encourage women to be honest and open or they may have the reverse effect. The interviews may also be affected by whether the researcher tells participants that she is a midwife

Q4. a) True – the researcher states that women preferred to be interviewed in their own homes
b) Maybe, but this may also have been affected by interviewer bias (see above)
c) This is unclear from the study, but it could have had a bearing on the findings and so additional information would have been useful

Q5. All of these are usually true, but bear in mind that there may be situations where the right to confidentiality needs to be waived; for example, if issues that involve child protection are uncovered

Q6. The term is *gatekeepers*. Gatekeepers provide access to the research area/participant. It is important to identify gatekeepers early in the research process as their support is essential to the success (or otherwise) of the research

Q7. Perhaps surprisingly, the answer is b). This is in part because it may be impossible to predict the possible harm that might occur. However, it may be that the benefits of obtaining the information outweigh any possible harm to participants. For example, an information leaflet that is trying to recruit parents who use drugs into a research study is unlikely to point out that the research may result in more babies being removed from their parents' care, even though this is a possible outcome. This is not to suggest that information leaflets should not highlight possible risks – clearly they should, but sometimes pragmatic decisions need to be made in order to get sometimes elusive but important information

Q8. Some examples include that:
- Tapes, field notes, and transcriptions of interviews should not include participants' names or any other identifying information
- Interview data should be stored in a locked, secure place
- Signed consent forms, which include participants' names, should be kept separately from interview data

Q9. In all the areas where I have worked as a community midwife, the discussion about place of birth begins at booking, even though women may change their minds at any point during the pregnancy. Excluding women of less than 32 weeks gestation risks excluding those who are dissuaded from having a home birth early in pregnancy

Q10. The answer is c)! The other types of sampling in this list are a) snowball, b) quota and d) convenience

Q11. a), b), c) and d) are all true

Q12. One definition of the iterative process might be: the repetitive, constant comparison of data and literature

Q13. a) No
b) Yes
c) No

d) Yes
e) Maybe
f) No

Q14. a) True
b) False
c) False
d) True
e) True

Q15. a) False
b) True
c) False
d) True
e) True

Q16. Points a), b) and d) should have been ticked. No matter how good the audit trail is, it does not 'prove' that the findings are correct. Nor does it demonstrate objectivity. In fact, it is an opportunity for the researcher to identify their own biases

Q17. There are two significant issues here. Under marital status, the numbers don't stack up – the totals are 25 in the home birth column and 8 in the hospital birth column. (Note from Sara: It looks to me as if the rows and columns have been transposed, so, although we cannot be certain, perhaps what they meant to say was that 10 women in the home birth group were married and 3 were single, whereas 15 in the hospital birth group were married and 5 were single. While I'm here this also makes me think – what about women (like me!) who are neither legally married nor single, and what about other women whose circumstances might not fit this criteria – lesbian women with partners, women who are married but not supported by their partners for any reason? It might be better in some studies to instead look at women 'with partners' or 'without partners'.) Also, data on education are ambiguous. It seems unlikely that 11 women finished their education at primary school level (aged 11), yet what the authors might mean by primary is not defined here

Q18. a) True
b) Maybe
c) True
d) Maybe

Q19. It is a leading statement as the researcher is suggesting that the reader *should* find this interesting. It also demonstrates the researcher's subjectivity. This is not necessarily a problem, but when reading a research paper it is really important to try and recognise these sorts of thing. It is quite OK to disagree with the researcher and to argue that this particular finding is not at all interesting to you!

Q20. Points a), c) and e) should all have been ticked. Point b) refers to reliability, and point d) to objectivity

DISCUSSION

Most women start making decisions about childbirth long before they ever become pregnant. Those decisions may change over time and are influenced by all sorts of factors, such as their social, cultural, spiritual and religious beliefs. One of the decisions they make is where to have their baby and, for most women in the UK, there seem to be just two stark choices: home or hospital.

One of the most startling findings of Madi and Crow's study – especially when you look at it in relation to the paper in Chapter 3 – is that some women did not know they *had* a choice about where their baby could be born. More than a decade after the publication of *Changing childbirth* (Department of Health 1993), with its mantra of choice, continuity and control, in reality some women appear to have little option about where they give birth.

I have often heard midwives complain that research simply states the obvious, that it proves something we 'knew' already. Of course, we 'knew' that it was safer to lie babies on their front to sleep until research demonstrated that the opposite was true. Similarly, I have heard midwives and other health professionals explain, with great conviction, that the rate of home birth in the UK is low because women do not want this choice. However, Madi and Crow's research suggests that in fact the reason is because women do not know that a choice exists. However, the maternity services have been shown to pay only lip service to the notion of informed choice, and in truth expect informed compliance from women. That is, the services are provided in such a way that women are coerced into making the 'right' choice, as decided by the care provider, rather than the choice that the woman herself might want. In contrast, the Albany Practice, a caseloading group of midwives in London, are proactive in offering women options around place of birth and, as a result, had a home birth rate of 57.4% in 2004 (Becky Reed, personal correspondence 2005).

So what are the strengths and weaknesses of Madi and Crow's study? Well, there are many positive aspects to the research. The authors have identified a wide range of literature that provides a compelling background to, and justification for, the research they have done. The point of the literature review is to demonstrate that this is an interesting and relevant subject to research and, most importantly, that the answer to the research question is not already known. They also give many multiple references; that is, they cite a range of authors to back up each point they wish to make, which adds strength to the plausibility of the claims they make. Effectively, they are saying 'Look, it's not only the two of us who think that this is the case, all these authors agree with us'.

The methods used for the research are also quite clearly explained and all the most important points, including ethical considerations, data collection and analysis, are covered, albeit briefly. Research articles published in midwifery and medical journals are always constrained by word limits. Most journals have an upper limit of 4000 words which, as those of you who have written dissertations will realise, is frustratingly little. As a result, important and useful information about the research process often gets condensed in order to leave sufficient words for the results and discussion.

In Madi and Crow's study I would have liked, in particular, to have known more about the process of data analysis. For example, they state (p 330) that emerging themes were identified 'as indicated by significant words and sentences' but we are not told who decided the significance of those words, nor on what basis. If I had been given the interview transcripts to review, would I have agreed with these findings? Similarly, they state (p 330) that a pictorial representation of all the categories and themes '…was drawn', but do not explain how this was decided or done. I accept that these omissions might have occurred because of the limited word allowance but one of the criticisms levelled against qualitative research is that authors simply give readers persuasive extracts from the data, without explaining in detail the context in which they occurred (Silverman 2000). It might have been more helpful if Madi and Crow had used fewer and/or shorter quotes from the participants and then given greater attention to discussing their possible significance and justifying the emerging themes in more detail.

Another criticism of qualitative research is that published reports might fail to acknowledge or analyse any examples of contradictory data, or fail to look for alternative explanations for what participants have said (Silverman 2000), but here Madi and Crow have shown the strength of their research. They point out that, while women appear to have been offered little information, most women were very happy with the options they had, and did not see themselves as disadvantaged in any way.

Madi and Crow's work would have been strengthened by triangulation of research methods. For example, they could have carried out interviews with midwives in order to try and understand why they might choose to withhold information about place of birth. They could also have videotaped some of the antenatal encounters between women and midwives, as this may have provided very rich data showing how information is shared and what this might say about power dynamics. As it is, the research feels rather one-dimensional but, of course, only one aspect of the study is being reported here and it may be that the authors collected other data that are not included in this relatively brief article.

I think the key limitation of this study is that, having demonstrated that midwives appear to be withholding information from women, Madi and Crow make little attempt to recommend how this problem might be addressed, simply suggesting that 'talking to women...about their rights and choices...could help' (p 334). Quite honestly, this feels like a cop-out. There is ample evidence in all areas of midwifery practice that flawed communication is the basis of most problems. Recognising that midwives need to talk to women more honestly and openly is really the easy part. It is far more problematic to try and understand *why* midwives fail to communicate properly and, having explored this, to then try and develop strategies to overcome the problem. I know that, if I were a midwifery manager, I could develop a policy whereby midwives have to discuss home birth with all women. However, this new policy might have no effect at all on the local home birth rate unless the midwives actually believe in and are committed to the choices they offer.

As with almost all research, Madi and Crow have generated more questions than answers. Those questions (how information about place of birth can be offered in a meaningful way that gives women the confidence to choose a home birth if this is what they want; how midwives can be inspired to believe in, and support, that choice) need to be addressed and answered with some urgency if the option of home birth is ever going to be anything more than a service available to a small number of extraordinarily determined women.

References

Department of Health 1993 Changing childbirth. Part 1: Report of the Expert Maternity Group. HMSO, London

Downe S 2004 Normal childbirth: evidence and debate. Churchill Livingstone, Edinburgh

Holloway I, Wheeler S 1996 Qualitative research for nurses. Blackwell Science, Oxford

Sarantakos S 2005 Social research. Palgrave Macmillan, Basingstoke

Silverman D 2000 Doing qualitative research. Sage Publications, London

Childbirth interventions

INTRODUCTION

The vast majority of the research that appears in medical journals these days is focused around testing interventions; setting out to find out whether pill A works better than pill B, or which of two procedures gives better outcomes. Whereas the articles in Section 1 looked at the intervention of giving informed choice leaflets to a group of women, the articles in this section consider the evaluation of other kinds of interventions. In Chapter 5, Julie Frohlich looks at a research study that considered whether eating fish in pregnancy led to better outcomes for babies, with a specific focus on preterm birth and low birth weight. Although the researchers could have asked some women to eat fish and some women to avoid eating fish, this might have been hard to do, for a number of reasons that I'm sure you can imagine! So, instead, they carried out a prospective cohort study, where they asked women to tell them (by way of a form) about how much fish they ate and then looked at whether there was a correlation, or relationship, between different levels of fish intake and neonatal outcomes.

In Chapter 6 we will return to the RCT and Ishvar Sheran and I will guide you through an RCT that set out to evaluate whether acupuncture could make a difference to nausea and vomiting in pregnancy. We have included this study not only because we wanted to look at a more complex RCT but also so that we can explore some of the issues that arise when you begin to evaluate some of the non-Western therapies with Western tools and frameworks like the RCT.

The kinds of research that test interventions, most especially the RCT, are often described as 'the gold standard' when it comes to research and are at the top of a hierarchy that, if it includes qualitative research at all, has this placed near the bottom. Is this because the RCT and other kinds of quantitative research are better ways of finding things out? Well...in my opinion, the reason that the RCT is considered the gold standard is partly because the experimental approach is the tool of science, and Western medicine likes to think of itself as scientific, and partly because this is the kind of study that is good at testing interventions, and interventions are the prime focus of Western medical care (or, perhaps more appropriately, Western medical cure). If you'd like a further illustration of this or need a bedtime story sometime, *The Practising Midwife* journal has kindly let us reprint a short article I wrote on this subject in the resources section at the back of this book (see p 160).

What you might well notice in this section is that, in contrast to Section 2, where the quantitative (Chapter 1) and qualitative (Chapter 2) arms of the study added value to each other, quantitative studies that look at interventions, although being good tools for their primary purpose, can sometimes leave us with a number of unanswered questions.

CHAPTER 5

Julie Frohlich

INTRODUCTION

In February 2005, a woman from Merseyside, Sara Griffin, age 25, gave birth to her first child, a boy, weighing 13 lbs 13 oz. He was declared the biggest British baby to be born since 1997 (BBC 2005). And to what did the stunned Ms Griffin attribute her son's prodigious weight? Her intense craving for seafood whilst she was pregnant! Sara is quoted as saying:

> I was eating cockles, mussels, roll mop herrings, crab claws – anything I could get my hands on. My partner Mike is a fishmonger, which meant I had a steady supply. There's no history of big babies in the family, so I can only think it must have been the seafood (BBC 2005 p 1)

The authors of the study we are considering here note in their introduction that high birth weights and long gestations have long been observed in the fish-eating community of the Faroe Islands, and Sara Griffin's experience would certainly appear to bear this out! They also cite two RCTs that report that fish oil can delay spontaneous birth and prevent recurrent preterm birth, as well as observational studies that have found seafood consumption during pregnancy to be directly associated with fetal growth rate. This raises the possibility that consuming fish, or fish oil, during pregnancy may reduce low birth weight and preterm birth. Conversely, low consumption may be a risk factor for low birth weight and preterm birth. So why could this be important?

Despite many improvements in the standard of neonatal intensive care in recent decades, prematurity and low birth weight continue to be the leading causes of perinatal death and morbidity (Nordentoft et al 1996). They are also significant causes of development problems in later life (Pryor et al 1995). These include perceptual and behavioural problems (Fitzhardinge & Steven 1972), difficulty with language (Walther & Ramaekers 1982), attentional deficits and failure at school (Allen 1984).

Several factors are associated with preterm birth including lower socio-economic status, young maternal age, cigarette smoking, multiple pregnancy, premature rupture of membranes, cervical incompetence, and having a previous preterm birth (Steer & Flint 1999). With the obvious exception of cigarette smoking, these risk factors are not easily modified and, consequently, there has been little change in preterm birth rates in recent years. In developed countries, rates vary between 5% and 10% (Meis et al 1995). In the UK, the preterm birth rate is around 7% (Steer & Flint 1999). Factors associated with low birth weight following intrauterine growth retardation include cigarette smoking, poor nutrition during pregnancy and low pre-pregnancy weight (Thompson et al 2001).

Reducing the risk of preterm birth and small-for-gestational-age babies, with their associated problems, would be desirable for any pregnant woman. Therefore, a study that seeks to assess a dietary factor in reducing the risk – in this case, the consumption of seafood – could have important and potentially life-saving consequences and is, therefore, a welcome addition to the literature.

The study reviewed here is a piece of quantitative research. It is described as a 'prospective cohort study', with the data being obtained through the administration of questionnaires at 16 and 30 weeks of pregnancy. (It is important to note that, although data were obtained at 16 and 30 weeks of pregnancy, questions relating to fish consumption were only included in the 16-week questionnaire – mention of the later questionnaire in the methods section of this paper is [if you'll pardon the use of an irresistible pun] something of a red herring.) Prospective cohort studies are commonly used in epidemiological research to determine the causes of disease (Bowling 2002 p 200). They are 'prospective' in that the data were obtained prior to the event they

Olsen SF, Secher NJ 2002 Low consumption of seafood in early pregnancy as a risk factor for preterm delivery: prospective cohort study. British Medical Journal 324:447–450 are designed to assess, i.e. the risk of preterm birth and low birth weight. However, it should be remembered that prospective studies rely on survey data might involve asking questions about the recent past, with the consequent risk of inaccurate or selective recall – recall bias (more on that later). A 'cohort' is simply a group who have something in common, in this case, pregnant women attending an antenatal clinic in Denmark. The thing is not to be put off by research terms – they can at first appear jargonistic, but they have a simple explanation that can easily be accessed from any good research book.

Papers

QUESTIONS FOR CHAPTER 5

1 a) The purpose of the abstract is to (True/False):
   i) Give a clear and succinct overview of the study
   ii) Be detailed enough to eliminate the need to read the article in full
   iii) Enable the reader to make an accurate judgement as to the importance and relevance of the study
   b) In this study, does the abstract fulfil the criteria of purpose? Yes/No/Maybe

2 a) What is the purpose of the introduction?
   b) In this study, does the introduction fulfil the criteria of purpose? Yes/No/Maybe
   c) The authors state that it is important to identify *modifiable* causes of preterm birth and fetal growth retardation:
   i) What is generally acknowledged as the single most important modifiable cause of preterm birth and fetal growth retardation?
   ii) Is this referred to in the introduction? Yes/No

3 a) What are the potential advantages of self-administered questionnaires?
   b) What are the potential disadvantages of self-administered questionnaires?

N1. It is not uncommon to be informed that the 'study base' or precise methodology has been described in detail elsewhere. This is because of limited publication space and unwillingness on the part of the author(s) and/or editor to 'waste' valuable lines repeating what has already been written elsewhere. It is usually fair to assume that the earlier publication referred to will describe the primary element of the study in question and that the later publication describes a secondary consideration of the research. Whatever the reason for omitting the full details of the study, it is clear that, without them, the reader is unable to make an accurate assessment of the research in question. This can be extremely frustrating (not to mention time-consuming) but the reader really has no alternative but to obtain a copy of the original paper. Where appropriate, I will highlight any relevant detail contained in the earlier publication (a copy of which I have obtained!) to help in assessing this current study.

N2. The time period 1992–6 was the second phase of the main study referred to in Note 1. In the main study, data were also collected between 1989 and 1991 but no questions about fish consumption were included in the 16-week survey at that time.

4 What is the justification for the inclusion criteria?

5 It is not always necessary to obtain ethical approval for a questionnaire survey of this type because anonymity can be assured. True/False

Low consumption of seafood in early pregnancy as a risk factor for preterm delivery: prospective cohort study

Sjúrður Fróði Olsen, Niels Jørgen Secher

Abstract

Objective To determine the relation between intake of seafood in pregnancy and risk of preterm delivery and low birth weight.
Design Prospective cohort study.
Setting Aarhus, Denmark.
Participants 8729 pregnant women.
Main outcome measures Preterm delivery and low birth weight.
Results The occurrence of preterm delivery differed significantly across four groups of seafood intake, falling progressively from 7.1% in the group never consuming fish to 1.9% in the group consuming fish as a hot meal and an open sandwich with fish at least once a week. Adjusted odds for preterm delivery were increased by a factor of 3.6 (95% confidence interval 1.2 to 11.2) in the zero consumption group compared with the highest consumption group. Analyses based on quantified intakes indicated that the working range of the dose-response relation is mainly from zero intake up to a daily intake of 15 g fish or 0.15 g n-3 fatty acids. Estimates of risk for low birth weight were similar to those for preterm delivery.
Conclusions Low consumption of fish was a strong risk factor for preterm delivery and low birth weight. In women with zero or low intake of fish, small amounts of n-3 fatty acids—provided as fish or fish oil—may confer protection against preterm delivery and low birth weight.

Introduction

It is important to identify modifiable causes of preterm delivery and fetal growth retardation, which are strong predictors of infants' later health and survival. Observations of high birth weights[1] and long gestations[2] in the fish eating community of the Faroe Islands suggested that intake of seafood rich in long chain n-3 fatty acids can increase birth weight by prolonging gestation[2] or by increasing the fetal growth rate.[3–6]

Fish oil has been shown in randomised trials[7 8] and animal experiments[9 10] to have the potential to delay spontaneous delivery and prevent preterm delivery, but the minimum amount of n-3 fatty acids needed to obtain this effect remains to be determined. No detectable effects on fetal growth rate were seen in these trials,[7 8] but fish oil was provided only in the second half

of pregnancy, and several observational studies have found direct associations between measures of seafood intake in pregnancy and fetal growth rate.[5 11–14]

We investigated these issues in a cohort of women in whom seafood intake in early pregnancy was assessed prospectively by a questionnaire method.[15] We tested whether a low intake of seafood in early pregnancy is a risk factor for preterm delivery and low birth weight and whether it is associated with a lower fetal growth rate. We related the findings to quantified intakes of fish and long chain n-3 fatty acids.

Methods

We invited all pregnant women receiving routine antenatal care in Aarhus, Denmark, to complete self administered questionnaires in weeks 16 and 30 of gestation. The study base has been described in detail elsewhere.[16] During 1992-6 the questionnaire administered at 16 weeks contained questions about intake of fish and fish oil. Only singleton, live born babies without detected malformations were included in the analysis. The local scientific-ethical committee approved the protocol, and we used an informed consent form.

Exposure variables

In Denmark fish is eaten mainly as part of a hot meal, in an open sandwich, or cold in a green salad or pasta salad.[15] Frequency of consumption of such meals has been shown to be a strong and independent predictor of variation in erythrocyte n-3 fatty acids, without taking into consideration whether the meals contained fat or lean fish.[15] We posed four questions: "How often did you eat: (a) fish in a hot meal, (b) bread with fish, (c) green salad or pasta salad with fish, and (d) fish oil as a supplement?" The women were asked to understand the term "fish" as including roe, prawn, crab, and mussel and to let the responses represent the period from when they first knew they were pregnant until completion of the questionnaire. Each question had six predefined response categories: never, less than once a month, 1-3 times a month, 1-2 times a week, 3-6 times a week, every day.

We quantified daily intakes of fish and long chain n-3 fatty acids on the basis of the following assumptions. (Contribution of long chain n-3 fatty aids from foods of non-marine origin—for example, offal meat—was considered negligible.) The six frequency

Papers

Low consumption of seafood in early pregnancy as a risk factor for preterm delivery: prospective cohort study

Sjúrður Fróði Olsen, Niels Jørgen Secher

Abstract

Objective To determine the relation between intake of seafood in pregnancy and risk of preterm delivery and low birth weight.

Design Prospective cohort study.

Setting Aarhus, Denmark.

Participants 8729 pregnant women.

Main outcome measures Preterm delivery and low birth weight.

Results The occurrence of preterm delivery differed significantly across four groups of seafood intake, falling progressively from 7.1% in the group never consuming fish to 1.9% in the group consuming fish as a hot meal and an open sandwich with fish at least once a week. Adjusted odds for preterm delivery were increased by a factor of 3.6 (95% confidence interval 1.2 to 11.2) in the zero consumption group compared with the highest consumption group. Analyses based on quantified intakes indicated that the working range of the dose-response relation is mainly from zero intake up to a daily intake of 15 g fish or 0.15 g n-3 fatty acids. Estimates of risk for low birth weight were similar to those for preterm delivery.

Conclusions Low consumption of fish was a strong risk factor for preterm delivery and low birth weight. In women with zero or low intake of fish, small amounts of n-3 fatty acids—provided as fish or fish oil—may confer protection against preterm delivery and low birth weight.

Introduction

It is important to identify modifiable causes of preterm delivery and fetal growth retardation, which are strong predictors of infants' later health and survival. Observations of high birth weights[1] and long gestations[2] in the fish eating community of the Faroe Islands suggested that intake of seafood rich in long chain n-3 fatty acids can increase birth weight by prolonging gestation[2] or by increasing the fetal growth rate.[3-6]

Fish oil has been shown in randomised trials[7 8] and animal experiments[9 10] to have the potential to delay spontaneous delivery and prevent preterm delivery, but the minimum amount of n-3 fatty acids needed to obtain this effect remains to be determined. No detectable effects on fetal growth rate were seen in these trials,[7 8] but fish oil was provided only in the second half

of pregnancy, and several observational studies have found direct associations between measures of seafood intake in pregnancy and fetal growth rate.[5 11-14]

We investigated these issues in a cohort of women in whom seafood intake in early pregnancy was assessed prospectively by a questionnaire method.[15] We tested whether a low intake of seafood in early pregnancy is a risk factor for preterm delivery and low birth weight and whether it is associated with a lower fetal growth rate. We related the findings to quantified intakes of fish and long chain n-3 fatty acids.

Methods

We invited all pregnant women receiving routine antenatal care in Aarhus, Denmark, to complete self administered questionnaires in weeks 16 and 30 of gestation. The study base has been described in detail elsewhere.[16] During 1992-6 the questionnaire administered at 16 weeks contained questions about intake of fish and fish oil. Only singleton, live born babies without detected malformations were included in the analysis. The local scientific-ethical committee approved the protocol, and we used an informed consent form.

Exposure variables

In Denmark fish is eaten mainly as part of a hot meal, in an open sandwich, or cold in a green salad or pasta salad.[15] Frequency of consumption of such meals has been shown to be a strong and independent predictor of variation in erythrocyte n-3 fatty acids, without taking into consideration whether the meals contained fat or lean fish.[15] We posed four questions: "How often did you eat: (a) fish in a hot meal, (b) bread with fish, (c) green salad or pasta salad with fish, and (d) fish oil as a supplement?" The women were asked to understand the term "fish" as including roe, prawn, crab, and mussel and to let the responses represent the period from when they first knew they were pregnant until completion of the questionnaire. Each question had six predefined response categories: never, less than once a month, 1-3 times a month, 1-2 times a week, 3-6 times a week, every day.

We quantified daily intakes of fish and long chain n-3 fatty acids on the basis of the following assumptions. (Contribution of long chain n-3 fatty aids from foods of non-marine origin—for example, offal meat—was considered negligible.) The six frequency

---

6
a) Is it safe to assume that the amount of fish consumed in each meal would be similar across and between categories? Yes/No/Maybe
b) How else might fish consumption be assessed?

7
a) The time-frame of the question about fish consumption was not the same for all women completing the questionnaire. This is because the time lapse from discovering they were pregnant until 16 weeks would have varied between women. How might this affect the study?
b) How else might the question have been worded?

8
a) The questionnaire used 'structured' or 'closed' questions and answers to assess fish consumption – respondents had to answer four questions using one of six pre-determined response categories. What are the advantages of structured questionnaires?
b) What are the disadvantages of structured questionnaires?
c) Where categories are used for respondents to answer structured questionnaires (True/False):
   i) The categories should be clear and unambiguous
   ii) The wording should be as simple as possible
   iii) A small degree of overlap between possible answers is acceptable
   iv) The answer must be either 'Yes' or 'No'

9 What are the potential problems with the assumptions made?

Table 1 Frequency of consumption of meals containing fish by 8729 women. Values are number (percentage). Women who took fish oil were excluded

Meal type	Never	<1 per month	1-3 per month	1-2 per week	3-6 per week	Every day	Total
Hot meal	999 (11.4)	2700 (30.9)	3851 (44.1)	1140 (13.1)	32 (0.4)	0	8722 (100)
Sandwich	601 (6.9)	1425 (16.3)	3196 (36.6)	2698 (30.9)	711 (8.1)	92 (1.1)	8723 (100)
Salad	3515 (40.3)	3111 (35.7)	1766 (20.2)	299 (3.4)	24 (0.3)	4 (0.0)	8719 (100)

9 (continued from previous page)

categories corresponded to 0, 0.5, 2, 4, 20, and 28 servings per 28 days. Each serving of a hot fish meal provided 144 g fish and 1627 µg n-3 fatty acids, a fish sandwich provided 29 g fish and 431 µg n-3 fatty acids, and a fish salad provided 50 g fish and 149 µg n-3 fatty acids. These values were mainly derived from work done by the Danish Veterinary and Food Administration on portion sizes, distributions of fish species in meals, and food tables for the Danish population.[17] [18] We defined six groups of exposure, with the lowest group consuming no fish and the other five groups being fifths of the remaining participants (designated QUANT0, QUANT1, QUANT2, QUANT3, QUANT4, QUANT5).

10 Was it reasonable to assume that limiting the number of variables in the alternative strategy would alleviate the uncertainties in Question 9? Yes/No/Maybe

To avoid the uncertainties of the above assumptions we adopted a priori an alternative analytical strategy, which was based solely on the raw food frequency variables ("food frequency strategy"), and which could still provide a strong test of the hypotheses. To limit the number of variables considered simultaneously, we restricted analyses to the 1304 women who had eaten no fish salad and who had consumed hot meals and open sandwiches with fish with the same frequency. To secure substantial exposure contrasts, we defined four comparison groups with reasonable sample sizes in such a way that both the defining variables increased progressively: women who had consumed fish as a hot meal and as open sandwiches (*a*) zero times, (*b*) more than zero but less than once a month, (*c*) 1-3 times a month, and (*d*) once or more often a week (designated FREQ0, FREQ1, FREQ2, and FREQ3).

Outcome variables

We assessed gestational age by early ultrasonography in 71% of participants, and otherwise from menstrual data or best clinical judgment. We defined low birth weight as <2500 g and preterm as delivery before 259 days. We assessed intrauterine growth retardation below the 10th centile and birth weight expected from gestational age from the infant's birth weight, gestational age, and sex, on the basis of a Danish standard.[19]

Covariates

We used covariates as previously described[16]: sex of infant (girl, boy); smoking (0, 1-9, ≥10 cigarettes a day) and alcohol consumption (<10 or ≥10 drinks a week) in pregnancy; maternal age (≤19, 20-29, 30-39, ≥40 years), parity (0, ≥1), height (≤159, 160-169, 170-179, ≥180 cm), and pre-pregnant weight (≤49, 50-59, 60-69, 70-79, ≥80 kg); length of education (≤7, 8-9, ≥10 years); and whether the mother had a cohabitant (0, 1).

Statistical analyses

The study hypothesis could be tested in many different ways with our data, so we decided all analytical conditions a priori. This avoided data dependent analyses and kept preconditions for interpreting P values and confidence intervals as valid as possible for an observational study with self selected rather than randomised allocation to levels of exposure. We used the χ^2 test, analysis of variance, and logistic regression. We included all suspected potential confounders (see covariate list) in the multivariate model simultaneously.

11 Was it equitable to assess gestational age in this way? Yes/No/Maybe

12 It could be argued that the definitions of low birth weight and preterm delivery (although technically correct) are somewhat crude. It might have been more informative to have included subcategories, or gradations of low birth weight and preterm delivery. For example, it cannot be assumed that preterm birth at 36 weeks would necessarily have the same causality or associations as preterm birth at 26 weeks

a) What is the likely reason for the choice of definitions in this study?
b) What would be required for more precise definitions of preterm delivery and low birth weight?

N3. The list of covariates (or potential confounders) varies slightly between the earlier description of the main study and this current paper. The earlier list includes some additional covariates: chronic diseases, previous preterm deliveries, caffeine intake, marital status (but not cohabiting as stated in this later paper so this may in fact be the same variable), and occupational status.

One can only speculate as to why they are not reported in the current paper, especially as they would appear to be important potential confounders.

Table 2 Occurrences of low birth weight, preterm delivery, and intrauterine growth retardation, and mean birth weight, gestation length, and birth weight adjusted for gestation length, according to quantified daily intake of long chain n-3 fatty acids

Group*	Dichotomous outcomes (No (%))			Continuous outcomes (mean (SD))		
	Low birth weight	Preterm delivery	Intrauterine growth retardation	Birth weight (g)	Gestation (days)	Adjusted birth weight (g)
QUANT0 (n=282)	20 (7.1)	20 (7.1)	23 (8.2)	3432 (589)	278.8 (14.3)	3466 (490)
QUANT1 (n=1723)	54 (3.1)	71 (4.1)	152 (8.8)	3543 (543)	281.7 (11.9)	3494 (486)
QUANT2 (n=1618)	52 (3.2)	61 (3.8)	116 (7.2)	3572 (559)	281.8 (12.4)	3521 (481)
QUANT3 (n=1890)	34 (1.8)	45 (2.4)	96 (5.1)	3592 (498)	282.2 (10.4)	3532 (446)
QUANT4 (n=1419)	35 (2.5)	50 (3.5)	91 (6.4)	3581 (521)	282.2 (11.3)	3520 (455)
QUANT5 (n=1775)	37 (2.1)	52 (2.9)	94 (5.3)	3617 (518)	282.4 (11.0)	3550 (457)
Statistical tests						
Between groups (P value)	<0.001†	0.001†	0.001†	0.001‡	0.001‡	0.004‡
Linear trend (P value)	<0.001	0.003	0.001	0.001	0.001	0.001

*See text for definitions of the six groups. †Pearson χ^2. ‡Analysis of variance.

Table 3 Occurrences of potential confounders according to quantified daily intake of long chain n-3 fatty acids. Values are percentages (numbers)

Group*	Smoker	High school	Primiparous	Single	<50 kg	<1.6 m	Teenager
QUANT0	40.7 (112/275)	34.2 (92/269)	58.5 (165/282)	7.6 (21/276)	6.5 (18/275)	10.1(27/268)	6.7 (19/282)
QUANT1	30.2 (508/1683)	44.1 (736/1669)	59.3 (1022/1723)	5.8 (98/1697)	5.2 (88/1700)	7.7 (131/1695)	1.9 (32/1723)
QUANT2	23.0 (363/1576)	56.2 (876/1560)	56.4 (912/1618)	4.9 (78/1593)	4.7 (75/1590)	6.2 (99/1604)	1.2 (19/1618)
QUANT3	19.0 (353/1851)	67.3 (1244/1849)	50.6 (956/1890)	3.9 (72/1865)	3.1 (57/1861)	5.1 (94/1861)	0.3 (6/1890)
QUANT4	21.1 (293/1391)	67.4 (931/1382)	47.9 (680/1419)	2.7 (38/1395)	3.3 (46/1399)	6.1 (85/1399)	0.6 (8/1419)
QUANT5	18.3 (315/1724)	69.9 (1201/1719)	49.6 (880/1775)	4.5 (78/1741)	4.2 (73/1749)	5.7 (100/1748)	0.4 (7/1775)

*See text for definitions of the six groups.

Table 1 Frequency of consumption of meals containing fish by 8729 women. Values are number (percentage). Women who took fish oil were excluded

Meal type	Never	<1 per month	1-3 per month	1-2 per week	3-6 per week	Every day	Total
Hot meal	999 (11.4)	2700 (30.9)	3851 (44.1)	1140 (13.1)	32 (0.4)	0	8722 (100)
Sandwich	601 (6.9)	1425 (16.3)	3196 (36.6)	2698 (30.9)	711 (8.1)	92 (1.1)	8723 (100)
Salad	3515 (40.3)	3111 (35.7)	1766 (20.2)	299 (3.4)	24 (0.3)	4 (0.0)	8719 (100)

categories corresponded to 0, 0.5, 2, 4, 20, and 28 servings per 28 days. Each serving of a hot fish meal provided 144 g fish and 1627 µg n-3 fatty acids, a fish sandwich provided 29 g fish and 431 µg n-3 fatty acids, and a fish salad provided 50 g fish and 149 µg n-3 fatty acids. These values were mainly derived from work done by the Danish Veterinary and Food Administration on portion sizes, distributions of fish species in meals, and food tables for the Danish population.[17][18] We defined six groups of exposure, with the lowest group consuming no fish and the other five groups being fifths of the remaining participants (designated QUANT0, QUANT1, QUANT2, QUANT3, QUANT4, QUANT5).

To avoid the uncertainties of the above assumptions we adopted a priori an alternative analytical strategy, which was based solely on the raw food frequency variables ("food frequency strategy"), and which could still provide a strong test of the hypotheses. To limit the number of variables considered simultaneously, we restricted analyses to the 1304 women who had eaten no fish salad and who had consumed hot meals and open sandwiches with fish with the same frequency. To secure substantial exposure contrasts, we defined four comparison groups with reasonable sample sizes in such a way that both the defining variables increased progressively: women who had consumed fish as a hot meal and as open sandwiches (a) zero times, (b) more than zero but less than once a month, (c) 1-3 times a month, and (d) once or more often a week (designated FREQ0, FREQ1, FREQ2, and FREQ3).

Outcome variables

We assessed gestational age by early ultrasonography in 71% of participants, and otherwise from menstrual data or best clinical judgment. We defined low birth weight as <2500 g and preterm as delivery before 259 days. We assessed intrauterine growth retardation below the 10th centile and birth weight expected from gestational age from the infant's birth weight, gestational age, and sex, on the basis of a Danish standard.[19]

Covariates

We used covariates as previously described[16]: sex of infant (girl, boy); smoking (0, 1-9, ≥10 cigarettes a day) and alcohol consumption (<10 or ≥10 drinks a week) in pregnancy; maternal age (≤19, 20-29, 30-39, ≥40 years), parity (0, ≥1), height (≤159, 160-169, 170-179, ≥180 cm), and pre-pregnant weight (≤49, 50-59, 60-69, 70-79, ≥80 kg); length of education (≤7, 8-9, ≥10 years); and whether the mother had a cohabitant (0, 1).

Statistical analyses

The study hypothesis could be tested in many different ways with our data, so we decided all analytical conditions a priori. This avoided data dependent analyses and kept preconditions for interpreting P values and confidence intervals as valid as possible for an observational study with self selected rather than randomised allocation to levels of exposure. We used the χ^2 test, analysis of variance, and logistic regression. We included all suspected potential confounders (see covariate list) in the multivariate model simultaneously.

N4. The term *a priori* is often used in research papers. It simply means 'prior to' or 'in advance'.

N5. Statistical analyses. The chi-square test is used to assess whether differences in proportions (e.g. preterm babies born to mothers who consumed no fish, compared to mothers who had a high intake of fish during pregnancy) are real, rather than simply due to chance. It is necessary to begin with a null hypothesis. In our example this would be 'There is no difference in the proportion of preterm babies born to mothers who don't consume fish during pregnancy and those who have a high intake'. In comparing the two proportions, the chi-square test compares *observed* numbers with those that would be *expected* if the null hypothesis were true.

Variance is a measure of spread of observations around the mean. It is based on the squared differences of each observation from the mean.

Logistic regression is a mathematical modelling procedure, commonly used for the analysis of epidemiological data. It can be used to describe the relationship of several independent (or predictor) variables to a dichotomous dependent (or outcome) variable. In this study, the independent variables are fish consumption and all the other factors in the list of covariates. The dependent variables are preterm birth and low birth weight.

What differentiates logistic regression from multiple regression is that it can be used to predict the probability of belonging to a particular category, or group. Results are given as odds ratios. For example, logistic regression could be used to compute the odds that a particular woman, with a known medical and obstetric history, will have a normal vaginal birth, or not (Frohlich 2004).

It is worth remembering that to fully appreciate research papers it is necessary to have a basic understanding of statistical tests and terms – but do not despair – it is not necessary to be a statistician. More information about statistics can be found in Section 6.

13 What appear to be the characteristics of those women who consumed no fish? (QUANT0)

Table 2 Occurrences of low birth weight, preterm delivery, and intrauterine growth retardation, and mean birth weight, gestation length, and birth weight adjusted for gestation length, according to quantified daily intake of long chain n-3 fatty acids

Group*	Dichotomous outcomes (No (%))			Continuous outcomes (mean (SD))		
	Low birth weight	Preterm delivery	Intrauterine growth retardation	Birth weight (g)	Gestation (days)	Adjusted birth weight (g)
QUANT0 (n=282)	20 (7.1)	20 (7.1)	23 (8.2)	3432 (589)	278.8 (14.3)	3466 (490)
QUANT1 (n=1723)	54 (3.1)	71 (4.1)	152 (8.8)	3543 (543)	281.7 (11.9)	3494 (486)
QUANT2 (n=1618)	52 (3.2)	61 (3.8)	116 (7.2)	3572 (559)	281.8 (12.4)	3521 (481)
QUANT3 (n=1890)	34 (1.8)	45 (2.4)	96 (5.1)	3592 (498)	282.2 (10.4)	3532 (446)
QUANT4 (n=1419)	35 (2.5)	50 (3.5)	91 (6.4)	3581 (521)	282.2 (11.3)	3520 (455)
QUANT5 (n=1775)	37 (2.1)	52 (2.9)	94 (5.3)	3617 (518)	282.4 (11.0)	3550 (457)
Statistical tests						
Between groups (P value)	<0.001†	0.001†	0.001†	0.001‡	0.001‡	0.004‡
Linear trend (P value)	<0.001	0.003	0.001	0.001	0.001	0.001

*See text for definitions of the six groups. †Pearson χ^2. ‡Analysis of variance.

Table 3 Occurrences of potential confounders according to quantified daily intake of long chain n-3 fatty acids. Values are percentages (numbers)

Group*	Smoker	High school	Primiparous	Single	<50 kg	<1.6 m	Teenager
QUANT0	40.7 (112/275)	34.2 (92/269)	58.5 (165/282)	7.6 (21/276)	6.5 (18/275)	10.1(27/268)	6.7 (19/282)
QUANT1	30.2 (508/1683)	44.1 (736/1669)	59.3 (1022/1723)	5.8 (98/1697)	5.2 (88/1700)	7.7 (131/1695)	1.9 (32/1723)
QUANT2	23.0 (363/1576)	56.2 (876/1560)	56.4 (912/1618)	4.9 (78/1593)	4.7 (75/1590)	6.2 (99/1604)	1.2 (19/1618)
QUANT3	19.0 (353/1851)	67.3 (1244/1849)	50.6 (956/1890)	3.9 (72/1865)	3.1 (57/1861)	5.1 (94/1861)	0.3 (6/1890)
QUANT4	21.1 (293/1391)	67.4 (931/1382)	47.9 (680/1419)	2.7 (38/1395)	3.3 (46/1399)	6.1 (85/1399)	0.6 (8/1419)
QUANT5	18.3 (315/1724)	69.9 (1201/1719)	49.6 (880/1775)	4.5 (78/1741)	4.2 (73/1749)	5.7 (100/1748)	0.4 (7/1775)

*See text for definitions of the six groups.

14 a) What piece of information is missing from this sentence?

b) What are the potential problems associated with low response rates in questionnaire surveys?

15 a) Why is it necessary to have a reference? (QUANT5)

b) What is meant by 'crude' and 'adjusted' odds ratios?

c) In simple terms, what do you understand by (95% CI) in this table?

16 The alternative strategy included only four groups with large differences in fish consumption. Do the results reported in Tables 6 and 7 appear to be consistent with those of the earlier analysis given in Table 4? Yes/No/Maybe

17 Bearing in mind the design of this study, in your opinion, is this a reasonable statement? Justify your answer.

18 Is it always necessary for the authors to highlight the strengths and weaknesses of the study in the discussion? Yes/No/Maybe

Results

Of 8998 women returning the 16 week questionnaire, 8729 (97%) had not consumed fish oil supplements—results refer to this restricted group. Mean birth weight was 3577 (SD 531) g, and duration of gestation was 280.0 (11.5) days. Low birth weight occurred in 2.7% (232/8707), preterm delivery in 3.4% (299/8707), and intrauterine growth retardation in 6.6% (572/8705) of participants. Table 1 shows unidimensional distributions of the three food frequency variables. On average, women consumed 15.8 (SD 13.9) g fish and 0.182 (0.161) g long chain n-3 fatty acids a day. Covariate distributions, assessed in a larger sample from the same population, have been published.[16]

Estimated mean daily intakes for the six exposure groups QUANT0 to QUANT5 were 0, 3.3, 8.0, 13.4, 18.0, and 38.4 g fish; and 0, 0.038, 0.092, 0.146, 0.216, and 0.445 g long chain n-3 fatty acids. Low birth weight, preterm birth, and intrauterine growth retardation all tended to decrease with increasing fish consumption, and mean birth weight, duration of gestation, and birth weight adjusted for gestational age tended to increase with increasing fish consumption (table 2). These associations were mainly apparent at the lower end of the exposure scale—this was particularly the case for preterm birth and mean duration of gestation.

Smokers, primiparous women, teenagers, and women with low weight, short stature, and without high school education and cohabitant occurred more frequently in the low exposure groups (table 3). The impression that the decline in risk occurred mainly at the lower end of the exposure distribution was confirmed on examination of adjusted odds ratios for low birth weight and preterm birth, with the highest intake group (QUANT5) as reference (table 4). The association between intake of fish and risk of fetal growth retardation weakened but was not always fully abolished after adjustment for potential confounding.

Alternative strategy

Table 5 defines the comparison groups of the food frequency strategy. Estimated mean daily intakes in the four groups FREQ0 to FREQ3 were 0, 3.1, 12.4, and 44.3 g fish; and 0, 0.037, 0.147, and 0.537 g long chain n-3 fatty acids. Occurrence of low birth weight and preterm delivery both decreased significantly and progressively across the four groups, as frequency of fish consumption increased (table 6). Intrauterine growth retardation exhibited a similar, but non-significant, pattern. Mean birth weight, duration of gestation, and birth weight adjusted for gestational age all increased significantly across the four groups.

Risks of low birth weight and preterm delivery were significantly increased in the lowest group compared with the highest group, even after adjustment for potential confounding, with odds ratios of 3.57 (95% confidence interval 1.14 to 11.14) for low birth weight and 3.60 (1.15 to 11.20) for preterm delivery, with the high intake group (FREQ3) as reference (table 7). The association between risk of intrauterine growth retardation and the dietary variable got much weaker and tended to be abolished after confounding.

Discussion

Low consumption of seafood was a strong risk factor for preterm delivery and low birth weight. The associations were strongest below a daily intake of 0.15 g long chain n-3 fatty acids or 15 g fish.

Strengths and weaknesses

Strengths of the study included that exposure data were collected in a concurrent fashion and long before

Table 4 Crude and adjusted* odds ratios (95% CI) for low birth weight, preterm delivery, and intrauterine growth retardation according to quantified daily intake of long chain n-3 fatty acids (n=7902). The highest intake group (QUANT5) is used as reference

Group†	Low birth weight	Preterm delivery	Intrauterine growth retardation
QUANT0:			
Crude	4.37 (2.43 to 7.87)	2.95 (1.67 to 5.20)	1.52 (0.91 to 2.55)
Adjusted	3.22 (4.73 to 6.00)	2.69 (1.49 to 4.84)	1.14 (0.67 to 1.98)
QUANT1:			
Crude	1.61 (1.02 to 2.55)	1.61 (1.09 to 2.37)	1.73 (1.31 to 2.28)
Adjusted	1.31 (0.82 to 2.10)	1.48 (0.99 to 2.21)	1.45 (1.09 to 1.94)
QUANT2:			
Crude	1.69 (1.07 to 2.68)	1.48 (0.99 to 2.21)	1.41 (1.05 to 1.90)
Adjusted	1.54 (0.97 to 2.46)	1.44 (0.96 to 2.16)	1.31 (0.97 to 1.77)
QUANT3:			
Crude	0.98 (0.60 to 1.61)	0.90 (0.59 to 1.38)	1.02 (0.76 to 1.38)
Adjusted	0.99 (0.60 to 1.63)	0.90 (0.59 to 1.39)	1.03 (0.76 to 1.40)
QUANT4:			
Crude	1.12 (0.67 to 1.88)	1.28 (0.83 to 1.96)	1.16 (0.85 to 1.59)
Adjusted	1.16 (0.69 to 1.94)	1.31 (0.85 to 2.01)	1.25 (0.91 to 1.72)
QUANT5:			
Reference	1.0	1.0	1.0
Statistical tests (dietary variable modelled as five indicator variables)			
Crude (P value)	0.0003	<0.0001	0.0003
Adjusted (P value)	0.004	0.003	0.09

*Adjusted for maternal smoking, alcohol consumption, age, parity, height, pre-pregnant weight, length of education, and cohabitant status (see text).
†See text for definitions of six groups.

Table 5 Frequencies of hot meals and sandwiches containing fish consumed by the 3515 women who never ate salad with fish (seven were missing on one or both of the other two variables) and definition of groups for comparison

Hot meals	Sandwiches						
	Never	<1 per month	1-3 per month	1-2 per week	3-6 per week	Every day	Total
Never	282*	143	186	99	14	4	728
<1 per month	100	301†	481	237	55	5	1179
1-3 per month	75	203	511‡	383	97	11	1280
1-2 per week	17	33	58	141§	51§	8§	308
3-6 per week	1	1	0	4§	6§	0§	12
Every day	0	0	0	0§	0§	0§	0
Total	475	681	1236	864	223	28	3507

*Group FREQ0. †Group FREQ1. ‡Group FREQ2. §Group FREQ3.

Table 6 Occurrences of low birth weight, preterm delivery, and intrauterine growth retardation, and mean birth weight, mean gestation length, and mean birth weight adjusted for length of gestation, according to frequency of fish intake

	Dichotomous outcomes (No (%))			Continuous outcomes (mean (SD))		
Group*	Low birth weight	Preterm delivery	Intrauterine growth retardation	Birth weight (g)	Gestation (days)	Adjusted birth weight (g)
FREQ0 (n=282)	20 (7.1)	20 (7.1)	23 (8.2)	3432 (589)	278.8 (14.3)	3466 (490)
FREQ1 (n=301)	12 (4.0)	14 (4.7)	27 (9.0)	3522 (576)	280.3 (12.8)	3513 (554)
FREQ2 (n=511)	13 (2.5)	18 (3.5)	30 (5.9)	3554 (512)	281.5 (10.9)	3512 (451)
FREQ3 (n=210)	4 (1.9)	4 (1.9)	13 (6.2)	3656 (536)	283.4 (10.8)	3561 (486)
Statistical tests						
Between groups (P value)	0.005†	0.03†	0.3†	<0.001‡	<0.001‡	0.2‡
Linear trend (P value)	0.001	0.003	0.2	<0.001	<0.001	0.04

*See text and table 5 for definitions of comparison groups. †Pearson χ^2. ‡Analysis of variance.

occurrence of outcome among more than 8000 women, that exposure categories and other analytical conditions were decided a priori, and that analyses took account of nine potential confounding factors.

The main weakness of the study, as with any observational study, was the possibility of confounding that was not adjusted for. Adjustment had little impact on measures of association, but confounding by unmeasured factors cannot be ruled out.

Another weakness was that the assumed values for portion sizes, distributions of fish species in meals, and food contents of nutrients are only approximations to the true values. Imprecise estimates of quantified intake of n-3 fatty acids are thus inevitable. Although this imprecision is unlikely to explain the steep decline in risk at the low end of the exposure distribution, it may contribute to the observed "bending" of the relation if imprecision increases with increasing exposure, a possibility that cannot be ruled out.

Alternative strategy

The alternative strategy was free of these assumptions as it simply used the questions on food frequency to define four groups with large differences in exposure; the questions had been shown to be strong and mutually independent predictors of n-3 fatty acids measured in erythrocytes in the same population.[15] It is therefore reassuring that this strategy corroborated the finding of a steep decline in risk across the lowest exposure groups, although with only four groups it was not pos-

What is already known on this topic

Long chain n-3 fatty acids in amounts above 2 g a day may delay spontaneous delivery and prevent recurrence of preterm delivery

Large studies have not been carried out to determine to what extent low consumption of n-3 fatty acids is a risk factor for preterm delivery

The dose-response relation has not been described

What this study adds

Low consumption of fish seems to be a strong risk factor for preterm delivery and low birth weight in Danish women

This relation is strongest below an estimated daily intake of 0.15 g long chain n-3 fatty acids or 15 g fish

sible to draw conclusions about levelling off at high exposures.

Comparisons with other studies

Overall, the findings agree with the randomised trials showing that consumption of fish oil in pregnancy can increase birth weight by prolonging gestation and reduce the risk of recurrence of preterm delivery.[7 8] The finding that the dose-response relations were strong at low exposures corroborates two earlier studies. A reduction in early delivery was seen in women who had received only 0.1 g n-3 fatty acids (along with other substances) a day from week 20 of gestation.[20-23] An association was seen between duration of pregnancy and a biomarker for intake of marine n-3 fatty acids (fatty acids measured in erythrocyte lipids) in Danish women, whereas no such association could be detected in Faroese women with a substantially higher intake, suggesting a stronger association at low exposures.[24]

A case-control study in the same population could not detect any association between seafood intake in pregnancy and risks of preterm birth[25]; unlike the present study, however, this study assessed dietary intake retrospectively after delivery, which may have distorted the results and led to the null finding.

Several observational studies have found associations between measures of maternal seafood intake and fetal growth rate.[5 11-14] In the randomised trials, where fish oil was provided after week 16-20 of

Table 7 Crude and adjusted* odds ratios (95% CI) for low birth weight, preterm delivery, and intrauterine growth retardation according to fish intake (n=1159). The highest intake group (FREQ3) is used as reference

Group†	Low birth weight	Preterm delivery	Intrauterine growth retardation
FREQ0:			
Crude	4.06 (1.34 to 12.01)	3.79 (1.26 to 11.38)	1.28 (0.61 to 2.71)
Adjusted	3.57 (1.14 to 11.14)	3.60 (1.15 to 11.20)	1.01 (0.45 to 2.26)
FREQ1:			
Crude	1.60 (0.49 to 5.27)	2.34 (0.75 to 7.30)	1.44 (0.70 to 2.96)
Adjusted	1.39 (0.41 to 4.67)	2.09 (0.66 to 6.62)	1.26 (0.59 to 2.66)
FREQ2:			
Crude	1.26 (0.40 to 3.96)	1.59 (0.52 to 4.85)	1.01 (0.51 to 2.03)
Adjusted	1.25 (0.39 to 3.94)	1.58 (0.52 to 4.83)	1.02 (0.50 to 2.08)
FREQ3:			
Reference	1.00	1.00	1.00
Statistical tests (dietary variable modelled as three indicator variables)			
Crude (P value)	0.004	0.03	0.5
Adjusted (P value)	0.02	0.06	0.8

*Adjusted for maternal smoking, alcohol consumption, age, parity, height, pre-pregnant weight, length of education, and cohabitant status (see text).
†See text and table 5 for definitions of comparison groups.

19 a) The authors conclude by recommending randomised controlled trials (RCTs) to further investigate the dose–response relationship between long-chain *n*-3 fatty acids and preterm birth. Considering the study overall, is this a valid recommendation? Yes/No/Maybe

b) The authors made no clinical recommendations. Again, considering the study overall, do you think they could have? Yes/No/Maybe

gestation, no effects were seen on fetal growth rate.[7 8] The observational data could therefore possibly be explained either by effects of n-3 fatty acids exerted before week 16-20 or by effects of other substances in seafood. Our study could substantiate neither of these two possibilities, as the associations between seafood consumption in early pregnancy and fetal growth rate tended to disappear after adjustment for potential confounders.

Randomised controlled trials to examine the dose-response relations between long chain n-3 fatty acids and timing of delivery and preterm risk are warranted.

NJS did part of this work during his current employment as chairman at the department of obstetrics and gynaecology, King Faisal Specialist Hospital and Research Center, Riyadh, Saudia Arabia. We thank Jakob Hjort, Ulrik Kesmodel, Janni Dalby Salvig, Kirsten Elise Højbjerg, Tine Brink Henriksen, and Morten Hedegaard for their help in producing the data set.

Contributors: SFO had the original idea for the study, formulated the questions about marine diets, was responsible for the statistical analyses, wrote the first draft of the paper, and is joint guarantor. NJS was responsible for initiating and building the cohort, contributed to the discussion of the results and the draft, and is joint guarantor.

Funding: Novo Nordisk Forskningsfond, Aage-Louis Hansens Fond, Danish National Research Foundation, March of Dimes Birth Defects Foundation, Danish Health Research Foundation, Egmont Fonden.

Competing interests: None declared.

1   Olsen SF, Joensen HD. High liveborn birth weights in the Faroes: a comparison between birth weights in the Faroes and in Denmark. *J Epidemiol Community Health* 1985;39:27-32.
2   Olsen SF, Hansen HS, Sorensen TI, Jensen B, Secher NJ, Sommer S, et al. Intake of marine fat, rich in (n-3)-polyunsaturated fatty acids, may increase birthweight by prolonging gestation. *Lancet* 1986;2:367-9.
3   Olsen SF, Hansen HS, Sorensen T, Jensen B, Secher NJ, Sommer S, et al. Hypothesis: dietary (N-3)-fatty acids prolong gestation in human beings. *Prog Clin Biol Res* 1987;242:51-6.
4   Olsen SF, Hansen HS. Marine fat, birthweight, and gestational age: a case report. *Agents Actions* 1987;22:373-4.
5   Olsen SF, Olsen J, Frische G. Does fish consumption during pregnancy increase fetal growth? A study of the size of the newborn, placental weight and gestational age in relation to fish consumption during pregnancy. *Int J Epidemiol* 1990;19:971-7.
6   Olsen SF. Marine n-3 fatty acids ingested in pregnancy as a possible determinant of birth weight [correction appears in *Am J Epidemiol* 1994;139:856]. *Epidemiol Rev* 1993;15:399-413.
7   Olsen SF, Sorensen JD, Secher NJ, Hedegaard M, Henriksen TB, Hansen HS, et al. Randomised controlled trial of effect of fish-oil supplementation on pregnancy duration. *Lancet* 1992;339:1003-7.
8   Olsen SF, Secher NJ, Tabor A, Weber T, Walker JJ, Gluud C. Randomised clinical trials of fish oil supplementation in high risk pregnancies. *Br J Obstet Gynaecol* 2000;107:382-95.
9   Olsen SF, Hansen HS, Jensen B. Fish oil versus arachis oil food supplementation in relation to pregnancy duration in rats. *Prostaglandins Leukot Essent Fatty Acids* 1990;40:255-60.
10 Baguma-Nibasheka M, Brenna JT, Nathanielsz PW. Delay of preterm delivery in sheep by omega-3 long-chain polyunsaturates. *Biol Reprod* 1999;60:698-701.
11 Olsen SF, Grandjean P, Weihe P, Videro T. Frequency of seafood intake in pregnancy as a determinant of birth weight: evidence for a dose dependent relationship. *J Epidemiol Community Health* 1993;47:436-40.
12 Olsen SF. Further on the association between retarded foetal growth and adult cardiovascular disease. Could low intake of marine diets be a common cause? *J Clin Epidemiol* 1994;47:565-9.
13 Dar E, Kanarek MS, Anderson HA, Sonzognu WC. Fish consumption and reproductive outcomes in Green Bay Wisconsin. *Environ Res* 1992;59:189-201.
14 Dagnelie PC, van Staveren WA, van Klaveren JD, Burema J. Do children on macrobiotic diets show catch-up growth? A population-based cross-sectional study in children aged 0-8 years. *Eur J Clin Nutr* 1988;42:1007-16.
15 Olsen SF, Hansen HS, Sandström M, Jensen B. Erythrocyte levels compared with reported dietary intake of marine n-3 fatty acids in pregnant women. *Br J Nutr* 1995;73:387-95.
16 Kesmodel U, Olsen SF, Secher NJ. Does alcohol increase the risk of preterm delivery? *Epidemiology* 2000;11:512-8.
17 Andersen LT, Jensen H, Haraldsdottir J. Typiske vægte for madvarer. *Scand J Nutr* 1996;40:S129-52.
18 Levnedsmiddelstyrelsen. Levnedsmiddeltabeller (The composition of foods). Copenhagen: Levnedsmiddelstyrelsen, 1996.
19 Secher NJ, Hansen PK, Lenstrup C, Pedersen-Bjergaard L, Eriksen PS, Thomsen BL, et al. Birthweight-for-gestational age charts based on early ultrasound estimation of gestational age. *Br J Obstet Gynaecol* 1986;93:128-34.
20 Olsen SF, Secher NJ. A possible preventive effect of low-dose fish oil on early delivery and pre-eclampsia: indications from a 50-year-old controlled trial. *Br J Nutr* 1990;64:599-609.
21 People's League of Health. Nutrition of expectant and nursing mothers. *Lancet* 1942;ii:10-2.
22 People's League of Health. The nutrition of expectant and nursing mothers in relation to maternal and infant mortality and morbidity. *J Obstet Gynaecol Br Emp* 1946;53:498-509.
23 People's League of Health. Nutrition of expectant and nursing mothers. *BMJ* 1942;ii:77-8.
24 Olsen SF, Hansen HS, Sommer S, Jensen B, Sørensen TIA, Secher NJ, et al. Gestational age in relation to marine n-3 fatty acids in maternal erythrocytes: a study of women in the Faroe Islands and Denmark. *Am J Obstet Gynecol* 1991;164:1203-9.
25 Kesmodel U, Olsen SF, Salvig JD. Marine n-3 fatty acid and calcium intake in relation to pregnancy induced hypertension, intrauterine growth retardation, and preterm delivery: a case-control study. *Acta Obstet Gynecol Scand* 1997;76:38-44.

(Accepted 5 November 2001)

ANSWERS

Q1. a) i) True
      ii) False
      iii) True
  b) Yes

Q2. a) i) Provide the background to the study
      ii) Set the study in the context of previous research in the area
      iii) Provide justification for conducting the study
      iv) Clearly state the intention of the study
  b) Yes – although more detail would be helpful
  c) i) Maternal cigarette smoking
      ii) No

Q3. a) i) Subjects will be familiar with the concept of a questionnaire – they are 'user-friendly'
      ii) They are relatively cheap to administer
      iii) There are no limits to sample size
      iv) They are easy to analyse, especially where 'closed' questions are used
      v) Subjects can be assured of anonymity
      vi) Large amounts of data can be generated relatively quickly
  b) i) Subjects may be disinclined to complete 'yet another questionnaire'
      ii) May have a low response rate
      iii) Closed questions may be perceived as not including an appropriate response for every individual – they can be too simplistic
      iv) They require the respondent to be literate
      v) Questions may be interpreted ambiguously
      vi) There is no way of clarifying anything contained within the questionnaire

Q4. To reduce potential confounding

Q5. False – ethical principles should always be applied when approaching pregnant women

Q6. a) No – it is likely that there is a great deal of variation, and portion sizes are by no means standardised
  b) Women could be asked to complete a daily food diary for a period of time

Q7. a) Some women will need to recall their fish consumption over many weeks, whereas some might have discovered they were pregnant very recently. This raises the question of recall bias, or memory bias, which is possible when surveys include questions about the past (Bowling 2002 p 305). Put simply, because of the time elapsed, the respondent cannot accurately recall the required information, possibly giving an inaccurate answer. Memory bias becomes more likely when longer time periods are involved. In general, the shorter the time period, the more accurate the response is likely to be. The representativeness of the time period under consideration is another potential problem of recall bias. For example, answers to questions about diet may vary according to the time of year. The question 'How often did you eat salad in the past week?' may elicit very different answers in winter compared to summer. Salad consumption during winter months may not be representative of salad consumption during the summer and vice versa
  b) A specific time frame could have been applied to the question, e.g. 'in the past week' or 'in the past month' how often did you eat fish?

Q8. a) i) Data can be easily collected
      ii) They are easy to analyse
      iii) Because of the ease of data collection and analysis, they are relatively cheap to administer
  b) i) They may not be precise enough to accommodate all possible responses
      ii) They may be misunderstood by some respondents

        iii) They may prompt respondents to answer in a way they may not otherwise have done, leading to bias

    c)   i) True

        ii) True

        iii) False

        iv) False

Q9. There is likely to be variation in size of portion as well as the type (and consequently fatty acid content) of fish in each portion

Q10. Maybe – it is likely to reduce uncertainties but does not rule them out altogether

Q11. No – to rule out potential inaccuracies, ultrasonography should have been carried out on *all* participants, especially in a study where gestational age at birth was a primary outcome

Q12. a) The amount of data available for analysis is limited by the total number of subjects. Preterm birth and low birth weight affect only a minority of babies. It is likely that differences between groups would therefore be small. Creating subdivisions for preterm birth and low birth weight would result in such small differences as to render them meaningless

    b) A much larger cohort

Q13. They appear more likely to be single, teenagers, less than 1.6 metres tall, have a pre-pregnancy weight of less than 50 kg and to smoke. They have a tendency to be primiparous compared to women who reported consuming most fish and appear less likely to have a high-school education

Q14. a) When describing the results of a questionnaire survey, it is usual to include the response rate, i.e. how many women were approached and how many returned their questionnaire. The questionnaire was given to eligible consenting women when they were attending the antenatal clinic for their 16-week check. In the earlier publication describing the methodology in full, it is stated that women were asked to fill in two self-administered questionnaires at 16 weeks: one for the medical record and a research questionnaire. Assuming that these were completed when at the antenatal clinic, it could be expected that most, if not all women who agreed to take part in the study would return their questionnaires before the end of their visit. This would imply a high response rate. It is generally accepted that a response rate above 75–80% is good for questionnaire surveys. This is because with higher response rates there is a lower risk of sample bias

    b) There is a greater risk of sample bias. Put simply, the effective sample size is reduced and there may be important differences between responders and non-responders that are not accounted for in the data

Q15. a) The reference is in effect used as a 'baseline' – logistic regression computes the odds ratios for having a low birthweight baby, preterm delivery, or intra-uterine growth retardation for each of the other five exposure groups

    b) Crude (or unadjusted) odds ratios take no account of potential confounders. Adjusted odds ratios are computed after data relating to potential confounders are included in the mathematical modelling

    c) The researchers are 95% confident that the true value (or true odds ratio) lies somewhere between the two levels shown in the brackets

Q16. Yes – women who had consumed no fish since finding out they were pregnant had a higher risk of preterm delivery and low birth weight compared to those who reported eating more fish

Q17. Please see the discussion that follows

Q18. Yes – it is essential to 'come clean' in the discussion, especially where weaknesses are concerned. Whatever the limitations of the study, it is far better for the author(s) to acknowledge these rather than be exposed to (possibly scathing) criticism later on

Q19. a) Maybe – even the best designed surveys are limited in that they can only provide estimates of association. In contrast, RCTs can be much more precise as to cause and effect. However, designing and conducting a RCT to assess fish consumption during pregnancy could be fraught with difficulty

b) Maybe – given the limitations of the study, making definite recommendations based on its findings would seem somewhat premature. However, that is not to say that pregnant women and their carers should not be made aware of the findings of this research, as individuals might wish to amend their own diet

DISCUSSION

When reviewing any research paper it is necessary to consider several aspects. These would include the appropriateness of the study (e.g. why it was carried out and how it fits within the literature), its strengths and weaknesses (in particular, concerning the methodology employed) and the relevance of its conclusions and recommendations for the future. When you have read the article in full and worked through the questions, you will already have developed a much clearer appreciation of this study. It would probably be helpful at this stage to make a list of the positive and negative attributes of the research as you see it.

It is worth mentioning, before we go any further, that the thoughts and comments of others who have also read and considered this article may well help you to gain a deeper insight as to its strengths and weaknesses. In this respect we are fortunate – the article was originally published in the *British Medical Journal* (*BMJ*). I have long been a fan of this journal for several reasons – not least that the *BMJ* has a 'rapid response' facility that encourages readers to submit their comments on articles published in the *BMJ* via its website. These can be easily accessed (along with the full text of each article) and downloaded by anyone – you do not need to subscribe or to have a password (http://www.bmj.bmjjournals.com). In discussing this paper, I will refer to a couple of the rapid responses but you can review them yourself at http://bmj.com/cgi/content/full/324/7335/447#responses

Strengths and weaknesses

The authors have compiled their own list of strengths and weaknesses in their discussion of the study. In addition to the strengths that they highlight, the fact that the questionnaire used closed questions and was administered during a visit to an antenatal clinic presumably means that it was relatively quick and straightforward to complete. From this, and the information given in the original paper describing the full methodology, it is reasonable to assume that there was a high response rate. This would reduce the likelihood of non-response bias, effectively increasing the accuracy of the survey estimates.

However, we also need to consider whether the setting of an antenatal clinic is appropriate for the administration of such a questionnaire. For example, are women likely to be relaxed and happy to comply with a request to take part in the study? Or are they more likely to be apprehensive and feel coerced into taking part, rushing through their answers without due consideration in order to 'get it over with' so that they can focus on the real reason they are attending the clinic? Are they also likely to feel there is a 'right' answer to the questions (especially concerning lifestyle or health behaviour) and modify their responses to give a better impression? We can only speculate, but the setting for any research is an important consideration when assessing its value.

The authors acknowledge two main weaknesses of the study. First, the possibility of confounding by factors that were not adjusted for, and second, the assumptions made about portion sizes and the fish content of meals. These are by no means minor weaknesses.

In the first case, confounding by covariates not controlled for in the analysis has the potential to completely distort the results of the study. Put simply, the apparent association between fish consumption, preterm birth and low birth weight could be a completely false finding.

In drawing up a list of potential confounders it is always necessary to consider known and possible factors of association with the subject under review. In my introduction, I highlighted some of the known risk factors for preterm birth and low birth weight. Although several of these were considered in the list of covariates to some extent, it could be argued that to include only nine potential confounders in this study is far too limited. For example, the only demographic data were length of education and whether or not the woman was cohabiting. Given the known association of low socio-economic status with preterm birth, this is not really good enough. Similarly, the only other dietary factor to be included as a potential confounder in this study was alcohol consumption. Again, given that poor nutrition is associated with low birth weight, other dietary factors should have been included in the list of covariates (Nagaraj 2005). As discussed in Note 6, the list of covariates described in the main study was more extensive than that reported here. As the additional covariates seem relevant, the reason they were not included in this analysis is something of a mystery. Although it is impossible in any observational study to ensure that every possible potential confounder is adjusted for, this particular study would have been enhanced by the inclusion of a much more comprehensive list of covariates.

The crux of the second main weakness of this study is: considering the accuracy of the available information on the intake of seafood during pregnancy, were the authors really able to 'relate the findings to quantified intakes of fish and long-chain n-3 fatty acids'? In essence, the answer seems to depend on your interpretation of 'quantified intakes'. Even the authors acknowledge their doubts. The data on fish intake depended entirely on women's recall, sometimes over several weeks prior to completing the questionnaire. They were asked neither to give any indication as to portion sizes nor to specify the type of fish included in their diet. Therefore a wide variation in portion sizes and fish oil content has to be expected (Harrison 2005). Given the design of the study, this was inevitable. That said, we should remember that women who reported consuming no fish (where there can be no doubt as to portion sizes) had a significantly increased risk of preterm birth and low birth weight compared to women who reported greater fish consumption.

Other methods could have been used to increase the accuracy of information on quantified fish intakes. For example, questions on seafood intake could have been more precise. Women could have been asked to specify the type of fish included in each meal (although recall beyond a certain time frame may be inaccurate and questions may need to be limited to short period of perhaps a week or so), and to give some indication as to portion sizes. A subgroup of women could also have been asked to complete a food diary which would give a 'snapshot' of each woman's diet over a given period of time. Data generated by the food diaries could be compared to the survey data.

One other significant weakness not acknowledged by the authors is the failure to confirm the gestation of every pregnancy by ultrasound scan (USS). This was only achieved in 71% of cases, leaving room for doubt in the remaining 29%. Although I would not wish to suggest that women themselves do not usually have an accurate idea of their own pregnancy dates, for the purposes of research it is important to treat every participant equally. This is especially so in this study because the outcome variables – preterm birth and low birth weight – are dependent on an accurate gestational age. Without it, the findings are open to question. Clearly, the authors should have ensured all women had agreed to have an USS in early pregnancy as part of the inclusion criteria.

Implications

So, overall, this is a useful study and does it have implications for the future? In conducting and publishing this research, the authors have certainly highlighted an area of potential significance. There is an increasing interest in 'healthy lifestyles' – ways of living that can affect health (Bowling 2002 p 33) and perhaps no more so than amongst pregnant women. We only have to consider the impact of recent television programmes such as 'You are what you eat', 'Our fat nation' and 'Jamie's school dinners' to realise that healthy eating is a hot topic. The findings of this study suggest that eating fish during pregnancy may be associated with certain health benefits, i.e. a lower risk of preterm birth and low birth weight, and many pregnant women would be receptive to such information. However, before we all rush out and recommend that women increase their fish intake during pregnancy, is it clear that fish consumption alone was responsible for an improved pregnancy outcome in this study, or might there have been other associations? Furthermore, might there be any disbenefits of increasing fish consumption during pregnancy?

Certainly, causality cannot be proven in a study of this type and, as stated earlier, even the best-designed surveys can only provide estimates of association. The concerns about potential confounders not included in the analysis, especially relating to other dietary factors and sociodemographic indicators, also limit the strength of the findings.

This study was not designed to assess any disbenefits of eating fish during pregnancy – it considered only two outcome variables and was of limited size. However, in recent years there have been concerns about the safety of eating fish during pregnancy, as some fish (including shark, swordfish and marlin) have been found to contain high levels of methylmercury, which could damage the nervous system of the fetus (Food Standards Agency 2002).

It seems, then, that the jury is still out on fish consumption during pregnancy. However, even given its limitations, this study has added to the research literature in the area and makes a strong case for further investigation. Future researchers will aim to build on its findings and design a more comprehensive study next time – one that avoids the current weaknesses and develops its strengths. That really is the nature of research – it chips away at a problem little by little, each study adding to our understanding of an area.

It is easy to be critical about individual studies but, again, we need to remember that researchers are often limited by time and resources and have to operate in the real world, sometimes having to compromise their methodology for practical reasons. As long as these are acknowledged, and researchers avoid making over-inflated claims for their findings, that is OK. Even the most seminal studies, including the largest multi-centre RCTs that have huge implications for our clinical practice, are rarely (if ever) perfect. The study reviewed here is certainly not perfect, but it has examined an interesting area and its findings are worthy of consideration.

References

Allen MC 1984 Developmental outcome and follow-up of small-for-gestational infants. Seminars in Perinatology 8:123–156

BBC 2005 'Biggest' newborn baby for years. Available online at: http://news.bbc.co.uk/1/hi/england/merseyside/4307669.stm [last accessed 7 March 2005]

Bowling A 2002 Research methods in health. Open University Press, Buckingham

Fitzhardinge PM, Steven EM 1972 The small-for-date infant. II. Neurological and intellectual sequalae. Pediatrics 50:50–57

Food Standards Agency 2002 Agency issues precautionary advice on eating shark, swordfish and marlin [press release]. Food Standards Agency, London

Frohlich J 2004 Maternal smoking during pregnancy and the outcome of labour and birth. Unpublished MSc thesis. University of Bristol

Harrison RA 2005 The safety of eating fish during pregnancy needs to be determined. Available online at: http://bmj.com/cgi/content/full/324/7335/447#responses [last accessed 2 May 2005]

Meis PJ, Michielutte R, Peters TJ et al 1995 Factors associated with preterm birth in Cardiff, Wales. I. Univariable and multivariable analysis. II. Indicated and spontaneous preterm birth. American Journal of Obstetrics and Gynecology 173(2):590–602

Nagaraj VK 2005 Is it really due to seafood? Available online at: http://bmj.com/cgi/content/full/324/7335/447#responses [last accessed 2 May 2005]

Nordentoft M, Lou HC, Hansen D et al 1996 Intrauterine growth retardation and premature delivery: the influence of maternal smoking and psychosocial factors. American Journal of Public Health 86:347–354

Pryor J, Silva PA, Brooke M 1995 Growth, development and behaviour in adolescents born small-for-gestational-age. Journal of Paediatric and Child Health 31:403–407

Steer P, Flint C 1999 Preterm labour and premature rupture of membranes. British Medical Journal 318:1059–1062

Thompson JMD, Clark PM, Robinson E et al 2001 Risk factors for small-for-gestational-age babies: the Auckland Birthweight Collaborative Study. Journal of Paediatrics and Child Health 37:369–375

Walther FJ, Ramaekers LH 1982 Language development at the age of 3 years of infants malnourished in utero. Neuropediatrics 13:77–81

Ishvar Sheran and Sara Wickham

Smith C, Crowther C, Beilby J 2002
Acupuncture to treat nausea and vomiting in
early pregnancy: a randomised controlled
trial. Birth 29(1):1–9

INTRODUCTION

Nausea and vomiting in early pregnancy is a common condition that, depending on whose data you use, affects between 50% and 90% of pregnant women (Erick 1997). We often use the term 'morning sickness', but this term can be misleading because many women report symptoms occurring throughout the day (Gadsby et al 1993). Despite being viewed as a normal and common occurrence in pregnancy (O'Brien & Naber 1992), the adverse effects on women's lives should not be underestimated. Many women experience considerable distress and temporary disability (Murphy 1998), which often curtails normal activities. As many as 25% (Vellacott et al 1988) to 33% (Gadsby et al 1993) of women experiencing nausea and vomiting in pregnancy report taking time off paid work, and 50% of women believe their work efficiency is reduced by these symptoms (Vellacott et al 1988). Indeed, the condition can become so severe that some women contemplate terminating their pregnancy (Mazzotta et al 2001).

In the past, pharmaceutical drugs have been the main treatment offered to women experiencing nausea and vomiting. However, these days, many women and physicians are cautious or even fearful about using drugs in pregnancy (e.g. Einarson et al 1998). This is hardly surprising since the thalidomide disaster and, subsequently, dietary and lifestyle changes are often the focus of treatment (Mazzotta et al 1999, Power et al 2001). Alternative medicine is in increasing demand and use by the general public (Long et al 2001), is often recommended by midwives (Allaire et al 2000), and may be able to provide alternative solutions for women experiencing nausea and vomiting during pregnancy. However, the current emphasis on evidence-based practice has led to the notion that we should evaluate non-Western therapies in the same way that we evaluate Western medical treatments.

The paper explored in this chapter looks at whether acupuncture can provide relief to women experiencing nausea and vomiting in pregnancy. Acupuncture treatments involve the insertion of slender needles into different parts of the body, at points where they can affect the flow of vital energy in the body. This energy is called 'chi' (pronounced chee) and it is fundamental to the concepts of Traditional Chinese Medicine, which sees everything in the universe as composed of energy (Kaptchuk 1983). Chi is often translated as breath, vitality or life-force energy. A wilting plant would be said to be lacking in chi, whereas a strong, lively, energetic person is full of chi: that is, without chi there is no life (Firebrace & Hill 1988). This idea of vital energy is not restricted to Traditional Chinese Medicine, or even Eastern medicine. In the West, many older traditions such as herbal medicine and naturopathy also speak of stimulating the vital force in the body to restore health (e.g. Newman Turner 1990).

Chinese people have used acupuncture to treat illness and restore health for thousands of years. A visit to the acupuncturist is as normal in the East as a visit to a doctor has become in the West (Firebrace & Hill 1988). Although acupuncture is often considered an alternative to Western medicine, to over 80% of the world's population, so-called 'alternative' medicine is the basis of the healthcare system (Larsson 1999).

However, while we might well think it wise to consider the efficacy of therapies such as acupuncture alongside the Western healing modalities that underpin midwifery practice, a number of challenges, difficulties and questions arise when alternative therapies are evaluated by the use of Western research methods. For instance, in Western medicine, certain groups of symptoms are usually perceived as leading to the diagnosis of a corresponding disease process. However, the diagnosis of problems and the treatments of them by alternative therapists are often far more complex than in Western medicine. In alternative approaches such as Traditional Chinese Medicine, the physical symptoms themselves are only one part of a complex diagnosis which takes account of many other individual factors that can affect health. Where the philosophy underpinning Western medicine would suggest that a group of people experiencing the same symptoms were probably experiencing the same condition, practitioners of other modalities such as Traditional Chinese Medicine might diagnose several different diseases – or causes of disease –within the same group of people (Hopwood & Lewith 2003). For example, Kaptchuk (1983) carried out a study with 112 people who had been diagnosed (with Western methods) as experiencing angina. A Traditional Chinese Medicine diagnosis of the same people uncovered five distinct patterns of illness, each of which would have been treated very differently by practitioners of Traditional Chinese Medicine. (In this study, 91% of the people treated with Traditional Chinese Medicine showed improvement.)

The very different style of diagnosis and individualised treatment in non-Western healing modalities presents serious issues when these therapies are evaluated by the use of research methods such as the RCT. RCTs are best used to evaluate single – and relatively simple – interventions, where symptom pattern A suggests diagnosis B and is treated by drug (or intervention) C. Because of the relative complexity of the belief systems which underpin non-Western approaches, the kinds of alternative approaches which women seek are not always supported by the kind of evidence of effectiveness that is seen as vital in Western society. The authors of this study have found creative ways around some of these problems, yet some bigger questions remain, to which we will return at the end of the paper.

Acupuncture To Treat Nausea and Vomiting in Early Pregnancy: A Randomized Controlled Trial

Caroline Smith, PhD, MSc, BSc, Lic Ac, Caroline Crowther, MD, FRCOG, FRANZCOG, CMFM, and Justin Beilby, MBBS, FRACGP, MPH

ABSTRACT: **Background:** *Nausea and vomiting in early pregnancy are troublesome symptoms for some women. We undertook a single blind randomized controlled trial to determine whether acupuncture reduced nausea, dry retching, and vomiting, and improved the health status of women in pregnancy.* **Methods:** *The trial was undertaken at a maternity teaching hospital in Adelaide, Australia, where 593 women less than 14 weeks' pregnant with symptoms of nausea or vomiting were randomized into 4 groups: traditional acupuncture, pericardium 6 (p6) acupuncture, sham acupuncture, or no acupuncture (control). Treatment was administered weekly for 4 weeks. The primary outcomes were nausea, dry retching, vomiting, and health status. Comparisons were made between groups over 4 consecutive weeks.* **Results:** *Women receiving traditional acupuncture reported less nausea (p < 0.01) throughout the trial and less dry retching (p < 0.01) from the second week compared with women in the no acupuncture control group. Women who received p6 acupuncture (p < 0.05) reported less nausea from the second week of the trial, and less dry retching (p < 0.001) from the third week compared with women in the no acupuncture control group. Women in the sham acupuncture group (p < 0.01) reported less nausea and dry retching (p < 0.001) from the third week compared with women in the no acupuncture group. No differences in vomiting were found among the groups at any time.* **Conclusion:** *Acupuncture is an effective treatment for women who experience nausea and dry retching in early pregnancy. A time-related placebo effect was found for some women. (BIRTH 29:1 March 2002)*

Caroline Smith is a postdoctoral research officer and Caroline Crowther is Associate Professor in the Department of Obstetrics & Gynaecology, Adelaide University; Justin Beilby is a Senior Lecturer in the Department of General Practice, Adelaide University, Adelaide, Australia.

The study was financially supported by the Department of Obstetrics and Gynaecology, Adelaide University, and the Women's and Children's Hospital Research Foundation, Adelaide, Australia. Needles were donated by Cathy Herbal Products, Sydney.

Address correspondence to Dr. Caroline Smith, PhD, MSc, BSc, Lic Ac, Department of Obstetrics & Gynaecology, Adelaide University, Women's & Children's Hospital, 72 King William Road, North Adelaide, SA 5006, Australia.

Nausea and vomiting are common troublesome symptoms experienced by some women in the first trimester of pregnancy, and affect 50 to 80 percent of all pregnant women (1–3). These symptoms can have a profound impact on women's general sense of well-being and day-to-day lives (4). Women often seek help from professionals and try numerous strategies to alleviate their symptoms, few of which suppress symptoms to their satisfaction.

In recent years the use of complementary medicine has become popular in many Western countries (5). Application of complementary therapies is more common among women of reproductive age, with almost one-half (49%) reporting use (6). It is possible that a significant proportion of women try these therapies during pregnancy. Interest in the antiemetic effect from using acupressure or acupuncture point pericardium 6 (p6) is increasing. Stimulation of point p6 has been proposed to have a specific effect on the upper digestive tract. The Cochrane systematic review of interventions to treat nausea and vomiting includes studies of acupressure point p6. The current Cochrane review contains no trials of acupuncture, and it concluded that acupressure may be helpful (7).

QUESTIONS FOR CHAPTER 6

1 The 50–80% figure relates to:

a) Incidence
b) Prevalence
c) Neither

2 Do the researcher's qualifications and background either:

a) Support this study and its objectives?
b) Detract from this study and its objectives?
c) Make no perceivable difference?
d) We can't tell

3 This statement should really have been supported with a reference. True/False

4 The phrase 'suppress symptoms to their satisfaction' seems to suggest that the researchers see symptom suppression as the aim of treatment. Do you think this could have an effect on the research? Why? Or why not?

5 Was the fact that literature review was limited to the trials in the Cochrane review:

a) An advantage?
b) A disadvantage?
c) Neither
d) Both

2

BIRTH 29:1 March 2002

However, the quality of the three acupuncture trials (8–10) included in the meta-analysis was not high. Data from a fourth trial contained data not in a form that could be included in the meta-analysis (11). The methodology of this trial was good; however, the trial found no beneficial effect from acupressure.

Case reports describe the effectiveness of traditional acupuncture for treating nausea and vomiting when applied in a traditional Chinese medicine framework (12,13). Such application may give improved results compared with use of the single antiemetic point p6.

One randomized controlled trial from the United Kingdom evaluated the use of acupuncture in early pregnancy (14). This trial, which randomized 55 women to receive acupuncture or sham acupuncture, reported no evidence that acupuncture was more effective than sham acupuncture to reduce nausea.

In the absence of high-quality randomized trials, skepticism remains with respect to the benefits of acupuncture to treat nausea and vomiting in early pregnancy. We undertook a single blind randomized controlled trial of acupuncture to determine whether acupuncture (both traditional acupuncture and p6 acupuncture) was better than sham (placebo) acupuncture or no acupuncture in reducing the frequency, duration, amount, and distress from nausea, dry retching, and vomiting, and improved the health status of women in early pregnancy.

Methods

Participants

Women were eligible for the trial if they were less than 14 weeks' pregnant with symptoms of nausea or vomiting. Women were excluded if they had clinical signs of dehydration, or if there was reason to suspect their symptoms were not due to pregnancy, for example, a recent episode of gastroenteritis. The previous use of antiemetics or any other comfort measure did not preclude entry into the trial. Women were able to continue with any existing measures during the trial, and a record of use was recorded at the start, during, and at the end of the trial.

Women were recruited to the trial at the Women's and Children's Hospital in Adelaide, Australia, between January 1997 and July 1999. The trial was promoted within the community using the media, and referrals were made by general practitioners and other hospital health practitioners. The study was approved by the hospital's research and ethics committee, and all women gave written informed consent before enrolling in the trial.

Procedure

Demographic information, history of nausea and vomiting, health status assessment, and a traditional Chinese medicine diagnosis were obtained from each woman before randomization. Women were randomly assigned to a study group controlled by a telephone randomization service at Adelaide University, Clinical Trials Unit. The randomization schedule used balanced variable blocks, and was prepared by a researcher not involved in the trial. Women were allocated into 1 of 4 study groups: traditional acupuncture, p6 acupuncture, sham acupuncture, or no acupuncture (control).

Acupuncture diagnosis and treatment were performed by the study investigator (CS) using a standardized protocol guiding the interaction with women, including diagnosis, acupuncture and sham acupuncture treatment, and needling techniques. The diagnosis included a tongue diagnosis (examination of color, shape, and coating) and an assessment of the quality of the pulse and a history of symptoms. Participation in the trial was for 4 weeks to provide information on the effectiveness of acupuncture and the nature of spontaneous remission of symptoms.

Women allocated to the 2 acupuncture groups and sham acupuncture group were advised to attend for treatment twice during the first week and then to attend weekly. The decision on treatment frequency was pragmatic, given the constraints of feeling unwell, traveling to the hospital, making provision for child care, and scheduling appointments around women's work commitments.

Serin (Japan) 0.2×30 mm needles were inserted using a guide tube. A maximum of 6 needles were used during a treatment session. Needles were stimulated after insertion by rotating them anticlockwise through 45 to 90 degrees, or by rotating clockwise through 180 degrees; further stimulation was minimal. Needles were inserted to a depth 0.5 to 1 cun (cun is a proportional unit of measurement relative to the subject), with *de qi*, a sensation associated with correct needling. Needles were retained over a 20-minute period.

Women allocated into the traditional acupuncture group were administered a treatment based on their traditional Chinese medicine diagnosis. A classically trained acupuncturist may treat individuals with nausea and vomiting in very different ways, according to the diagnosis made. Treatment was guided by the approach described by Maciocia (15). Treatment used acupuncture points on the mid and upper abdomen, located on the energy pathways (meridians) in this area; for example, stomach meridian on

---

6 'Single blind' means that:

a) The researchers didn't know who was in which group but the women did

b) The women didn't know who was in which group but the researchers did

c) No one knew who was in which group

d) None of the above

7 Do you feel these exclusion criteria were justified? Yes/No/Maybe/We can't tell

8 Could a participant's use of anti-emetics have a possible influence on any outcome? Yes/No/Maybe

9 What are some of the things that women need to know about in this kind of trial before their informed consent can be gained?

N1. Acupuncture research presents some fundamental problems due to the different approaches to diagnosis and treatment found in Western medicine and Traditional Chinese Medicine, which does not have a rigid recipe of set acupuncture point treatments for specific biomedically classified diseases (Hopwood & Lewith 2003). Traditional Chinese Medicine treats people very differently and individually depending on factors other than their pathology (as defined in Western medicine). By incorporating a group receiving Traditional Chinese Medicine acupuncture the authors have made a good attempt to account for this approach to diagnosis and treatment.

10 What are benefits of randomisation and why is a randomisation service seen as an advantage in a study such as this?

11 List at least two advantages of using four study groups in this trial

12 Why do you think the researchers chose to undertake a Traditional Chinese Medicine diagnosis of all of the women taken before randomisation, when only one group would go on to have traditional acupuncture treatment?

13 Was 4 weeks long enough? Yes/No/We can't tell

BIRTH 29:1 March 2002

3

acupuncture points stomach 19, 20, 21; kidney meridian, kidney points 21 and 20; and conception vessel points 14, 13, 12, 11, or 10. Acupuncture points were also selected to treat the traditional Chinese medicine diagnosis: *liver qi stagnation* (conception vessel 12 on the mid abdomen, p6 on the medial surface of forearm, gallbladder 34 below the knee, conception vessel 13 mid abdomen, kidney 21 upper abdomen, stomach 34 superior to the patella, stomach 36 below the knee); *stomach* or *spleen qi deficiency* (stomach 36, p6, conception vessel 12); *stomach heat* (stomach 44 on top of the foot, conception vessel 11 mid abdomen, stomach 34, stomach 21 mid abdomen, p6 and pericardium 3 on the forearm); *phlegm* (stomach 40 lateral to tibia, spleen 9 medial surface of lower leg, stomach19 mid abdomen, bladder 20 [on the back] kidney 21); *heart qi deficiency* (heart 5 forearm, p6, stomach 36, conception vessel 14 mid abdomen); or *heart fire* (p6, conception vessel 14, bladder 15 on the back).

Women allocated to the p6 study group received this single point only. This point is located on the anterior surface of the forearm. Women allocated to the sham acupuncture group received acupuncture needles inserted into an area close to, but not on, acupuncture points. Specific points were located on the upper limb between the pericardium and lung meridian at 6 cun, a point on the ankle area between the stomach and gallbladder meridians, a point on the foot between the third and fourth metatarsals, and a point on the lower leg between gallbladder and stomach channel 3 cun below stomach 36.

A no acupuncture control group was included to control for the effect of spontaneous remission of symptoms. To reduce disappointment when women were allocated to this group, a standardized information sheet was made available about advice on diet, lifestyle, and the use of vitamin B6 during the 4-week study period. Women in this group received a weekly 10-minute telephone call from the study investigator to assess their general sense of well-being and to encourage compliance with participating in the trial.

The primary outcomes were experience from nausea, dry retching, and vomiting at days 7, 14, 21, and 26 measured by the Rhodes Index of Nausea and Vomiting Form 2 (16), a 5-point Likert scale. Women's health status was measured by the MOS 36 Short Form Health Survey (SF36) (17). The SF36 is a general outcome measure consisting of an 8 multi-item scale measuring physical functioning, physical role functioning, emotional role functioning, social functioning, bodily pain, mental health, vitality, general health perceptions, and a rating of their health compared with a year ago. The responses to each SF36 domain are summed to provide 8 scores,

and transformed into a multi-item scale between 0 and 100, with 0 indicating poor health and 100 suggesting good health. An assessment of health status was made at days 1, 14, and 28.

Statistical Analysis

Sufficient women were randomized to provide reliable evidence of the effect of acupuncture on nausea and vomiting. It was an entry requirement that women experienced nausea at trial entry. A trial of 114 women would have an 80% power to detect a treatment effect of a 35 percent reduction in the number of women reporting nausea from 99 to 64 percent ($p = 0.05$, beta 0.2). The prevalence of vomiting is reported at 50 percent (18), and to detect a treatment effect of a 35 percent (10,11) reduction in vomiting from 50 to 32.5 percent ($p = 0.05$, beta 0.2), a sample size of 592 women was required. The sample size allowed for a 10 percent loss to follow-up (pregnancy loss or withdrawal from the trial).

To detect changes in health status, sample size calculations were made for each SF36 domain, and were based on an improvement of 25 percent for each score. Sample size varied from 29 women per group for the mental health domain to 143 women for the vitality domain. At the time of designing the trial, no data were available to guide a sample size calculation to demonstrate a difference between acupuncture and a placebo effect.

Women recorded their own primary outcome scores, and data were entered by an experienced data entry operator blinded to study group allocation. Analysis was by intention to treat using SPSS 9.0 for Windows (19). Each symptom of nausea, dry retching, and vomiting was summed into a subscale describing women's experience (based on a recording of the frequency or amount, duration, and distress). Differences in the mean experience subscales were examined using analysis of variance (ANOVA) for normally distributed data, and the Kruskal-Wallis 1-way ANOVA by ranks for data not normally distributed. Mean SF36 domain scores were explored using ANOVA for repeated measurements between traditional acupuncture and p6 acupuncture and the two control groups. Multiple comparisons among study groups were adjusted using the Tukey means comparisons. The chi-square test was used for binary variables. A p value of less than 0.05 was used to demonstrate differences in primary outcomes. Relative risks and 95% confidence intervals (CI) and the number needed to treat with 95% confidence intervals were reported for the primary outcomes. The number needed to treat is based on the number

---

14 Can you think of any disadvantages of using sham acupuncture?

15 This means that the control group were not a control group as such. True/False

16 Discuss some of the advantages and disadvantages of using the SF36 and of asking women to fill this out themselves.

17 Was the 10% loss to follow-up rate allowed for in the power calculation acceptable? Yes/No/Maybe/We can't tell

18 This means that (more than one answer may be correct):

a) The researchers wanted all of the primary outcomes to have significance of 0.05 or less

b) The researchers planned to consider the results relating to the primary outcomes to be significant only if the p value was 0.05 or less

c) The researchers used 0.05 as the starting point for their data analysis and were only interested in analysing results which fell at or below this value

4

BIRTH 29:1 March 2002

of people who will benefit within a certain period of time who otherwise would not benefit (it is calculated as 1/control event rate-experimental event rate).

Results

A total of 593 women were randomized to the trial. Figure 1 summarizes recruitment and return of data forms. We received data from 534 (90%) of women at the end of the first week of the trial, and data from 443 (75%) at the end of the fourth week of the trial (Fig.1). No differences in baseline characteristics, including demographic characteristics (Table 1), nausea, dry retching, and vomiting experience scores (Table 2) and SF36 domain scores (Table 3), were found among study groups. A lower response rate to the SF36 was obtained from women in the no acupuncture control group at baseline ($p < 0.05$) compared with other groups; however, no differences were found in SF36 scores among groups at baseline (Table 3).

Effect of Acupuncture on Nausea

Women's experience of nausea differed among study groups at the end of the first week in the trial ($p < 0.05$) (Table 2). Women receiving traditional acupuncture reported less frequent and shorter periods of nausea, which caused less distress, compared with women in the no acupuncture group ($p < 0.05$). Women in the traditional acupuncture group (13, 9%) were more likely to be free from nausea compared with women in the no acupuncture control group (4, 3%) (relative risk 0.93, 95% CI 0.88–0.99) at the end of their first week of treatment. Fifteen women (95% CI 8–166) receiving traditional acupuncture would need to be treated for 1 woman to report complete relief from nausea at the end of the first week of the trial.

During the second week of the trial, women who received traditional acupuncture ($p < 0.001$), and p6 acupuncture ($p < 0.05$) reported lower nausea scores compared with women in the no acupuncture control group. This improvement in nausea continued for women receiving traditional acupuncture ($p < 0.001$) and p6 acupuncture ($p < 0.01$) into the third week compared with women in the no acupuncture control group. From the third week, women in the sham acupuncture group ($p < 0.01$) also reported lower nausea scores compared with women in the no acupuncture control group. In the final week of the study, improvements in nausea continued for women in the traditional acupuncture ($p < 001$), p6 acupuncture

19 This is a useful diagram which clearly shows the progression of women through the study. True/False

20 This is most likely to be due to (more than one answer may be correct):

a) The placebo effect
b) Poor study design
c) Incorrect use of sham acupuncture by the researcher(s)
d) Sham acupuncture being ineffective as a control method
e) We can't tell

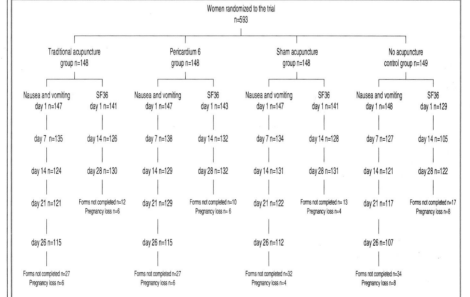

Fig. 1.   *Trial profile: Return of nausea and vomiting and SF36 questionnaires at days 1, 7, 14, 21, and 26.*

21 The characteristics of the women in all four groups were similar enough to say that randomisation worked effectively. True/False

BIRTH 29:1 March 2002   5

Table 1. Comparison of Women by Treatment Group

Characteristics	Traditional Acupuncture (n = 148)	P6 Acupuncture (n = 148)	Sham Acupuncture (n = 148)	No Acupuncture Control (n = 149)
Age (yr) (mean ± SD)	29.5 (4.7)	30.1 (4.8)	29.6 (4.6)	30.0 (5.2)
BMI (kg.m²) (mean ± SD)	24.7 (4.6)	24.0 (4.4)	24.2 (4.6)	23.7 (4.4)
Gestational age (wk) (median and range)	8.3 (5–13)	8.3 (4–14)	8.0 (4–13)	8.4 (5–14)
Parity (≥ 20 wk) (No. and %)				
0	59 (40)	51 (35)	51 (34)	50 (34)
1 or more	89 (60)	97 (65)	97 (66)	99 (67)
Smoked at trial entry (No. and %)	7 (4)	7 (4)	4 (12)	5 (3)
Previous use of acupuncture* (No. and %)	28 (19)	29 (20)	17 (12)	32 (21)
Private patient† (No. and %)	34 (24)	47 (32)	39 (26)	52 (35)
Employed outside the home (No. and %)	97 (66)	95 (64)	102 (69)	105 (70)

*Not significant ($p > 0.12$).
†Not significant ($p > 0.13$).
BMI = body mass index.

Table 2. Experience of Nausea, Dry Retching and Vomiting by Treatment Group

Experience of Symptoms	Traditional Acupuncture (n = 148)	P6 Acupuncture (n = 148)	Sham Acupuncture (n = 148)	No Acupuncture Control (n = 149)	p
Nausea (range 0–12) (mean ± SD)					
Baseline	8.3 (2.5)	8.2 (2.6)	8.6 (2.5)	8.4 (2.3)	ns
Day 7	5.0 (3.0)	5.4 (3.3)	5.7 (2.8)	6.1 (2.9)	0.05
Day 14	4.6 (3.1)	4.8 (3.6)	5.0 (3.0)	6.0 (3.1)	0.01
Day 21	3.8 (3.1)	4.3 (3.3)	4.4 (2.7)	5.8 (3.1)	0.001
Day 26	3.4 (3.0)	4.0 (3.3)	3.7 (2.8)	5.0 (3.0)	0.001
Dry retching (range 0–8) (mean ± SD)					
Baseline	2.5 (1.9)	2.5 (2.2)	2.4 (2.1)	2.6 (1.8)	ns
Day 7	1.3 (1.4)	1.6 (1.7)	1.5 (1.8)	1.7 (1.7)	ns
Day 14	0.9 (1.3)	1.3 (1.5)	1.3 (1.7)	1.6 (1.7)	0.01
Day 21	0.9 (1.4)	0.9 (1.3)	0.9 (1.3)	1.6 (1.7)	0.001
Day 26	0.8 (1.4)	0.9 (1.3)	0.9 (1.4)	1.6 (1.7)	0.001
Vomiting (range 0–12) (mean ± SD)					
Baseline	2.3 (2.7)	2.1 (2.8)	2.4 (2.8)	2.1 (2.7)	ns
Day 7	1.4 (2.0)	1.2 (2.0)	1.5 (2.2)	1.5 (2.1)	ns
Day 14	1.1 (1.8)	1.3 (2.2)	1.4 (2.1)	1.6 (2.2)	ns
Day 21	0.9 (1.6)	1.2 (2.1)	1.0 (1.7)	1.1 (2.1)	ns
Day 26	0.9 (1.5)	0.9 (1.8)	1.0 (1.6)	1.4 (2.0)	ns

22 Which of these *p* values denotes the most statistically significant result?

a) 0.05
b) 0.01
c) 0.001

Table 3. Change in Mean SF36 Domain Over Trial Period

SF36 Domain	Traditional Acupuncture (n = 148)	P6 Acupuncture (n = 148)	Sham Acupuncture (n = 148)	No Acupuncture Control (n = 149)	p
Social function					
Day	48.3 (28.6)	45.1 (30.3)	42.9 (28.5)	45.3 (28.5)	0.01*
Day 14	51.9 (29.0)	50.7 (28.4)	48.5 (28.1)	45.1 (28.7)	0.01†
Day 28	54.0 (27.1)	51.4 (32.0)	48.9 (28.0)	37.8 (22.5)	0.001‡
Vitality					
Day 1	23.4 (18.0)	21.6 (17.7)	22.6 (18.3)	24.1 (15.4)	ns*
Day 14	30.0 (19.7)	27.4 (23.1)	25.8 (18.0)	22.8 (15.1)	0.001†
Day 28	31.9 (20.4)	27.0 (18.9)	27.0 (19.0)	26.0 (17.0)	0.05‡
Physical function					
Day 1	63.7 (24.0)	58.7 (26.5)	63.1 (25.0)	63.0 (25.2)	ns*
Day 14	68.5 (26.1)	63.3 (23.1)	66.0 (24.5)	59.4 (27.3)	0.01†
Day 28	68.0 (21.0)	64.0 (23.5)	66.0 (21.0)	63.3 (25.0)	0.05‡
Physical role function					
Day 1	12.6 (26.4)	11.7 (27.0)	11.4 (26.8)	9.3 (23.0)	ns*
Day 14	7.3 (14.6)	6.3 (13.5)	6.0 (11.9)	4.1 (10.4)	0.001†
Day 28	8.7 (15.5)	6.6 (14.1)	5.0 (11.7)	11.9 (25.0)	0.05‡
Bodily pain					
Day 1	60.0 (24.5)	60.7 (26.7)	59.0 (26.1)	64.3 (24.7)	ns*
Day 14	65.9 (22.5)	66.5 (24.7)	60.0 (24.5)	65.9 (23.0)	0.001†
Day 28	65.2 (22.8)	68.0 (23.0)	65.0 (25.1)	66.6 (22.7)	ns‡
Mental health					
Day 1	59.2 (18.0)	56.6 (18.4)	57.3 (18.1)	58.0 (19.7)	0.05*
Day 14	66.2 (20.2)	60.0 (20.1)	62.0 (17.7)	58.2 (19.9)	0.001†
Day 28	64.7 (18.8)	62.0 (19.1)	64.6 (17.7)	58.6 (20.0)	0.01‡
Emotional role function					
Day 1	54.9 (45.5)	47.4 (44.5)	54.0 (46.6)	52.7 (45.4)	ns*
Day 14	61.4 (44.7)	49.1 (45.8)	59.7 (45.8)	54.7 (45.3)	0.001†
Day 28	68.7 (43.0)	57.2 (52.0)	60.7 (44.4)	53.2 (45.0)	ns‡
General health perception					
Day 1	67.9 (19.1)	64.1 (21.0)	67.7 (20.9)	67.7 (7.5)	ns*
Day 14	65.3 (19.4)	62.6 (19.0)	64.7 (19.4)	63.4 (18.7)	0.001†
Day 28	67.0 (20.6)	63.8 (20.3)	66.1 (19.5)	65.3 (21.6)	ns‡

Figures are mean and standard deviation (SD).
Group: differences in SF36 scores across groups.
†*Time observation of the SF 36 score at days 1, 14, 28.*
‡*Differences in SF 36 scores across all groups over time.*

($p < 0.05$), and sham acupuncture ($p < 0.01$) groups compared with women in the no acupuncture group.

Effect of Acupuncture on Dry Retching

Differences in women's experience of dry retching were first demonstrated among study groups by the end of the second week of the trial ($p < 0.01$) (Table 2). Women receiving traditional acupuncture experienced fewer periods and less distress from dry retching compared with women in the no acupuncture control group ($p < 0.01$). During the third week of the trial, differences in women's experience from dry retching were evident again among study groups ($p < 0.001$).

Women in the traditional acupuncture ($p < 0.001$), p6 acupuncture ($p < 0.01$), and sham acupuncture ($p < 0.001$) groups all experienced fewer periods of, and less distress from, dry retching compared with women in the no acupuncture control group. Sixty eight (56%) women in the traditional acupuncture group were free from dry retching compared with 46 (39%) women in the no acupuncture control group by the end of the third week (relative risk 0.72, 95% CI 0.56–0.93, $p < 0.01$; number needed to treat = 6, 95% CI 3–22). In the sham acupuncture group, 72 (59%) women were free from dry retching compared with 46 (39%) women in the no acupuncture control group (relative risk 0.68, 95% CI 0.52–0.87, $p < 0.001$; number needed to treat = 6, 95% CI 3–13). These improvements continued to the end of the trial. In the p6 acupuncture group, no difference occurred in women free from

BIRTH 29:1 March 2002

dry retching compared with women in the no acupuncture control group.

Effect of Acupuncture on Vomiting

No differences in women's experience from vomiting were found among study groups at any stage in the trial (Table 2).

Effect of Acupuncture on Women's Health Status

At the end of the trial, evidence was seen of a study group effect on the social function ($p < 0.01$) and mental health ($p < 0.05$) SF36 domains. A time effect was seen on all SF36 domains and a study group time effect on five SF36 domains. Women in the traditional acupuncture group showed an improved health status on five SF36 domains over time (Table 3) compared with improvements on two domains for women receiving p6 or sham acupuncture, and an improvement on one domain for women in the no acupuncture control group.

Women receiving traditional acupuncture reported higher vitality ($p < 0.05$), social function ($p < 0.001$), physical function ($p < 0.01$), mental health ($p < 0.01$), and emotional role function ($p < 0.05$) scores compared with women in the no acupuncture control group at the end of the trial. Women in the traditional acupuncture group also reported higher vitality scores compared with women in the p6 acupuncture ($p < 0.05$) and sham acupuncture ($p < 0.05$) groups. Improvements were also reported midway through the study on the vitality ($p < 0.01$), physical function ($p < 0.001$), and mental health ($p < 0.01$) domains for women receiving traditional acupuncture compared with women receiving no acupuncture. An improvement was also observed midway through the study for women receiving traditional acupuncture compared with women receiving p6 acupuncture ($p < 0.05$) for the emotional role functioning domain. At the end of the study, women receiving p6 acupuncture and sham acupuncture reported improved scores on the social function domain ($p < 0.001$) and mental health domain ($p < 0.01$) compared with women in the no acupuncture control group. Women in the latter group reported higher physical role function scores compared with women in the p6 ($p < 0.05$) and sham acupuncture ($p < 0.001$) groups. No other differences among study groups and SF36 domains were found.

Discussion and Conclusions

Women who took part in this trial reported a range of health benefits. Traditional acupuncture was shown to be an effective treatment for women who experience nausea and dry retching in early pregnancy. Pericardium 6 acupuncture reduced nausea and dry retching, although the therapeutic response occurred a week later compared with women receiving traditional acupuncture, and a time-related placebo effect occurred for some women receiving sham acupuncture.

Findings from our trial cannot easily be compared with those of other trials that used acupressure for nausea and vomiting in early pregnancy. Acupuncture and acupressure are different treatment modalities and cannot be compared directly. One trial that compared acupuncture with sham acupuncture among women presenting with nausea showed that acupuncture had no effect (14). The data collection tools used in our trial and the trial by Knight et al (14) were different, and the data were not comparable. Our sample size was sufficiently large to detect changes in nausea, vomiting, and health status, and it included a control group to take account of spontaneous remission of nausea and vomiting, which may explain the difference in results.

Acupuncture failed to reduce vomiting at any time—a lack of beneficial treatment response that some might consider to be disappointing. The observation of a time difference in the efficacy of traditional acupuncture to reduce nausea and dry retching suggests that the frequency of treatments might need to be greater than two treatments in the first week followed by weekly treatments. In trials of acupressure, bands are worn continuously. Two trials of acupressure described its beneficial effect on reducing vomiting during pregnancy (8,9). However, two trials failed to show any therapeutic effect on vomiting (9,11). The optimum frequency of acupuncture treatments for vomiting has not been documented in the literature, but it is possible that increasing the frequency of treatment may reduce the frequency and severity of vomiting. Daily treatments of acupuncture have been recommended for women with severe vomiting (15). Future research may consider evaluating the impact of daily acupuncture treatments to assess its efficacy with reducing vomiting.

No published research has measured the effect of acupuncture for nausea and vomiting on women's health status during early pregnancy. Our results showed that women's health status improved with time. In addition, there was strong evidence of a treatment effect over time that differed between study groups. This time effect was greater for women receiving traditional acupuncture with improvements on five SF36 domains, improvements on two domains for p6 acupuncture and sham acupuncture, and improvements on one domain for

N2. Acupressure is sometimes referred to as 'needle-less acupuncture' because both forms of treatment use the same points to achieve the desired results. The main difference is that an acupuncturist stimulates points by inserting needles, whereas an acupressurist stimulates the same points using finger pressure (Acupuncture Today 2003). The researchers say that acupressure and acupuncture are different modalities and cannot be compared directly. However, this is debatable since stimulation to P6 by either acupressure or acupuncture is equally regarded as a treatment for nausea (e.g. Tiran 2002), and it could also be argued that both modalities have the same effect.

23 Do you consider this to be disappointing? Write a sentence or two of reflection on how you feel about this and what it might mean

N3. The author's results indicated that increased frequency of treatment could help reduce nausea and vomiting, with recommendations made for more than two treatments in the first week. This is an important point as, in the Eastern tradition, acupuncture treatments are often carried out daily. Because of this, and as the authors note here, any future research that can inform on optimum frequency or dosage of treatment is to be welcomed since few data exist for this (Sherman & Cherkin 2003).

24 The differences between efficacy and effectiveness are that (more than one answer may be correct):

a) Effectiveness is about theory and efficacy is either about practice, or about research based on practice
b) Efficacy is about how something works in a research or laboratory setting and effectiveness is about how it works in the real world
c) Effectiveness is about systems and efficacy is about people
d) This is a trick question – they actually mean the same thing

25 List two reasons why women might have found this particular kind of trial a source of support (compared with other kinds of trials).

26 Why were women asked about 'the credibility of the treatment'?

27 What's the other name given to the effect whereby simply being in a research trial can have an effect on participants' experiences?

a) The Halo effect
b) The Kartz–Reimer effect
c) The Hawthorne effect
d) The Blinovitch limitation effect

28 Do you agree with this conclusion based on what you now know about the details of the trial?

---

no acupuncture. These results again demonstrate the efficacy of traditional acupuncture in improving women's physical and emotional well-being compared with women receiving no acupuncture, and improving women's vitality compared with the use of p6 and sham acupuncture. Evidence of a placebo effect was demonstrated with sham acupuncture, which improved women's emotional well-being and social function.

The use of traditional acupuncture as a treatment for nausea and vomiting provided an opportunity to practice acupuncture in a traditional Chinese medicine framework compared with the use of a single acupuncture point p6. The study findings support the validity of the traditional Chinese medicine approach compared with the sole use of p6 acupuncture point.

The existence of a placebo effect in health care is well established, multifaceted, and composed of several nonspecific effects. Recent work by Hrobjartsson and Gotzsche found little evidence that placebo effects had any powerful clinical influence (20). We suggest that the placebo effect demonstrated in our trial may have been affected by women finding the trial a source of support. Moreover, the weekly treatments provided an opportunity for the development of a relationship between study participants and the practitioner. It would not be unreasonable to assume that these nonspecific effects would become greater with time and contribute toward a placebo effect. No external observation of the treatment administered between study participants and practitioner was performed, and practitioner bias cannot be excluded. However, women were asked to comment on the "credibility of the treatment" to assess the effectiveness of blinding. Women were blinded to their group allocation, and these findings will be reported elsewhere. With increasing evidence of a time-related placebo effect (14), further research is warranted to understand the placebo effect and to recognize its contributions to an individual's sense of well-being.

Evidence from trials using pharmacological and nonpharmacological methods to treat nausea and vomiting in early pregnancy suggest that many effective interventions reduce the severity of symptoms rather than relieve symptoms completely (21).

Nausea and vomiting in early pregnancy remains a significant public health problem that results in physiological, emotional, social, and economic consequences on women, their families, and society. For women looking for relief from these symptoms and desiring an overall improvement in well-being, the use of acupuncture in early pregnancy will reduce or resolve symptoms earlier than simply waiting for them to improve spontaneously. Based on these findings, acupuncture can be considered an effective, nonpharmacological treatment option for women who experience nausea and dry retching in early pregnancy.

Acknowledgments

We thank the women for participating in this trial; the general practitioners, obstetricians, and midwives at the Women's and Children's Hospital for referring women to the trial; and the staff in the Maternal and Perinatal Clinical Trials Unit.

References

1. Tierson FD, Olsen CC, Hook EB. Nausea and vomiting of pregnancy: An association with pregnancy outcome. *Am J Obstet Gynecol* 1986;155:1017–1022.
2. Soules MR, Hughes CL, Garcia JA, et al. Nausea and vomiting of pregnancy: Role of human chorionic gonadotrophin and 17 hydroxyprogesterone. *Obstet Gynecol* 1980; 55:696–700.
3. Lacroix R, Eason E, Melzack R. Nausea and vomiting during pregnancy: A prospective study of its frequency, intensity and pattern of change. *Am J Obstet Gynecol* 2000; 182:931–937.
4. Smith C, Crowther C, Beilby J, Dandeaux J. The impact of nausea and vomiting on women: A burden of early pregnancy. *Aust N Z J Obstet Gynaecol* 2000;4:397–401.
5. MacLennan A, Wilson DH, Taylor AW. Prevalence and cost of alternative medicine in Australia. *Lancet 1996;347:* 569–573.
6. Eisenberg DM, Kessler RC, Foster C, et al. Unconventional medicine in the United States: Prevalence, costs and patterns of use. *N Engl J Med* 1993;328:246–352.
7. Jewell MD, Young G. Interventions for nausea and vomiting in early pregnancy. In: *The Cochrane Library*. Issue 2. Oxford: Update Software, 2001.
8. Dundee JW, Sourial FB, Ghaly RG, Bell PF. P6 acupressure reduces morning sickness. *J R Soc Med* 1988;81:456–457.
9. Belluomini J, Litt RC, Lee KA, Katz M. Acupressure for nausea and vomiting in pregnancy: A randomized blinded study. *Obstet Gynecol* 1994;84:245–248.
10. De Aloysio D, Penacchioni P. Morning sickness control in early pregnancy by Neiguan point acupressure. *Obstet Gynecol* 1992;80:852–854.
11. O'Brien B, Relyea MJ, Taerum T. Efficacy of P6 acupressure in the treatment of nausea and vomiting during pregnancy. *Am J Obstet Gynecol* 1996;174:708–715.
12. Rongjun Z. 39 Cases of morning sickness treated with acupuncture. *J Trad Chin Med* 1987;7:25–26.
13. Changxin Z. Acupuncture treatment of morning sickness. *J Trad Chin Med* 1988;8:228–229.
14. Knight B, Mudge C, Openshaw S, White A. Effect of acupuncture on nausea of pregnancy: A randomized, controlled trial. *Obstet Gynecol* 2001;9:184–188.
15. Maciocia G. *Obstetrics and Gynecology in Chinese Medicine.* New York: Churchill Livingstone, 1998:451–463.
16. Rhodes VA, Watson PM, Johnson MH. Development of a reliable and valid measure for nausea and vomiting. *Cancer Nurs* 1984;7:33–41.

BIRTH 29:1 March 2002

9

17. Ware JE, Sherbourne CD. The MOS 36 Item Short Form Health Survey (SF-36): Conceptual framework and item selection. *Med Care* 1992;30:473–483.

18. Klebanoff MA, Koslowe PA, Kaslow R, Rhoads GG. Epidemiology of vomiting in early pregnancy. *Obstet Gynecol* 1985;66:612–616.

19. SPSS, Inc. *Statistical Package for the Social Sciences [Version 10.0]*. Chicago: 1988.

20. Hrobjartsson A, Gotzsche PC. Is the placebo powerless? An analysis of clinical trials comparing placebo with no treatment. *N Engl J Med* 2001:344:1594–1602.

21. O'Brien B, Zhou Q. Variables related to nausea and vomiting during pregnancy. *Birth* 1995;22:93–100.

ANSWERS

Q1. b) Prevalence, which is the measure of a condition or disease (nausea and vomiting) in a given population (pregnant women) at a point in time. Incidence is the number of new cases of a disease which occur over a given period of time

Q2. We can't really tell, and this is a difficult question to answer partly because we don't know very much about the researchers and partly because we need to be careful in making assumptions about a person's ability from his or her name, background and qualifications! The fact that at least one researcher is interested in and has experience of treating people with acupuncture might support the study, although it might also lead to potential bias, and the fact that they may have grown up in the Western hemisphere (although we don't know this either) might lead them to have a philosophy that doesn't totally embrace Eastern healing modalities and/or might allow them to be less biased than if they did!

Q3. Well, it depends on your perspective! It is useful to support statements like this with references because it evidences that this is not simply the writer's opinion or personal experience. However, this doesn't mean that experience isn't valuable and, sometimes, it is impossible to provide references because no-one else has documented what you want to say. It is also possible to become a slave to referencing and this is not necessarily useful. In this case, it might have been helpful if the authors had clarified whether this statement was made from their personal experience or the general experience of the profession

Q4. We feel this could have an impact on the research because Traditional Chinese Medicine doesn't seek to suppress symptoms but to help bring about rebalance!

Q5. d) Both. Given that this research was an RCT, it made sense for the researchers to review the other RCTs before beginning. However, the Cochrane review focuses on well-designed, experimental research, and it is possible that other studies, which may not have been included in the Cochrane review, could still have been valuable in helping to design the study and/or enabling exploration of other aspects of clinical questions

Q6. b) Although with this trial it is more questionable whether the participants really didn't know, or whether they could have worked it out from what they experienced. The researchers tried to deal with this potential problem by including sham acupuncture and they also explored this issue by asking women about credibility, which they discuss later in the paper

Q7. Yes, we feel they were. Women were admitted to the trial if they were less than 14 weeks into their pregnancy and suffering from nausea or vomiting. Those experiencing dehydration were excluded, or if there was a chance that the symptoms were not due to pregnancy. This ensured that only women with nausea and vomiting in pregnancy were studied. Treatment for nausea and vomiting may not have been successful for women with complications such as dehydration, or symptoms of different aetiology, and their inclusion could have affected results by showing a higher negative response rate to treatment. If the assessments of women's symptoms were correct then these exclusions were justified to reduce the possibility of bias entering into the trial by eliminating potentially confounding variables

Q8. Maybe – women using anti-emetic drugs or other measures to prevent nausea and vomiting were not screened out of the trial, which may be a potential source of bias. There is a need to balance the ethical implications of asking women to refrain from such measures with the potential impact of this kind of additional variable on trial results, as it is possible that a better improvement rate may have been attributed to acupuncture when it was partially due to anti-emetics

Q9. To obtain informed consent it is important that those participating in the trial are made fully aware of the nature of the research and the demands it will make upon them, including the potential costs, time and inconvenience and any risks or disbenefits as well as any potential benefits. Issues such as confidentiality and the assurance that women's care will not otherwise be affected should also be discussed

Q10. Randomisation itself is a crucial feature of any good RCT, which guarantees that the differences in the attributes of the sample emerge by chance. This decreases the probability of selecting a sample that is unrepresentative of the population. Random assignment of the sample into groups means each group tends to have participants with equivalent traits, so that any trends identified in the results can be attributed to the experimental treatment. The women were randomised into four groups by a researcher who was independent of the study. Using an independent service gives the best chance of eliminating bias and should have allowed for a good distribution of demographic and other characteristics across all four groups

Q11. In this trial, having four groups meant that it would be possible to analyse some of the differences between different approaches to treating nausea and vomiting, e.g. comparing traditional and P6 acupuncture. There is merit in allocating groups for both traditional as well as P6 acupuncture since Traditional Chinese Medicine is a far more individualised treatment than the single P6 point acupuncture, and this allowed for pragmatic results that mirror real-world acupuncture treatment (MacPherson 2000). It also provided for a control group – in the form of the sham acupuncture group – who, at least in theory, would have been 'blind' to whether they were having real or sham acupuncture. By including four groups the researchers were employing a fair test of the efficacy of Traditional Chinese Medicine

Q12. This is about attempting to reduce bias. There are two big advantages of the researcher/acupuncturist assessing everybody before she knew which group they would go into. One is that the assessment does not then act as a confounding variable; although it seems unlikely, it might be that the assessment itself could have made a difference to women's nausea and vomiting but as everybody experienced the assessment, the potential for confounding in this part of the study is removed. Perhaps more importantly, the researcher's assessment of each woman was performed without knowing which group she would go into, which reduces the risk of researcher bias in this aspect of the study method. As the researcher continued to perform the treatment for all those receiving traditional acupuncture, P6 acupuncture and sham acupuncture, the question of researcher bias entering the trial cannot be removed completely, but the a priori assessment is a step towards reducing it

Q13. We can't tell. It may well have been long enough, or the results may have been different if the treatment had continued for another 2 or 4 weeks. For many pregnant women, nausea and vomiting do not last for an enormously long time (which is not to underestimate the effect they can have while they do last) and so, with this in mind, there is the question of whether women would want to use a treatment that took 8 weeks to have a significant impact. It is a question of balancing what is practical and what is acceptable, while giving the treatment a 'fair chance' of accurate evaluation

Q14. This method of placebo treatment, while admirable in that it seeks to make the study 'single blind' (and thus reduce the potential placebo effect), is far from ideal. Needling near an acupuncture point is problematic since some people argue that acupuncture point selection is not precise enough to guarantee that the point chosen is not an active point (e.g. Aird et al 2000). The approach used by medical acupuncturists often involves inserting needles for general pain relief to an area without regard to specific points, and this does produce a physiological effect (Mann 1992) and any kind of needle insertion may trigger reactions in the skin and tissues similar to, or the same as, those achieved by true acupuncture, particularly when near a specific point (Gaw et al 1975). It is, therefore, virtually impossible to guarantee that this type of control treatment is inert (Hopwood & Lewith 2003). This method may have mimicked the effects of real acupuncture by producing an increased reduction in symptoms in the sham group, thus preventing an unbiased comparison of the sham group's results with the other groups

The potential effects of invasive sham acupuncture are of such significance that this could be a serious methodological flaw in the study design (Birch 2003) which means the trial may be inadequately constructed to answer the question posed by the researchers. A non-specific control such as that used here is one of the great challenges of research into acupuncture (Sherman et al 2002)

Q15. Well… this is another of those grey areas to which there is no absolute answer, so we were a bit naughty to ask you to choose between 'true' and 'false' – sorry! We need to bear in mind that, as it says in the line above the paragraph relating to this question, the control group were included to control for the effect of spontaneous remission of symptoms. However, the women in the no acupuncture/control group were given dietary advice and advice on using pyridoxine (vitamin B6) during the 4-week study period. This is a potential pitfall since at least two trials have shown positive effects from taking pyridoxine for NVP (Vutyavanich et al 1995, Sahakian et al 1991), with a reduction noted in severity of nausea and vomiting. This could have influenced the results in this group – and may not give us an accurate measure of spontaneous remission of symptoms – although it is not clear if some or all participants took pyridoxine or not. However, the researchers were keen to ensure that the women in the control group were not disappointed or they may not have remained in the trial. It could also have been seen as unethical to offer no advice or treatment to these women who were, after all, experiencing nausea and vomiting as well

Q16. The SF36 (or any other numerical tool) can be a relatively quick and simple way of recording well-being. However, there is an argument for an element of qualitative data collection to be included here since the questions on the SF36 may not have had the scope to represent each woman's individual experience of nausea and vomiting. One advantage of the women being asked to record their own scores would be the elimination of any bias that might have arisen in the interaction with the researcher, or misinterpretation by the researcher. It also saves the researchers' time, money and effort and may enable women to feel that they are true participants in the research. However, women may not have understood some of the questions and/or may have filled the SF36 out quickly; let's not forget that they were all experiencing nausea, which might not cause you to want – or be able – to spend lots of time on filling out forms!

Q17. Yes and No. Yes, because the 10% loss to follow-up rate allowed for in the power calculation was within the normal range for a study of this kind, so it was not an unreasonable choice for the researchers to make at the onset of the study. However, if you look at Figure 1 and the corresponding text, you will see that only 75% of women returned data at the end of the trial, leading to a 25% loss to follow-up rate, which may affect the significance of the results obtained

Q18. b). The reason c) is not true (although it might look like it could be!) is that the p value is not the starting point for data analysis

Q19. In our opinion, false, because it is not clear to us from the diagram how the numbers in each successive box are calculated. Have a look at the line showing the return of nausea and vomiting questionnaires in the traditional acupuncture group – the boxes on the left, as they go from top to bottom. 147 out of 148 women returned them on day 1, and 135 on day 7. But does this mean that the researchers removed the woman who didn't return the form on day 1 from the study, or was she still in the study? Also, if you look at the total number of forms not completed (27) and pregnancy losses (6) in this group, this does not seem to tally with the numbers of forms not returned at each stage of the research. (If you want to check this for yourself, subtract the number of forms not returned each day from 148 and then add those numbers together – you certainly don't get a number anywhere near 27 + 6!) The suggestion that women might have been removed from the study if they didn't complete forms seems to fall down when you look at the vertical line of boxes relating to the SF36 questionnaires in the sham acupuncture group, because more women returned these on day 28 than day 14. All in all, it is rather difficult to make sense of what this figure is actually telling us, and how it relates to the brief statement about response rates in the text

Q20. e) We can't tell, although it could be due to a), c) and/or d)! The reason why we can't tell is not because the study is poorly designed (although we have discussed the problems raised by the use of sham acupuncture above) but because this kind of research can only tell us what happened, not why or how it happened

Q21. True. We, like the researchers, noticed that, although the four groups are similar in most characteristics, there appeared to be more of a difference in the numbers of women who had experienced acupuncture before and, to a lesser extent, in the number of women who were private 'patients'. However, the researchers carried out statistical tests to see if the differences between the groups in these categories were statistically significant (hence the little footnotes under the table relating to these two categories) and found that they were not

Q22. c) 0.001, because this means that there is a one in a thousand chance that the result came about by chance alone, compared to a one in a hundred chance with a p value of 0.01 and a one in 20 chance with a p value of 0.05. See the guide to statistics in Section 6 for more on this

Q23. This is all about bias! If you find the results disappointing, this might be because you wanted acupuncture to be beneficial in reducing vomiting, or it might be because you have a personal interest in finding a treatment which is helpful. If you are not disappointed, or surprised, this might reflect that you didn't feel acupuncture was that useful in the first place, or perhaps that you were really open-minded about the question. Both responses might give you an insight into how our own bias – and that of researchers – can affect the way we write and think about research and different treatments

Q24. b)

Q25. Most of the possible reasons for this are linked with the fact that women in some or all of the study groups would have received more attention than they might normally have done. Women in the trial may have been able to spend more time with the practitioner than they might have with a midwife or doctor with a Western approach, or in a different kind of trial, which would give them more time to ask questions. The fact that they were filling out questionnaires relatively frequently might mean that some women were reflecting on how they felt more than usual, which could have had a positive effect. Also, participants might have had more time to discuss and/or explore the way they were feeling (both physically and emotionally) with someone else in a trial involving Traditional Chinese Medicine than in trials involving drugs or other kinds of Western treatments

Q26. In order to further explore the placebo effect. This might also help determine whether the women in the trial really were 'blind' to the treatment they had experienced, i.e. whether the sham or P6 acupuncture was perceived differently from the traditional acupuncture. Because the results of this part of the trial are reported elsewhere, we don't know anything else about this from the paper, but if you are interested in this area, you may like to look this up and see if you can find further work from the same authors

Q27. c) The Hawthorne effect, which was named after the Hawthorne plant in Illinois. This factory was the setting of a study to assess whether changes in the environment improved workers' productivity and the results showed that, no matter what the researchers did to manipulate the environment, productivity improved. The conclusion was drawn that the mere presence of the researchers and the attention that was paid to workers had a positive effect on productivity

Q28. The answer to this one is up to you, although you'll be able to read our thoughts in the discussion that follows these answers

DISCUSSION

Those of us in the West live in a culture that requires medical treatments to be 'proven' to gain validation (Seale et al 2001). However, a wealth of anecdotal evidence supports the effectiveness of acupuncture and Aldridge (2000) believes that anecdotal stories are both reliable and rich in useful information. However, Western medicine considers these unreliable as 'evidence' and the successes of acupuncture are often dismissed as merely a placebo effect (White et al 2001) or psychosomatic cure (Kaptchuk 1983). Mann (2000) disagrees with this, suggesting that suffers of migraine or sciatica would find little relief from visiting a psychiatrist whereas acupuncture could help them in most cases.

There are clearly differences of opinion in the West but one of the biggest issues raised here is whether we can judge modalities like acupuncture and Traditional Chinese Medicine solely by Western standards:

> Chinese medicine is a coherent system of thought that does not require validation by the West as an intellectual construct. Intellectually, the way to approach Chinese concepts is to see whether they are internally logical and consistent, not to dismiss them because they do not conform to Western notions. (Kaptchuk 1983 p 52)

Most of the RCTs conducted in this area have focused on outcomes that are easier to measure by Western standards, such as pain management and the relief of nausea and sickness, and acupuncture has often been shown to be effective (Hopwood & Lewith 2003). However, by searching for one specific effect, such as relief from nausea and vomiting, researchers don't always consider that a cure might be the consequence of a number of different influences. In fact, the Chinese would consider Western medicine to be out of balance in seeking one specific aspect that created a cure (Kaptchuk 1983).

Traditional Chinese Medicine and acupuncture are uniquely different from Western biomedicine *because* of the reliance on the practitioner–patient interaction (Lao & Ezzo 2003). Yet this is the very kind of thing that makes the RCT a debatable tool for researching non-Western healing modalities – it is based on the idea of separation (e.g. of groups, of different influences), yet how do you separate out the difference between the effect of the needles, the effect of how the person feels during the treatment (which can be very soothing, relaxing or energising) and the effect of the practitioner? The researchers have attempted to separate out the effect of the specific acupuncture points by including a sham acupuncture group but, as we have suggested in the 'answers' section above, this is not without its problems. We also wondered whether the women receiving traditional acupuncture would have possibly had longer sessions than those receiving P6 acupuncture, and may additionally have had more faith in an approach that employed more needles?

The time-related placebo effect is another interesting issue to think about a bit further. The researchers note that women in the traditional acupuncture group reported less frequent and shorter periods of nausea at the end of the first week. This was a feature in the second week for those in the P6 acupuncture group as well as for the women in the traditional acupuncture group, and by the third week those women in the sham acupuncture group also reported improvement compared with the no acupuncture control group. This may be because of the placebo effect – which we know is an issue in health care generally – but it could also indicate that sham acupuncture does have a non-specific effect and could therefore be a confounding factor.

You might have noticed that most of the issues we have raised were not necessarily huge failings of this study or of the researchers – who found some very creative ways to get around the problems they faced – but are wider issues raised by the question of whether we can use Western frameworks to research and evaluate non-Western healing modalities. We are hopeful that, in the future, we will see a movement towards designing research methods that can be used to evaluate and explore non-Western approaches in ways that align with and are respectful of their underpinning philosophies, rather than trying to force non-Western healing modalities into Western evaluative frameworks. However, in the meantime, there is no reason to disregard further research into other areas of acupuncture or other non-Western modalities – the key is to be cognisant of the issues and challenges that such research faces. Despite the complicated issues that we are raising for discussion here, the research in this chapter has attempted to include the Traditional Chinese Medicine approach within a study which uses Western research methods and provides a useful example of how this can be done.

This study does seem to show that traditional acupuncture is more beneficial than single point acupuncture for nausea, although it doesn't show a difference for vomiting. Before reading this study, we both believed (from both experience and earlier research) that acupuncture was one of a range of treatments that could be helpful to women experiencing nausea and vomiting in pregnancy. As a result of the study, should we change our view to incorporate the evidence that acupuncture is useful for nausea but not for vomiting? We think not – although the study shows no difference in vomiting when you compared the traditional acupuncture group to the other three groups, this was because all of the women in *all* of the groups experienced less vomiting by the end of the study. Consequently, the lack of difference between the groups might be because of spontaneous remission, or might be because all of the treatments worked, whether this was because of a treatment effect, placebo effect or, in the 'control' group, because the women took the advice offered and used other alternative treatments.

What will you take away from this study and the discussion around it? Individual practitioners have a decision to make when it comes to suggesting that women look into treatments which do not come under the Western medical umbrella. Do you feel it is preferable to warn women that some so-called alternative treatments have not been well evaluated (by Western methods) and advise them to steer clear of them? Or do you feel it is better to offer women as many options as possible, which might include things that seem to have helped others but that have not been well evaluated by Western research methods? A dilemma may exist for practitioners who are wary of embracing treatments that are, by current Western standards, unproven, yet are aware that those same treatments appear to offer positive experiences and outcomes to people who have used them. The key issue for us is the need to tailor suggestions for treatment to the individual woman, perhaps along with some discussion around the kinds of issues we have raised here. This returns us very neatly to the importance of the therapeutic relationship, which is simultaneously the cornerstone of holistic practice *and* the reason why it is so difficult to evaluate some kinds of treatment which form a part of that practice.

References

Acupuncture Today 2003 Available online at: http://www.acupuncturetoday.com/abc/acupressure.html [accessed 8 December 2003]

Aird M, Cobbin DM, Zaslawski C 2000 A study of the comparative accuracy of two methods of locating acupuncture points. Acupuncture and Medicine 18:15–21

Aldridge D 2000 Spirituality, healing and medicine: return to the silence. Jessica Kingsley Publishers, London

Allaire AD, Moos MK, Wells SR 2000 Complementary and alternative medicine in pregnancy: a survey of North Carolina certified nurse-midwives. Alternative Medicine in Pregnancy 5(1):19–23

Birch S 2003 Overview of models used in controlled acupuncture studies and thoughts about questions answerable by each. Clinical Acupuncture and Oriental Medicine 3:207–217

Einarson TR, Koren G, Bergman U 1998 Nausea and vomiting in pregnancy: a comparative European study. European Journal of Obstetrics and Gynaecology and Reproductive Biology 76:1–3

Erick M 1997 Nausea and vomiting in pregnancy. ACOG Clinical Review Volume 2, Issue 3. American College of Obstetricians and Gynecologists, Washington DC

Firebrace P, Hill S 1988 A guide to acupuncture. Hamlyn Publishing, London

Gadsby R, Barnie-Adshead AM, Jagger C 1993 A prospective study of nausea and vomiting during pregnancy. British Journal of General Practice 43(373):325

Gaw AC, Chang LW, Shaw LC 1975 Efficacy of acupuncture on osteoarthritic pain. A controlled, double blind study. New England Journal of Medicine 293:375–378

Hopwood V, Lewith G 2003 Acupuncture trials and methodological considerations. Clinical Acupuncture and Oriental Medicine 3:192–199

Kaptchuk TJ 1983 The web that has no weaver: understanding Chinese medicine. Congdon & Weed, Chicago

Lao L, Ezzo J 2003 Designing acupuncture trials: one size does not fit all. Clinical Acupuncture and Oriental Medicine 3:218–221

Larsson HJ 1999 Alternative medicine: why so popular? Health News, Issue 93, September 1999. 1320 Point Street Victoria, BC, Canada V8S 1A5

Long L, Huntley A, Ernst E 2001 Which complementary and alternative therapies benefit which conditions? A survey of the opinions of 223 professional organizations. Complementary Therapies in Medicine 9:178–185

MacPherson H 2000 Out of the laboratory and into the clinic: acupuncture research in the real world. Clinical Acupuncture and Oriental Medicine 1(2):97–100

Mann F 1992 Reinventing acupuncture. Butterworth-Heinemann, Oxford

Mazzotta P, Magee LA, Maltepe C et al 1999 The perception of teratogenic risk by women with nausea and vomiting of pregnancy. Reproductive Toxicology 13:313–319

Mazzotta P, Stewart DE, Koren G, Magee LA 2001 Factors associated with elective termination of pregnancy among Canadian and American women with nausea and vomiting of pregnancy. Journal of Psychosomatic Obstetrics and Gynaecology 22(1):7–12

Newman Turner R 1990 Naturopathic medicine; treating the whole person. Thorsons, Wellingborough, Northamptonshire

O'Brien B, Naber S 1992 Nausea and vomiting during pregnancy: effects on the quality of women's lives. Birth 19(3):138–143

Power ML, Holzman GB, Schulkin J 2001 A survey on the management of nausea and vomiting in pregnancy by obstetrician/gynecologists. Primary Care Update for Obstetrics and Gynecology 8(2):69–72

Sahakian V, Rouse D, Sipes S et al 1991 Vitamin B6 is effective for nausea and vomiting of pregnancy: a randomised, double-blind, placebo-controlled study. Obstetrics and Gynaecology 78(1):33–36

Seale C, Pattison S, Davey B 2001 Medical knowledge: doubt and certainty. Open University Press, Buckingham

Sherman KJ, Cherkin DC 2003 Challenges of acupuncture research: study design considerations. Clinical Acupuncture and Oriental Medicine 3:200–206

Sherman KJ, Lao L, MacPherson H et al 2002 Matching acupuncture clinical study designs to research questions. Clinical Acupuncture and Oriental Medicine 3:12–15

Tiran D 2002 Nausea and vomiting in pregnancy: safety and efficacy of self-administered complementary therapies. Complementary Therapies in Nursing and Midwifery 8:191–196

Vellacott ID, Cooke EJ, James CE 1988 Nausea and vomiting in early pregnancy. International Journal of Obstetrics and Gynaecology 27:57–62

Vutyavanich T, Wongtra-ngan S, Ruangsri R 1995 Pyridoxine for nausea and vomiting of pregnancy: a randomised, double-blind, placebo-controlled trial. American Journal of Obstetrics and Gynecology 173(3 Part 1):881–884

White AR, Filshie J, Cummings TM 2001 Clinical trials of acupuncture: consensus recommendations for optimal treatment, sham controls and blinding. Complementary Therapies in Medicine 9:237–245

Women's experiences

INTRODUCTION

As we spent the last section looking in more depth at quantitative studies, it seems like a good point to return to qualitative research. Qualitative approaches are becoming increasingly popular in birth-related research, not least because, while you almost always need your study to be at least partially quantitative if you want to evaluate an intervention, you equally almost always need your study to be qualitative if you want to explore women's experiences in depth. And, at the end of the day, childbirth and midwifery are all about women's experiences, and how those experiences are grounded in both women's lives and the bigger sociocultural picture.

The two papers in this section look in depth at these issues. In Chapter 7, Ruth Deery looks at a study that used a phenomenological approach to explore women's encounters with their midwife during childbirth. In Chapter 8, Tricia Anderson critiques an ethnographic study that, again, looks at women's experiences but also goes on to analyse these in relation to existing anthropological theories.

These are the final papers in this book and, after you have worked through these, you will have explored four very different areas of birth-related research and a number of research approaches. Of course, there are other approaches that we haven't looked at here, but the principles of appraisal are similar no matter what kind of research you are looking at. One of the key questions to consider as you are working through this section is this: Given what we can learn from women's experiences of childbirth from the kinds of research that appear in this section, is the research we are doing in the area of childbirth based on women's needs, and are our service agendas and research priorities built on what we can learn about women's experiences?

Ruth Deery

INTRODUCTION

Berg M, Lundgren I, Hermansson E 1996 Women's experience of the encounter with the midwife during childbirth. Midwifery 12(1):11–15

Qualitative research is an approach to research that claims to be holistic, humanistic and person centred. The researcher focuses on the uniqueness of the participants, valuing their contribution to the research process and their different experiences and interpretations of social situations. Researchers who work within the qualitative paradigm use subjective experiences (of their participants and/or themselves) to further understand complex and difficult human situations or problems (Patton 2002) with a view to developing and generating theory. This approach to research is therefore particularly suitable for midwifery, where women's and midwives' experiences of the maternity services are to be explored with a view to seeking better understanding of these experiences. We are fortunate in midwifery to have access to research that now has international standing. When evaluating such research it is important to remember that the first language of the researchers may not be English.

So, what is phenomenology? What does phenomenology have to offer in order that you can develop your midwifery practice further? How can you evaluate the appropriateness of this phenomenological study? Should you incorporate the findings of this study into your midwifery practice? These are questions that I hope you will be able to answer after reading this chapter so that you can make an informed decision.

Phenomenology (a difficult word to pronounce!) is a qualitative approach to research where the nature and meaning of an experience are the focus of the research. Over the years, however, phenomenology has become harder to define. This is because it has become more and more popular with researchers and definitions have become confused and diluted (Patton 2002). Several authors have suggested that phenomenological researchers have misinterpreted phenomenology (Crotty 1996, Paley 1997, 1998) because it can refer either to a philosophy or to a research methods framework. Walters (1995) believes this confusion has led researchers to refer to phenomenology as if it was a 'homogenous philosophical school' (p 791). Crotty (1996) challenged the interpretation and conduct of phenomenological research in nursing, referring to it as 'so-called phenomenology'. He accused English nurse researchers of being descriptive, uncritical and subjective. Barkway (2001), writing in support of Michael Crotty, explores this phenomenological debate further, stating that Crotty wanted researchers not to uncritically accept what their research participants told them – because their perceptions could be distorted or mistaken.

In terms of a philosophical tradition, phenomenology was developed by the German philosopher Edmund Husserl. He believed that people could only know what they experienced, and that this happened by paying attention to perceptions and meanings that might increase a person's conscious awareness. Husserlian phenomenology therefore deals with the nature of reality and researchers had to become in touch with their own conscious awareness, be able to interpret this experience and therefore the 'essence' of the experience.

To interpret these 'essences' or 'lived experiences', researchers had to engage in reduction or 'bracketing' (Paley 1997). Reduction involves reducing a complex problem (let's use stress in midwifery as an example) into basic components by eliminating the researcher's own prejudices about stress. Husserl believed that this would ensure a focused understanding of what was being investigated by 'putting on hold every assumption that is normally made in the "natural attitude" – the habits of mind which are characteristic of everyday understanding...' (Paley 1997 p 188). This is an important point to grasp because being able to suspend all judgements about the external world is not something that a researcher 'can just do' because 'essences' do not exist in isolation from conscious experience (Walters 1995). If this were possible, then the researcher would be immediately removed from the social world. Yet within the literature 'bracketing' is a technique that is claimed to reduce bias and preconception (Paley 1997, Patton 2002). Husserl's philosophy sought to give phenomenology the same recognition that was given to rigorous science, thereby studying phenomena in a detached, unemotional way (Gadamer 1976, Reed 1994). This approach can also be referred to as Cartesian subject–object dualism (Walters 1995). A contradiction immediately comes to mind in that a woman-centred approach is encouraged in midwifery that fosters trusting relationships and the notion of equal partners (Department of Health 1993). This might not be possible if the researcher has to study in a detached, unemotional way.

Heideggarian phenomenology represents a scientific or theoretical approach to the world (Paley 1998, Patton 2002) where it is deemed impossible to create an understanding of the world through a rigorous scientific approach. Rather, Heidegger's phenomenology is based on an existential perspective, where understanding a stressed midwife's experience could not take place without an understanding of the midwifery workplace. As such, the researcher would concentrate on the phenomenon under investigation (for example, stress in midwifery) and then try to make sense of this so that a worldview (or a midwifery view) could be developed. The notion of a single reality is not possible in Heideggarian phenomenology and would take into account that every midwife can experience stress differently, thus creating multiple realties of stress in the workplace.

Heidegger therefore attempted to reinterpret Husserlian phenomenology by arguing that it was impossible to bracket everyday understanding because human reality could not be objectified. Instead, Heidegger believed that understanding the ordinary everyday existence of people was essential and that people are in and of the world, rather than subjects in a world of objects (Reed 1994). The phenomenological method that Heidegger used for analysis was a hermeneutic (or interpretive) approach that presupposes prior understanding on the part of the researcher (Walters 1995). 'Bracketing' therefore is not congruent with all phenomenological research.

Nevertheless, at the end of the day, phenomenology aims to focus on exploring how research participants make sense of experience (Patton 2002). This is a highly suitable approach for midwifery research where women and/or midwives are often encouraged to perceive, describe, judge, remember and make sense of their experiences within the maternity services. Thus, phenomenological research provides an approach that enables women and/or midwives who have directly experienced or have 'lived experience' of a phenomenon (for example, caesarean section, home birth, stress, midwifery work or the culture of midwifery) to provide further insights and bring their experiences and understanding to the research process.

Women's experience of the encounter with the midwife during childbirth

Marie Berg, Ingela Lundgren, Evelyn Hermansson and Vivian Wahlberg

Marie Berg
RNM, BNSc, Midwife,
Obstetric Medicine Ward,
Department of Obstetrics
and Gynecology, Sahlgrenska
University Hospital, 413 45
Gothenburg

Ingela Lundgren
RNM, BNSc, Midwife
ABC-Centre, Department of
Obstetrics and Gynecology,
Sahlgrenska University
Hospital, Gothenburg

Evelyn Hermansson
RNM, BA, Dipl Ed.
Post-graduate Student
Department of Advanced
Nursing Education, Göteborg
University

Vivian Wahlberg
RNM, Dr. MedSci, Professor
The Nordic School of Public
Health, Gothenburg, Sweden

(Requests for offprints to MB)
Manuscript accepted
15 December 1995

Objective: to describe women's experience of the encounter with the midwife during childbirth.
Design: a qualitative study using a phenomenological approach. Data were collected via tape-recorded interviews.
Setting: the Alternative Birth Care Centre, Sahlgrenska University Hospital, Gothenburg, Sweden in 1994.
Participants: 18 women, six primiparous and 12 multiparous who were two to four days post delivery.
Key findings: the essential structure of the studied phenomenon was described as 'presence' and included three themes: to be seen as an individual, to have a trusting relationship and to be supported and guided on one's own terms.
Implications for practice: the need to be seen as an individual can be realised by affirmation and familiarity with the midwife and surroundings. A trusting relationship can be obtained by good communication and proficient behaviour. By providing a sense of control the women can be supported and guided on their own terms. Above all they must feel that the midwife is present.

INTRODUCTION

It should be the aim of each midwife to provide individualised care and to develop a close and co-operative relationship with each woman. During this century maternity care in the developed world has undergone massive change. Deliveries which previously took place at home with a familiar attendant, now occur in institutions, and are characterised by protocols and increased alienation. Today nearly all deliveries take place in hospitals and many women have expressed feelings of alienation during their hospital stay. According to Macintyre (1982) some women felt that their body and baby were owned by the hospital. A number of studies show communication difficulties to be one of the biggest complaints among childbearing and birthing women (Cartwright 1979, Kirke 1980, Macintyre 1982, MacIntosh 1988). The encounter between client/patient and care provider is of central importance in all care situations and a necessary condition for practising good care is to establish a good relationship. This is valid in maternity care as well, where the midwife plays a vital role.

The science of nursing has its origins in a humanistic approach. Each person is seen as a unique, open creature with freedom of choice in every situation and with an ability to be responsible for his or her own choices (von Wright 1988). Paterson and Zderad (1976) describe a 'humanistic nursing practice theory' which focuses on the encounter. In their theory, nursing is an experience lived between human beings, it is a lived human dialogue, a nurturing, inter-subjective transaction in which there is a real sharing which involves both a mode of being and doing.

This approach is of special importance at the Alternative Birth Care centre (ABC-centre). The characteristics of ABC-centres are continuity of care, restriction of medical technology, parental responsibility and self-care. There have been two such centres in Sweden since the late 1980s. An ABC-centre was started in Gothenburg 1988. As antenatal care is not provided in the centre but by other agencies a preparatory visit before the delivery is integrated in this service.

The aim of the study reported in this paper was to describe the encounter between the birthing women and the midwife during childbirth.

METHODS

To be able to describe fully the dialogue between a birthing woman and midwife, we need to enter deeply into this encounter. This is possible with a phenomenological approach. Phenomenology is a philosophy as well as a research method. The word 'phenomena' is derived from a greek verb 'phainomenon' which means to show or appear. The philosopher from

QUESTIONS FOR CHAPTER 7

1 The purpose of the abstract is to:
a) Provide a description of the participants
b) Provide a clear and succinct outline of the study
c) Highlight the headings within the study
d) Identify the research question

2 Do you feel this is a useful abstract? Yes/No/Maybe

3 Background information about the authors/researchers is important. True/False

4 The purpose of including a literature review is to:
a) Inform the reader what is already known about the research area
b) Describe and summarise previous research
c) Provide a systematic, critical and comparative review of previous research
d) Identify literature from one discipline only

5 Do the researchers make it clear which phenomenological tradition they are using? Yes/No/Maybe

6 Can you say, in your own words, what is meant by 'intersubjectivity'?

which phenomenology emerged is Edmund Husserl (1965) who challenged individuals to 'go back to the things themselves' (p.102), and see the everyday world as it appears varied and complex, i.e. the life world perspective. The philosopher Merleau-Ponty (1976) describes intersubjectivity and co-existence with others as *central concepts* in the life world perspective. The phenomenological method began to crystallise in reaction to the denigration of philosophical knowledge and the objectification of humans (Omery 1983). It affords a new way to interpret the nature of consciousness of an individual's involvement in the world (Beck 1994). The purpose of phenomenological research is to describe experiences as they are lived and it is an *attempt to understand a phenomenon from the* perspective of those individuals being studied. The method seeks to uncover the meaning of humanly experienced phenomena through the analysis of subjects' descriptions (Parse et al 1985). The analysis of the data, through abstracting the words of those interviewed, discovers the essence of the experience, which responds to the research question (Oiler 1982, Burns & Grove 1993).

Phenomenology involves four basic steps: bracketing, intuition, analysing and describing (Spiegelberg 1965). Bracketing means that the researcher holds in abeyance theoretical and experiential knowledge, preconceived notions or expectations about the phenomenon. Through intuition the researcher examines the phenomenon with wide open eyes, absorbs it without being possessed by it. During analysis the descriptions are compared and contrasted, and recurring elements are noticed. In the final operation a description of what has been revealed is formulated. Here the researcher discovers, describes and discusses the essence of the lived experience (Oiler 1982).

Inclusion and exclusion criteria

Women were invited to participate if they had had a normal delivery and had a good knowledge of the Swedish language. Both primiparous and multiparous women were included. Women were not invited to participate if they had been cared for by any of the researchers or had been discharged from the centre less then two days after delivery.

Conduct of the study

The women were invited to participate after delivery and one to two days before the interview. Permission to conduct and tape-record the interviews was obtained from each woman and each was assured that all information would be treated confidentially. Two to four days after

7 List two advantages and disadvantages of using interviews as a method of data collection in this kind of study

8 List three other means of collecting qualitative data

9 It is ethically acceptable to simply inform women that information will be treated 'confidentially'. True/False

delivery the women were interviewed on one occasion by one of two interviewers (MB, IL). The interviews lasted 45 to 75 minutes and were made in a private setting. A tape-recorder was used to record the interviews. The initial question was 'Can you tell me about the encounter with the midwife/midwives during delivery?'. The woman was encouraged to describe all her feelings and experiences fully and without interruption.

Data analysis

The interviews were transcribed and analysed according to the phenomenological approach. Each interview was read through to gain a feeling of entirety. The descriptions were again read and essential meaning units were marked. The meanings were then organised into different themes by relating them to each other. After reading through once again and reflecting on the emerging themes, the descriptions of the women were abstracted to a more concept-defined vocabulary. Finally, the essential structure of the phenomenon was formulated.

Ethical approval and permission to undertake the study was obtained from the physician in charge of the maternity ward, Sahlgrenska University Hospital.

FINDINGS

The sample consisted of 18 women who had given birth at the ABC-centre, Sahlgrenska Hospital in 1994. Six of the women were primiparous, seven had had their second baby, four their third and one her fourth baby. The women's ages varied between 23 and 38 years. Three-quarters of them had upper secondary school or university education.

The meaning units were organised in three different themes: to be seen as an individual, to have a trusting relationship and to be supported and guided on one's own terms. The themes do not have clear boundaries but there are some overlaps. Women who had a negative delivery experience described disturbances in one or more of the themes.

To be seen as an individual

The women emphasised the importance of being met on an equal level and with respect, and to be seen for oneself without having to feel ashamed of their behaviour. The midwife should see their needs:

> She treated me with respect, not looking down from a superior position but on the same level. (Interview 9)

10 What is the purpose of informed consent?

11 Was written informed consent obtained from the participants? Yes/No/Maybe/We can't tell

12 Was the study approved by a research ethics committee? Yes/No/Maybe/We can't tell

13 Do you think that they went through appropriate ethical procedures? Yes/No/Maybe/We can't tell

14 List four ways in which researchers can ensure rigour within their research

I think it's important that she can see a little more … my needs. You are afraid that she'll think you are mean, that you cry too much … you want to feel that you can do as you want and that she (the midwife) understands you. (Interview 7)

This was the first time I felt that someone listened to me and not just to the baby's heartbeat. (Interview 9)

One woman felt she was not seen as an individual. This is shown in this quotation:

But I felt as she always came just two minutes too late … I felt as if half of her was still in the other room. (Interview 5)

To have a trusting relationship

The women wanted the midwife to be friendly and gentle.

She was so very nice and gentle and I felt that she understood. (Interview 15)

Other qualities of importance were openness and conveyance of safety. This mediated a feeling of tranquillity and security, and the woman could relax and feel she was participating in decisions. In this way she gained control of the situation:

It was very important to feel secure. Then I could listen to my body and wasn't so frightened. I gained control over the whole plan and it worked. (Interview 1)

Many women expressed the importance of interpersonal congruity:

Then I felt that she suited me very well and there was a balance. (Interview 5)

The midwife's intuition and availability was important. This was expressed when she saw the needs and assisted the woman without a verbal request from her:

She helped when she saw that maybe I had back-pain … I never had to say anything. I don't know if it was done consciously. (Interview 2)

She was able to stay in the background without letting slip of us … I never felt deserted, someone was always there. (Interview 3)

If any of these characteristics was lacking the women felt a lack of confidence in the midwife which resulted in communication problems. One woman said:

I felt that we didn't talk, we were not on the same wavelength. We had no direct communication. (Interview 16)

To be supported and guided on one's own terms

The women wanted support and encouragement. When it was necessary they wanted to be guided by the midwife, but on their own terms. There was a greater need for guidance during the more intensive part of the labour:

To be advised but not forced … she encouraged at the right time and she believed that I was able to manage. (Interview 12)

There was a need to be encouraged to listen to the innermost feelings. It was also important to be left in peace when this was desired:

I wanted to listen to myself. (Interview 4)

No one could touch me and it was good that I had a midwife with whom I could relate and I could be in my own world and remain there. (Interview 7)

Sometimes when the women wanted to have control over the birth it was just to let the labour itself take control and to comply with it. One woman expressed it like this:

The labour was so powerful that it was impossible to control, it was just a question of following. (Interview 2)

Another said:

What enormous power! One can't control the contractions, just follow, merely drift and try to navigate a boat in storm. (Interview 18)

When the midwife needed to guide, it was important that the woman was given time in order to be able to have control over giving birth. A dialogue was required:

We discussed what we should do … eye contact, wait for my comments. (Interview 6)

Even if I received expert help … it wasn't the intention of someone else that dominated, but my own desire. (Interview 8)

If the guidance was too predominant the women had negative feelings such as fear, stress, aggression or disturbance:

But I was already so scared and it got worse and worse. Finally I was totally disturbed … I had to let her know that I wanted to remain untouched. (Interview 16)

The essential structure

The essential structure of women's encounter during childbirth was formulated in three themes. 'To be seen as an individual' was expressed as being met with respect and seen for oneself. 'To have a trusting relationship' described the midwife's character, professional knowledge and proficiency as well as the women's feeling of security. Keywords here were: friendliness, openness, safety, interpersonal congruity, intuition and availability. 'To be supported and guided' on one's own terms expressed the women's need for control, to listen to their innermost feelings and to be given time. But most of all the presence of the midwife was recognised as a main theme. The essential structure therefore could be summarised as presence. If any of the mentioned features was lacking, the women felt that the midwife was 'absently present'.

DISCUSSION

This study was undertaken with a small group of women delivered in one Birth Care Centre in Sweden. Whilst Waldenström (1993a) found that women birthing at an ABC-centre in Stockholm were older, better educated, had better physical health and tended to be less anxious when contemplating the approaching birth and motherhood than the control group we cannot claim that the women in this study are representative of all women using birth centres, let alone all women giving birth in Sweden. However, there are some lessons which can be learnt from the findings. Knowledge about the relationship between the birthing woman and the midwife is acquired over the years. It is a tacit knowledge embedded in practice. This kind of knowledge can be described as to know how to do something only by relying on our awareness of it, attending to a record activity (Polanyi 1967). By analysing this knowledge as it relates to maternity care, we hope to develop a more consistent professional approach, in order to meet the women's needs. The basis of our study was to begin to understand the phenomenon of women's encounter with the midwife during childbirth. The phenomenological approach enabled us to describe this complex subject by providing the participants with enough time to express their feelings and reactions at each phase of their labour. By interviewing women who delivered at an ABC-centre, we concentrated on the encounter between woman and midwife compared to a traditional delivery with different categories of professionals.

In our analysis of the findings we initially put 'presence' under different themes until we realised that it was an expression that permeated all the themes. According to Paterson and Zderad, presence is a main concept in the encounter. 'For genuine dialogue to occur there must be a certain openness, a receptivity, readiness or availability. The open or available person reveals himself as present' (Paterson & Zderad 1976, p.28)

Unfortunately some women felt that the midwife was 'absently present'. There are heavy demands on the midwives and other attendants on birthing women and a positive relationship has to be created during a painful and tough phase of the birth. However, in this study we found that it is not only what is done during labour and at delivery or how it is done, but just the calm presence of the midwife that seems to constitute the essential value itself.

'To be seen as an individual' means that the birthing woman wants to be recognised by the midwife and that the midwife is interested in her as an individual. The woman wants to feel that she is significant, and not just anyone of the numerous women cared for by the midwife. This postulates that the midwife shows respect for the woman by trying to understand who the woman is, her personality, her background and life experience. The women described that they wanted to be able to listen to themselves. Affirmation seems to be an essential part of this theme. Buber (1957) states that every person has a wish to be affirmed as what he is, even as what he can become, by humanity. In a study of hospitalised adults in surgical and obstetric units care givers were described as either emotionally warm and caring or cold and uninterested (Drew 1989). Care giver behaviour that was warm and nurturing produced feelings of comfort, strength and relaxation for them. This category was labelled affirmation.

Hodnett (1989) interviewed women choosing hospital birth and women choosing home birth in the US. Those who chose home birth had a greater degree of affiliation with their care giver and more freedom of exploration and self-expression, while those who gave birth in hospital experienced more aversive stimuli as intrusive procedures and unfamiliar people. Our ABC-centre is organised to be as homelike as possible within the confines of the hospital. In this way it is easier for the women to dare to be themselves by being seen as they are.

Under the theme 'To have a trusting relationship', the need for good communication and proficiency was revealed. The importance of communication in this study confirms earlier findings (Cartwright 1979, Kirke 1980, Macintyre 1982, MacIntosh 1988). According to Merleau-Ponty (1976) the intersubjectivity of the interpersonal sphere expresses the fact that people co-exist with other human beings. In the interhuman dimension we cross the border of our worlds. This is what the relation deals with and what the interviewed women expressed. The organisation of ABC-centres facilitates a good relationship since the women become familiar with the centre and the midwives before childbirth (Waldenström 1993b).

The women expressed that they wanted 'to be supported and guided on their own terms'. This represents the third main theme in our study. They searched for hospital care, because they needed the available professional knowledge. But the women themselves wanted to be the authority at birth. They emphasised the importance of participating in the delivery process, not only to go through a great deal of suffering and handle the labour, but to have control and be involved in decision-making. Waldenström (1993a) shows that women birthing at an ABC-centre were far more interested in playing an active part in decisions

---

15 What do you think about the statement, 'women felt...'?

Women's experience of the encounter with the midwife during childbirth   15

related to pregnancy and birth than the control group giving birth in the hospital. A study of 825 birthing women in England shows that information and feeling in control were consistently associated with positive psychological outcomes (Green et al 1990). Bluff and Holloway (1994) found that the birthing women in their study trusted midwives as experts who knew best. Nevertheless, these women wanted to play an active role in the control of labour.

In our interviews the multiparous women often mentioned former deliveries spontaneously, even if we did not ask about them. Some of our interviewees had chosen the ABC-centre because they felt they had missed something in the individual caretaking during the previous births. They described negative experiences when they had lost control of the situation and had not been able to participate in decision-making. Staff had taken control without giving the woman time to be involved. Even in emergency situations the women wanted the staff to stop even for just a second and communicate with them. Eye contact and explanation of the reason for interventions, followed by a moment of thinking, were desired in order to maintain the control and feel part of the birthing process.

Many factors influence the relationship between birthing women and midwives, and these include midwives' views? McCrea (1993) found that for 'special' relationships to develop between women and midwives important conditions were necessary. These were that midwives needed to be in full control of decision-making, their authority and decisions needed to be respected and accepted by other staff, and women had to be confident in the midwives' abilities and therefore trust their authority.

As midwives it is helpful to analyse our encounters with birthing women so that we can learn from these situations. Paterson and Zderad (1976) suggest that the nurse should always think about her relationship with patients and analyse them in the light of previous 'I–Thou relations'.

In summary, an analysis of the birthing experience facilitated by a midwife for 18 women revealed that a presence is required for a positive interaction to take place between woman and midwife. Presence permeates the three basic themes of the encounter: to be seen as an individual, to have a trusting relationship and to be supported and guided on one's own terms. The need to be seen as an individual can be realised by affirmation and familiarity with the midwife and surroundings. A trusting relationship can be obtained by good communication and proficient behaviour. By providing a sense of control the women can be supported and guided on their own terms. Above all they must feel that the midwife is present.

REFERENCES

Beck CT 1994 Phenomenology: its use in nursing research. International Journal of Nursing Studies 31 (6): 499–510

Bluff R, Holloway I 1994 They know best: women's perspective of midwifery care during labour and childbirth. Midwifery 10: 157–164

Buber M 1957 Distance and relation. Psychiatry 20: 97–104

Burns N, Grove S 1993 The practice of nursing research. Saunders Company, Philadelphia

Cartwright A 1979 The dignity of labour? Tavistock Publications, Cambridge

Drew N 1989 The interviewer's experience as data in phenomenological research. Western Journal of Nursing Research 11 (4): 431–439

Green J, Coupland V, Kitzinger J 1990 Expectations, experiences, and psychological outcomes of childbirth. Birth 17: 15–24

Hodnett 1989 Personal control and the birth environment. Comparison between home and hospital settings. Journal of Environment Psychology 9: 207–216

Husserl E 1965 Phenomenology and the crisis of philosophy: philosophy as rigorous science, and philosophy and the crisis of European Man, translated by Quentin Lauer. Harper & Row, New York

Kirke P N 1980 Mother's views of obstetric care. British Journal of Obstetrics and Gynaecology 87: 1029–1033

Macintyre S 1982 Communications between pregnant women and their medical and midwifery attendant. Midwives Chronicle 95 (1138): 387–394

McCrea H 1993 Valuing the midwife's role in the midwife/client relationship. Journal of Clinical Nursing 2: 47–52

McIntosh J 1988 Women's views of communication during labour and delivery. Midwifery 4: 166–170

Merleau-Ponty M 1976 Phenomenology of perception, translated by C. Smith. The Humanitis Press, New Jersey

Oiler C 1982 The phenomenological approach in nursing research. Nursing Research 3: 178–181

Omery A 1983 Phenomenology: a method for nursing research. Advances in Nursing Science 5: 49–63

Parse R R, Coyne A B, Smith M J 1985 Nursing research – qualitative methods. Brady Communications Company, Bowie, Maryland

Paterson J G, Zderad L T 1976 Humanistic nursing. Wiley, New York

Polanyi M 1967 The tacit dimension. Routledge and Kegan Paul, London

Spiegelberg H 1965 The phenomenological movement, Vol 2. Martinus Nijhoff, The Hague

von Wright G H 1988 Humanismen som livshållning och andra essayer. Raben & Sjögren, Stockholm

Waldenström U 1993a Characteristics of women choosing birth center care. Acta Obstetrica Gynecologica Scandinavia 72: 181–188

Waldenström U 1993b Föda barn på ABC. Team Offset, Malmö

ANSWERS

Q1. Possibly (b). By reading the abstract you should be able to obtain a clear picture of the research study. A good abstract can be extremely helpful and 'time-saving' during literature 'searches' especially when you are preparing for essays/assignments/report writing

Q2. Only you can answer this, but it seems fairly clear and succinct, thus meeting the criteria in Question 1

Q3. True. I am a great believer in working across professional boundaries and believe we have much to learn from researchers/authors from other disciplines. Therefore professional and educational background information is relevant. I like to see collaboration between researchers/authors. However, I would be critical/curious about researchers/authors that demonstrate no midwifery background

Q4. a) and c)

Q5. No – more on this in the discussion that follows these answers

Q6. Subjectivity pervades the whole qualitative research process and I believe this is advantageous. Researchers can sometimes experience thoughts of 'this is me' or intersubjectivity (Klein 1983) when collecting data. When such experiences are shared with participants the research relationship has potential to become more equal

Ann Oakley (1981) in her seminal (although now dated) paper on interviewing refers to intersubjectivity as a positive experience and where the researcher can invest their own personal identity in the research relationship (p 81)

Hollway & Jefferson (2001) refer to 'unconscious intersubjectivity' (p 45) that can come into play during the interview process. This unconscious dimension of interviewing accepts that the researcher and participant have feelings and that they are of value and significance in understanding the dynamics of the research relationship. This can lead to the co-production of data within interviews

Q7. Possible advantages include that:
1. The researcher can use a conversational style in order to make the interview interactive and encourage the participant to tell their own story
2. Interviewing can foster an equal relationship between the researcher and the participant. This is congruent with women being encouraged to become equal partners in the planning and delivery of maternity care (Department of Health 1993)

Possible disadvantages include that:
1. Interviews can be time-consuming if the researcher decides to use a more conversational style
2. Copious amounts of data can be generated, which have then to be transcribed and analysed. Transcribing can be tedious and can take many hours

Q8. There are countless ways in which qualitative data can be collected, as you will see in other qualitative studies in this book. It is important that the data collection method is congruent with the research method

Q9. False – I don't think it is enough to simply inform women that information will be treated confidentially. Participants need to know that any information they divulge to the researcher will be kept anonymous and that information will not be able to be traced back to them. The participants also need to know that their care will not be affected in any way if they decide not to participate. I don't think confidentiality can be guaranteed by the researcher because they should have informed the participants that data may be used in conference presentations and in the writing up of reports. Participants will need to be reassured that pseudonyms will be used. Therefore, anonymity can be guaranteed but not confidentiality

Q10. The purpose of informed consent is to safeguard the privacy and welfare of the participants. Informed consent also provides an opportunity to make a choice about whether or not to take part in the study. Increasingly research ethics committees, in accordance with research governance, are requesting that written informed consent is obtained from research participants. This is to ensure that the participants know what they are consenting to and that the role of the researcher and research is clearly understood. Researchers usually have to provide evidence of this when they attend local research ethics committees. Informed consent in action research is problematic because the amorphous quality of this approach does not allow for the prediction of what the participants have to consent to

Q11. It may well have been but we can't tell from the information provided

Q12. No. Approval was sought from a doctor but there is no indication of the ethics/research background of this person

Q13. Not by UK standards, which would entail getting written informed consent from participants and getting approval from an ethical committee rather than one person, but it is important to remember that this study was carried out in a different cultural context, where the 'rules' may be different

Q14. 1. The accuracy of interview transcripts can be checked by the participants
  2. The researcher keeps a research/reflective diary in order to self-evaluate their input to the research process
  3. Research peers and critical friends can help in the validation and interpretation of the data
  4. Seeking ethical approval and guaranteeing anonymity and confidentiality

Q15. I don't think that researchers can ever truly know what their research participants are feeling. I therefore feel uncomfortable when I see researchers writing comments like 'women felt...'. When writing up research I think it is more appropriate to write things like 'the data suggest...' or 'their words suggested that...'

DISCUSSION

Undertaking a critique of this paper has been both enlightening and provocative for me. This remains one of my favourite research papers, especially as it relates to the relationship between the midwife and the woman. However, I have had to come to terms with the fact that it has several limitations. Although it has been easy for me to identify more weaknesses than strengths, I am reminded only too well of the editing processes that research papers have to go through when they are submitted to journals for publication. Indeed, the requirements to modify the original submission might have been so drastic that some of the ethos of the paper was lost through editorial demands.

This leads me to recount a recent experience a colleague and I had in submitting a paper to an academic journal that insisted we use traditional headings for our paper. We had suggested within the body of the paper that 'potential data can be rendered redundant and much of the research story lost as complexities are omitted from the established publication format' (Deery & Hughes 2004 p 52). Although we are explicitly commenting on action research, this reinforces the point I make in the opening paragraph and also highlights that different ways of writing up research stories can be used in order to present a fuller and more accurate story.

It is important when writing up phenomenological research that researchers do not blur the different philosophical traditions and that they make their standpoint clear. This is not clear in the paper by Berg et al (1996), where there is no discrimination between the two philosophical traditions. The authors do, however, raise important theoretical points relating to phenomenology. Perhaps this paper uses what Crotty (1996) refers to as 'new' phenomenology. This is where the subjective understanding of the experience of the phenomenon, from the participant's perspective, is sought. This subjective experience is then objectively scrutinised (Barkway 2001).

I was unable to assess how the researchers had ensured rigour within their study and although I refer to reliability and validity in the suggested list for evaluating qualitative research in Section 1, there are other ways of assessing this. Reliability and validity are concerned with bias (Reed & Biott 1995) and how this is controlled. Interestingly, Miles & Huberman (1994) provide an account of internal and external validity in qualitative research where they transfer the notion of quantitative validity (for example, triangulation and sample selection) to qualitative research. Annells (1999) states that using traditional criteria such as reliability and validity is inappropriate for phenomenology because, as an approach, phenomenology does not use 'procedural precision' within the research process.

Lincoln & Guba (1985) offer different 'criteria', stating that trustworthiness of the data and their interpretation must be demonstrated. They offer four alternative approaches to demonstrate trustworthiness: credibility instead of internal validity, transferability instead of external validity, dependability instead of reliability and confirmability instead of objectivity. This approach plus terms such as reflexivity, rigour, authenticity and resonance seem more appropriate within qualitative research.

Usher & Edwards (1994) use the term 'resonance' to refer to something important happening within the research process. Does the research story related by Berg et al (1996) have resonance for you personally and perhaps other midwives in the UK?

The relationship between women and midwives now has a growing body of literature (Deery 2003, Edwards 2001, Kirkham & Stapleton 2000, 2001) and this paper adds to that body of knowledge. This paper asks us to analyse our encounters with women so that we can learn from these situations. However, this is easier said than done in a culture where midwives have expressed feeling unsupported (Kirkham & Stapleton 2001) and where the relational aspects of midwifery are neglected (Deery 2003). If midwives are to become able, or even begin, to understand the emerging dynamics of the midwife–mother relationship, there needs to be an increasing emphasis placed on the development of self-awareness (see Deery 2003, 2005). This is crucial for effective mother–midwife relationships where midwives give physically intimate care within an emotionally close relationship.

References

Annells M 1999 Evaluating phenomenology: usefulness, quality and philosophical foundations. Nurse Researcher 6(3):5–19

Barkway P 2001 Michael Crotty and nursing phenomenology: criticism or critique? Nursing Inquiry 8(3):191–195

Crotty M 1996 Phenomenology and nursing research. Churchill Livingstone, London

Deery R 2003 Engaging with clinical supervision in a community midwifery setting: an action research study. Unpublished PhD, University of Sheffield

Deery R 2005 An action research study exploring midwives' support needs and the impact of group clinical supervision. Midwifery (in press)

Deery R, Hughes D 2004 Supporting midwife-led care through action research: a tale of mess, muddle and birth balls. Evidence-Based Midwifery 2(2):52–58

Department of Health (DoH) 1993 Changing childbirth, part 1 (Report of the Expert Maternity Group). HMSO, London

Edwards N 2001 Women's experiences of planning home births in Scotland, birthing autonomy. Unpublished PhD thesis, University of Sheffield

Gadamer HG 1976 Philosophical hermeneutics. University of California Press, Berkeley

Hollway W, Jefferson T 2002 Doing qualitative research differently. Free association, narrative and the interview method. Sage Publications, London

Kirkham M, Stapleton H 2000 Midwives' support needs as childbirth changes. Journal of Advanced Nursing 32(2):465–472

Kirkham M, Stapleton H 2001 Informed choice in maternity care: an evaluation of evidence based leaflets. Women's Informed Childbearing and Health Research Group, School of Nursing and Midwifery, The University of Sheffield/NHS Centre for Reviews and Dissemination, University of York

Klein RD 1983 How do we do what we want to do: thoughts about feminist methodology. In: Bowles G, Klein RD eds Theories of women's studies. Routledge and Kegan Paul, Boston, p 88–104

Lincoln Y, Guba E 1985 Naturalistic inquiry. Sage Publications, California

Miles M, Huberman M 1994 Qualitative data analysis: an expanded sourcebook. Sage Publications, London

Oakley A 1981 Interviewing women: a contradiction in terms. In: Roberts H ed Doing feminist research. Routledge and Kegan Paul, London, p 30–61

Paley J 1997 Husserl, phenomenology and nursing. Journal of Advanced Nursing 26:187–193

Paley J 1998 Misinterpretive phenomenology: Heidegger, ontology and nursing research. Journal of Advanced Nursing 27:817–824

Patton MQ 2002 Qualitative research and evaluation methods, 3rd edn. Sage Publications, London

Reed J 1994 Phenomenology without phenomena: a discussion of the use of phenomenology to examine expertise in long-term care of elderly patients. Journal of Advanced Nursing 19:336–341

Reed J, Biott C 1995 Evaluating and developing practitioner research. In: Reed J, Procter S eds Practitioner research in health care. The insider story. Chapman and Hall, London, p 189–204

Usher R, Edwards R 1994 Postmodernism and education. Routledge, London

Walters AJ 1995 The phenomenological movement: implications for nursing research. Journal of Advanced Nursing 22:791–799

CHAPTER 8

Tricia Anderson

Machin D, Scamell M 1997 The experience of labour using ethnography to explore the irresistible nature of the bio-medical metaphor during labour. Midwifery 13:78–84

INTRODUCTION

'No man is an island', somebody famous once said. Or, to put it into our context: 'no midwife works in a vacuum'. Midwives are part of a culture of midwifery and midwifery is part of a culture of NHS maternity care, into which women come – for a short time in their lives – to have their babies. This culture is complex, messy, contradictory and all the other things that mark out the real world from the clean, orderly world of textbooks. As most readers will know, this culture is also powerful and influential; it affects how people behave – how they act, how they talk, how they interrelate and so on.

Most research methods just look at one small thing. As we have already seen, quantitative methods study a dose or type of drug, for example, a particular disease or treatment, or an intervention in health care (like increasing the number of visits). This type of study tells us the '*what*'. Qualitative studies, such as interviews with small groups of women about their birth experiences, will often tell us the '*how*'. All these studies are very useful and can often tell us what we '*should*' be doing, and how we '*should*' be doing it, according to the latest good-quality research evidence. But you and I know that there's a vast amount of research that tells us what we 'should' be doing (no routine CTGs, women not lying on their backs, no coached pushing, just to name a few). And there's equally lots of research telling us how we should be doing it (respectfully, calmly, professionally, treating each woman as an individual and so on). And you and I know that an awful lot of people ignore all this and healthy women continue to be put on monitors, lie on their backs and hold their breath to push their babies out. We need to understand what's going on, and that means understanding the culture in which midwives work and in which most women in the UK give birth. This study by Machin & Scammell uses ethnography to try to unpick what happens to so many women on the labour ward: why most of the women who say they want a natural, unmedicated birth end up embracing all the technology with gusto.

Ethnography stands right back and looks at the whole thing. Its aim is to be holistic: to study and understand a distinct, naturally occurring culture or 'people' and describe them 'in the round'. In health-care research it might be a large culture, such as 'midwifery', or a smaller subculture such as a GP practice or a labour ward. The method derives from anthropology, where researchers 'go into the field' and try to describe through a detailed process of careful observation and systematic recording what people in a certain culture do, what they believe, how they interact, what rules and social norms they abide by, the objects they surround themselves with and so on. In order to increase understanding, they may compare two differing cultures and, in situations where two cultures or subgroups clash, they might explore the reasons for the conflict. It is a slow and painstaking process: good ethnography takes a great deal of time. There might be an overlap with other qualitative methods in terms of similar data collection methods (such as interviews and observation) but, unlike phenomenology (which tries to capture the essence of a phenomenon) or grounded theory (which tries to generate new theory about a specific experience), ethnography specifically looks at a 'whole culture'. The researchers might try to 'map' what they see against existing theories to try and explain or understand it better, but the aim is not to generate new theory. So, unlike much other research, ethnography is not aiming to test or generate a particular theory but it is very useful for trying to understand why people in a certain group or subculture speak, act and behave the way they do. In health-care ethnography, there is also commonly an intention to use the insights derived from the research to improve health-care provision and practice.

Unless we understand all the forces at play within the culture of childbirth, midwifery and maternity care, we will not be successful in bringing in changes. That's why ethnographic research is such a useful tool: it can help visitors or newcomers to the culture understand the 'rules' ('Oh so *that's* why they behave the way they do!'); and it can help long-standing group members step back and see their culture with new eyes. Marsden Wagner (2001) wrote a brilliant paper called 'Fish can't see water' in which he discusses how members of a culture (midwives) are so immersed in their own world (the 'medical model') that they can't even see it any more. Ethnography can also help anyone trying to bring in change or innovation to devise workable, appropriate and culturally specific strategies that will work 'on the ground'.

There are lots of pitfalls with undertaking ethnographic research. As an ethnographic researcher, it takes a lot of time to 'immerse' yourself in a culture and there's always the danger of 'going native' and starting to take on board the study group's norms and values yourself. Do you reveal yourself as a researcher to the group (in which case, are the group members likely to change their behaviour in front of you), or do you masquerade as a group member (but how ethical is this?) Do you try and retain 'outsider' status, in which case the group might not 'let you in' and you will receive the expected (misleading) responses they give to outsiders? Or do you try to become an 'insider', in which case your objectivity may falter, you may suffer role conflict as you try to both observe what is happening and participate in it, and you may focus more on the dramatic events rather than the everyday.

Ethnography can be tricky to evaluate, yet it is important that it is assessed carefully because, as we have seen, there is the possibility of researcher misinterpretation, bias and so on, as well as some major ethical issues. So how do we tell good ethnography from bad?

There are four guiding principles to bear in mind when evaluating ethnographic research. Is the paper:

- *contributory* in advancing wider knowledge or research?
- *defensible in design* by providing a research strategy which can address the evaluation questions posed?
- *rigorous in conduct* through the systematic and transparent collection, analysis and interpretation of data?
- *credible in claim* through offering well-founded and plausible arguments about the significance of the data generated? (Cabinet Office 2003).

1 Are the objectives of this study clearly stated?
a) Yes
b) No
c) Don't know

The experience of labour: using ethnography to explore the irresistible nature of the bio-medical metaphor during labour

David Machin and Mandie Scamell

Objective: taking evidence provided by an ethnographic study based on women's experiences of pregnancy and childbirth, and using ritual theory in the analysis of the relationship between the medical metaphor, inherent in contemporary birth settings, and the views and expectations of childbirth which the women bring with them to that setting.

Design: small scale qualitative study using ethnographic research techniques.

Setting: GP surgeries, two consultant-led, hospital-based antenatal units, labour suites and postnatal wards, plus the homes of the women involved from the north east of England.

Participants: 40 primigravid women providing two sample groups. Half of the women were actively involved in antenatal class programmes run by the National Childbirth Trust and the NHS and the other half did not attend any antenatal classes.

Main findings: within the sample there was a clear cultural diversity which carried significant implications on how the women assembled their understanding of pregnancy and birth antenatally. However, this division lost clarity at the onset of labour, rendering delivery experiences more similar than might have been expected. Ritual theory offers significant insight into this phenomenon, analysing birth as a rite of passage provided a necessary tool to explain why this pattern emerged in the data.

Key conclusions and implications for practice: cultural diversity suggests an element of caution should be used when advocating the notion of 'informed choice' across the board, sensitivity to existing cultural values is imperative. Despite an emphasis on informed choice, midwifery practice continues to offer the medical metaphor as the dominant cultural prop in the labour ward.

David Machin
BA, PhD, PGCE, Lecturer
Anthropology Department,
Goldsmith's College,
University of London,
40 Lewisham Way,
New Cross, London SE 14,
UK

Mandie Scamell
BA, MA, Post graduate
researcher, Department of
Anthropology, University of
Durham. Old Elvet,
Durham City, UK

Correspondence to: DM
Manuscript accepted
30 January 1997

INTRODUCTION

'Informed choice' is a central theme to which midwifery practice in the UK is aspiring following the publication of the Winterton (House of Commons Health Committee 1992) and *Changing Childbirth* reports (Department of Health 1993). By definition informed choice would constitute women receiving information about the possibilities of different birth environments, providing them with the confidence to make a choice about where they would like to deliver their baby. Despite this priority and a barrage of litera-ture challenging the assumption that the hospital environment, with its tendency for interventionist practices, is the only safe place to give birth (Haire 1976, Chard 1977, Cartwright 1979, Arms 1984, Brackbill 1984, Inch 1984, Zander 1984, Campell & Macfarlane 1990, Tew & Richards 1990) plus the consistent pressure from groups such as the Active Birth Center and the National Childbirth Trust (NCT), hospital confinements continue to dominate birth behaviour in the UK. This trend suggests that the radical changes advocated in *Changing Childbirth* (Department of Health 1993) will not happen overnight.

2 What was the researchers' interest in the area?

a) They were commissioned by the Department of Health following the publication of *Changing childbirth*
b) They both have a research background in childbirth anthropology
c) Don't know

3 Is an ethnographic method appropriate for what they are trying to study?

a) Yes
b) No
c) Don't know

4 Is this an example of:

a) Descriptive ethnography?
b) Critical ethnography?

5 The funding for the study was from the Richard Stapely Trust. This could be a source of bias. True/False

Existing research, which partly fueled the Winterton (House of Commons Health Committee 1992) and *Changing Childbirth* (DoH 1993) reports, argues that reform is needed since women are universally rejecting the dominant medicalised childbirth culture (Topliss 1970, Kitzinger 1978, Cartwright 1979, Graham & Oakley 1991). Other authors suggest that this might not be quite the case, since women from lower socio-economic groups tend not to oppose medical intervention (Reid 1983, Nelson 1983, McIntosh 1989). Both these schools of thought fail to address the problem of why a large proportion of those primigravid women who do talk about rejecting medical intervention, still have a tendency to revert to the dominant medical childbirth culture at the time of their labour and birth. There is the assumption that women from higher socio-economic groups are naturally in accord with informed choice, and with that are more likely to espouse the natural birth ideology. It is this paradox that is analysed in the study reported here.

Using ethnographic evidence it is argued that a more sensitive approach is necessary in order to gain an understanding of birth behaviour. To achieve this the interaction between the ideological perceptions women bring to labour and birth, and the inherent messages in that setting must be examined, as merely analysing women's views of childbirth fails to provide a solution. Using evidence from an ethnography carried out on women's experiences of pregnancy and childbirth in 1994–1995, we will demonstrate that the key to the problem lies in the way the dominant medicalised birth culture is presented to the women during their emotionally charged intrapartum period. We will show that with the onset of labour the setting changes. Women become vulnerable as they feel themselves move over a boundary into a domain where the medicalised procedures, once associated with safety become overwhelming. Normality is interrupted, the norms, rules and values of everyday life become temporarily suspended (Leach 1961), the power of setting, thus, takes on a new dimension. The implications of this change should never be underestimated and the analytical tool which we felt could best explain this power was ritual theory. In this article the possibilities of using ritual theory are explored, to explain why birth behaviour in the UK continues to be dominated by medical, and often interventionist, practices.

The ethnographic study from which the data are drawn was funded by the Richard Stapely Trust, and focused on the experiences of 40 women living in the north east of England. The basis of the research was an investigation of the way in which women assemble their understanding of pregnancy and delivery through the materials of culture, namely, the available folk-themes, medical advice and experience. Data were collected through recordings of conversations; interviews, which were transcribed verbatim; observation; photographs; and generally from fieldnotes made while 'hanging out' with the women (Malinowski 1966, Oakely & Callaway 1992, Carrithers 1992). The women were followed from early in pregnancy until several months after delivery.

METHODS

We wanted a comparative element to our ethnography and so wanted to include both women who sought out formal advice through antenatal classes, pregnancy and childbirth literature, and through the services provided by the NCT, and women who did not feel these sources of information were relevant to their experience. We felt that the number of women used should allow for the in-depth qualitative analysis characteristic of ethnographic research, and give a sense of the range of different experiences which women might have.

The sample consisted of two groups of women: 20 contacted through the NHS, from classes four and five who, therefore, shared relatively low socio-economic status (this group will be referred to in this article as the NHS group); and 20 from classes one and two contacted through the local NCT, all who shared a relatively high socio-economic status (these women will be referred to as the NCT group). The first women we contacted were the women who did not seek formal information routes. These women were approached through the NHS after clearance by the South Durham Health Authority Research Ethics Committee. The women were selected on a random basis from a specially formulated client list, this list was made up of women put forward by their midwives because of their apparent lack of interest in the NHS antenatal class programme offered to them. After arranging an initial interview with these women at their home to establish contact (this followed semi-structured interview guidelines and was taped), we accompanied them into all the settings associated with their pregnancy: hospital antenatal clinics; GP's surgery antenatal clinics; labour ward; and postnatal ward. As time went by our visits became less formal and we were introduced to their local networks of friends and family, and, importantly, other women who were also pregnant.

6 Why did they want two different groups of women to compare? (More than one answer might be correct)

a) To introduce a comparative element into the study
b) To compare women's experiences across all social classes
c) To compare women who sought out antenatal education with those who did not
d) To compare women from different geographical areas

7 What 'culture' are they studying?

a) Pregnant women
b) Labour wards
c) Childbearing women

8 What type of sample did they study?

a) Homogenous sample
b) Heterogenous sample
c) Total population sample

9 Would you describe the sample as:

a) Purposive?
b) Random?
c) Representative?
d) Convenience?

10 Is the sample size appropriate for this study?

a) Yes
b) No
c) Don't know

11 Who were the key informants in this study?

a) Childbearing women
b) Midwives
c) Obstetricians
d) Don't know

12 Why do you think the researchers chose to study only primigravid women? Would it have made a difference to the results if they had studied multiparous women?

13 Do you feel overall that this was an ethically conducted study?

a) Yes, because the study got ethical approval from a health authority research ethics committee
b) Yes, because the researchers are academics from a good university of high repute
c) Don't know, because the researchers do not give enough information about the conduct of the study
d) No, because the researchers did not give details of how the women were consented to take part

Existing research, which partly fueled the Winterton (House of Commons Health Committee 1992) and *Changing Childbirth* (DoH 1993) reports, argues that reform is needed since women are universally rejecting the dominant medicalised childbirth culture (Topliss 1970, Kitzinger 1978, Cartwright 1979, Graham & Oakley 1991). Other authors suggest that this might not be quite the case, since women from lower socio-economic groups tend not to oppose medical intervention (Reid 1983, Nelson 1983, McIntosh 1989). Both these schools of thought fail to address the problem of why a large proportion of those primigravid women who do talk about rejecting medical intervention, still have a tendency to revert to the dominant medical childbirth culture at the time of their labour and birth. There is the assumption that women from higher socio-economic groups are naturally in accord with informed choice, and with that are more likely to espouse the natural birth ideology. It is this paradox that is analysed in the study reported here.

Using ethnographic evidence it is argued that a more sensitive approach is necessary in order to gain an understanding of birth behaviour. To achieve this the interaction between the ideological perceptions women bring to labour and birth, and the inherent messages in that setting must be examined, as merely analysing women's views of childbirth fails to provide a solution. Using evidence from an ethnography carried out on women's experiences of pregnancy and childbirth in 1994–1995, we will demonstrate that the key to the problem lies in the way the dominant medicalised birth culture is presented to the women during their emotionally charged intrapartum period. We will show that with the onset of labour the setting changes. Women become vulnerable as they feel themselves move over a boundary into a domain where the medicalised procedures, once associated with safety become overwhelming. Normality is interrupted, the norms, rules and values of everyday life become temporarily suspended (Leach 1961), the power of setting, thus, takes on a new dimension. The implications of this change should never be underestimated and the analytical tool which we felt could best explain this power was ritual theory. In this article the possibilities of using ritual theory are explored, to explain why birth behaviour in the UK continues to be dominated by medical, and often interventionist, practices.

The ethnographic study from which the data are drawn was funded by the Richard Stapely Trust, and focused on the experiences of 40 women living in the north east of England. The basis of the research was an investigation of the way in which women assemble their understanding of pregnancy and delivery through the materials of culture, namely, the available folk-themes, medical advice and experience. Data were collected through recordings of conversations; interviews, which were transcribed verbatim; observation; photographs; and generally from fieldnotes made while 'hanging out' with the women (Malinowski 1966, Oakely & Callaway 1992, Carrithers 1992). The women were followed from early in pregnancy until several months after delivery.

METHODS

We wanted a comparative element to our ethnography and so wanted to include both women who sought out formal advice through antenatal classes, pregnancy and childbirth literature, and through the services provided by the NCT, and women who did not feel these sources of information were relevant to their experience. We felt that the number of women used should allow for the in-depth qualitative analysis characteristic of ethnographic research, and give a sense of the range of different experiences which women might have.

The sample consisted of two groups of women: 20 contacted through the NHS, from classes four and five who, therefore, shared relatively low socio-economic status (this group will be referred to in this article as the NHS group); and 20 from classes one and two contacted through the local NCT, all who shared a relatively high socio-economic status (these women will be referred to as the NCT group). The first women we contacted were the women who did not seek formal information routes. These women were approached through the NHS after clearance by the South Durham Health Authority Research Ethics Committee. The women were selected on a random basis from a specially formulated client list, this list was made up of women put forward by their midwives because of their apparent lack of interest in the NHS antenatal class programme offered to them. After arranging an initial interview with these women at their home to establish contact (this followed semi-structured interview guidelines and was taped), we accompanied them into all the settings associated with their pregnancy: hospital antenatal clinics; GP's surgery antenatal clinics; labour ward; and postnatal ward. As time went by our visits became less formal and we were introduced to their local networks of friends and family, and, importantly, other women who were also pregnant.

We met with the group of women who did seek out various kinds of formal guidance through the local NCT. These women were chosen randomly from enrolment lists and then approached. The procedure we followed with this group was the same as with our NHS sample. We conducted an initial semi-structured interview, which lasted anything up to two hours, and used this as a spring board for contact.

While participant and non-participant observation was the main emphasis of our methodological approach, we supplemented this technique with two tape recorded, semi-structured interviews with each woman (Morse & Harrison 1992). The initial inter-

14 What consent procedure was followed? (More than one answer might be correct)

a) The women were given written information to read about the study
b) The women were given exact details of the aims of the study
c) The women were given time to think about whether they wished to take part before they had to make their decision
d) Don't know

15 How many women declined to take part?

a) 10
b) 20
c) Don't know

16 Did the researchers attend the labours of the 40 women in the study?

a) Yes
b) No
c) Don't know.

17 Why did they use semi-structured interviews? (More than one answer may be correct)

a) To check the validity of their observational findings
b) To ensure that they asked all the women the same questions
c) To limit the time taken for each interview
d) To gain baseline information from women in pregnancy

18 Was a scheme of questions or topics followed in the semi-structured interviews?

a) Yes
b) No
c) Don't know

19 Which of the following are major ethical issues that arise when undertaking participant observation? (More than one answer may be correct)

a) It can lead to the researcher getting inaccurate data from the group
b) It can lead to group members 'letting their guard down' and forgetting they are being studied
c) It can lead to the researcher 'going native' and taking on the biases of the group
d) It can include covert observation, of which those being researched are not aware

20 They chose a mix of participant and non-participant observation because... (More than one answer may be correct)

a) As non-health professionals it would have been impossible for them to be complete participants in the labour ward setting
b) Participant and non-participant observation each give complementary, different perspectives
c) Using only non-participant observation would have possibly inhibited the women and thus limited the richness of the data

21 The researchers say that they used a mix of participant and non-participant observation but do not give more details. Which of the following is most likely to be true? (More than one answer may be correct)

a) They undertook participant observation on the labour ward
b) They undertook non-participant observation 'hanging out' with women
c) They undertook participant observation in the GP antenatal clinics
d) They undertook non-participant observation on the labour ward

22 How confident are you that the analysis process was rigorous and robust?

a) Very confident
b) Reasonably confident
c) Not at all confident

23 Which of the following is true?

a) The emic perspective is the viewpoint of the outsider to the culture
b) The emic perspective is the viewpoint of the insider
c) The etic perspective is the analysis provided by an objective third party (neither insider or outsider)
d) The etic perspective is a theoretical dilemma observed by the researcher

view, already mentioned, was conducted during pregnancy while the second was conducted postnataly.

From our initial lists we successfully contacted 18 women, but the numbers of women in the study expanded, through the snow-ball sampling technique, to 40 women, 20 for each group. This happened as some women became interested in our activities and others became naturally involved owing to our interactions with their friends who were already participating. The women were told that we were anthropologists interested in their experiences of childbirth.

Analysis

Analysis was an ongoing procedure which is indicative to this kind of qualitative style of research. Fieldnotes were written up daily during the research, and were discussed amongst the researchers on a weekly basis. In this way we were able to reassess our priorities, check our techniques and address any problems arising from the data (Rainbow 1977, Clifford & Marcus 1986, Okley 1992, Davies 1995).

The semi-structured interviews were tape recorded and then transcribed verbatim and exchanged amongst the researchers. The findings from these interviews were directly compared to establish patterns emerging from the material (Morse 1992). These findings were then followed up using our less formal research techniques, what ethnographers often refer to as 'hanging out'.

Further input was contributed towards this ongoing analysis and discussion of our findings, by staff from The Institute of Health Studies and The Department of Anthropology in the University of Durham. Reviews of this nature were held on a monthly basis and offered invaluable insight into the analysis of the data.

FINDINGS

The first pattern, which soon became apparent from the analysis of the ethnographic data, was that we were dealing with distinct cultural differences between the NHS and NCT groups. This cultural dichotomy made a marked impression upon the concepts from which the women drew to talk about their expectations and experiences of pregnancy and childbirth (Machin & Scamell forthcoming). These were the cultural differences we had expected to see, since they confirmed the findings produced by an abundance of previous research (Nelson & Newson 1963, Reid 1983, McIntosh 1989, Lumley 1993, Hancock 1994, Nolan 1995); however, this turned out to be only half of the story. Although there was a clear division in outlooks between the two groups of women which coincided with their social class differences, this division blurred with the onset of labour.

The 20 women in our study who attended NCT classes were, according to the *Changing Childbirth*

(Department of Health 1993) model, in the position to make an 'informed choice'. What we mean by this is that they were fluent in their knowledge of both the medical and alternative non-medicalised childbirth methods, and seemed to be extremely confident that they knew what they themselves wanted from their own deliveries. Wanting natural birth without the use of drugs and with the minimum of medical contact possible was a very common theme in their discourse. What stood out in the discourse of these women was the expression of control and self empowerment. The women said they were compelled to take responsibility for their pregnancies and births. They felt that they could maintain this level of personal autonomy via an informed choice approach (Machin & Scamell forthcoming).

The other 20 women in the study attended no antenatal classes and tended to use friendship networks for their information, advice and support. They did not generally challenge the interventionist medical model, having little concern for any alternatives. Their priorities tended to be only for a painless delivery and a healthy baby. According to the NHS group this was to be achieved through handing responsibility over to the professionals. While making a preferred choice it seems unlikely that these women could be described as making an 'informed choice' in the *Changing Childbirth* (Department of Health 1993) interpretation of the term (Machin & Scamell forthcoming). They were not interested in accessing information, being informed was irrelevant to their experience, similarly, they did not see any need for decision making since they had no choices.

The two groups of women were, thus, highly contrasted. The outstanding themes in the NCT group were control and self empowerment. None of the women from the NHS group ever mentioned these concepts, they simply did not form part of their discourse. The emphasis in this group was on the professionals' ability to take care of everything. There was no need, therefore, for 'informed choice', the concept was irrelevant to their experience. Any information the NHS group women needed tended to come from local social networks rather than the professionals. These extracts show the cultural division in the convictions expressed by the two groups of women.

It seemed logical that such huge differences between the kind of themes these two groups of women covered, in their discussions of pregnancy and childbirth, would have an impact on their behaviour during labour. We expected there to be a difference in where and how these women delivered their babies; but as our research unfolded, and the women involved had their babies, these differences did not transpire. What the findings from our ethnography suggest is, that while NCT women were able to use cultural themes about empowering and alternative approaches to childbirth as they went about their everyday lives, at the commencement of labour the setting changed. They were no longer independent people standing up to needless interference in what should be the beautiful and spiritual experience of childbirth. They became vulnerable and felt themselves moving into a different category of person. The setting changed and with that so did the rules of the setting.

On the other hand the NHS women had never aspired to the notions of control, responsibility and personal autonomy, they had been prepared to hand over full responsibility to the medical staff. In this way this group of women had anticipated this crucial setting change.

Our problem is to offer an explanation of why, with this marked difference in expressed expectations of childbirth where some women are clearly informed to make choices to the contrary, hospital confinements still continue to dominate birth behaviour in this county. The dominant childbirth culture in the UK society is a medical one, what we need to explain is why the NCT women involved in our research managed to resist this interpretation of childbirth throughout their pregnancies, only to rely on it in the same fashion as the NHS women at the time of their deliveries. Analysing our data using ritual theory clarifies how this process occurs.

It is necessary to look more carefully at the transformation, since it is through analysis at this point that we can see where the ideological perceptions women bring with them to the birth setting interact with the symbolic messages of that setting. First we need to introduce the analytical tool-kit necessary to do this. This will allow us to move through the transitional stages, providing an explanation at each salient point. Our tool-kit is drawn from the ritual theory in the Social Sciences.

The ritual theory tool-kit

The pioneering work of van Gennep (1960) provides the specific tools necessary for analysis. He describes the behaviour that surrounds childbirth as a rite of passage. Women, according to van Gennep, make a journey during labour and childbirth from pregnancy to motherhood, and the fetus a journey to becoming an independent being. These journeys involve the individuals moving from one socially prescribed category to another, a movement which threatens the fabric of those categorisations (van Gennep 1960). Drawing on the same structuralist school of thought in her work on purity and danger, Douglas (1980) argues that such a social movement which involves a biological component, as is the case in childbirth, is particularly dangerous to both those experiencing it and those around:

The ideal order of society is guarded by dangers which threaten transgressors… At this level the laws of nature are dragged in to the sanction of the moral code. (Douglas 1980, p.3)

According to van Gennep (1960), culturally specific ceremonies are devised to protect all those involved from the perceived dangers of these journeys. Thus, the potentially dangerous biological processes of childbirth can be cacooned into the safety of cultural manipulation. In the case of a rite of passage, this cultural manipulation involves three crucial stages: separation, transition and reintegration.

More contemporary structuralist writers such as Lomas (1978) have shown how ritual theory can be applied in the analysis of contemporary, cultural manipulation of childbirth. He argues that:

Behaviour in hospitals is not always as rational and scientific as it would seem. Much that occurs in obstetrics is heavily ritualised… We do not regard the practices surrounding childbirth in our society as ceremonial or ritualistic, but may the ritual be hidden from us only because we are so hypnotised by the apparently rational assumptions behind them that we do not even begin to seek a further explanation? (Lomas 1978, p.174)

In the same vein Davis-Floyd (1990) has applied the three stages of van Gennep's (1960) model to explain hospitalised childbirth practices in the West (Davis-Floyd 1990). The hospital confinement, with its medicalised procedures, can, thus, be treated as ritualistic behaviour.

By looking at the onset of labour using the analytical tools provided by the structuralist's theory of ritual, we are able to examine the interaction between the ideology the women bring with them into the birth situation and the symbolic messages shrouding that environment. It is through using this perspective in our analysis that we are able to explain the clouding of the cultural divide between the two groups of women. Ritual theory, thus, provides the specific tool necessary to appreciate the setting change inherent in labour.

With the analytical tool-kit we will introduce some of the women involved in this research. Using primary data we will move through the stages of childbirth as a rite of passage providing explanation of each stage. Consider these examples (all names and identifying features have been altered to protect anonimity) taken from both groups of women, as representations of the first stage.

Separation

The physical and emotional movement from the profane (normal) into the sacred (special):

Tracy (NHS): Well you don't give birth now every day do ya? I mean it's not like pegging out the washing or sommat… It's something special and you should go out of your home to do it. You know go somewhere special to do something special.

Trisha (NCT): I actually found that in the end I rather liked the hospital environment. I grew rather fond of it in fact. When I was there… because I

---

24 What theory did they use to explain their findings? Was this well justified and did it 'fit'?

25 Which of the following is true? In ethnography… (More than one answer may be correct):
a) 'Thick description' is too densely presented to read and understand
b) 'Thin description' is when the meaning is teased out to the greatest possible depth
c) 'Thick description' is theoretical and analytical and gives meaning to the data described
d) A 'thin description' is a brief, condensed summary of the findings

26 Is there sufficient 'thick' description in this study? Have the researchers analysed and interpreted their data convincingly, or is it simply presented in a descriptive way ('thin' description)?

27 Where do the quotations come from?
a) Field notes
b) Antenatal semi-structured interviews
c) Postnatal semi-structured interviews
d) Don't know

was there really it felt like a special event. I went into hospital to have my baby. Everything was taken care of there for me… Where as every day is the same at home, sort of thing.

These comments represent the type of things said by all the women. They clearly show that the women talked in terms of moving away from their normal (the profane) lives into a special environment (the sacred). The setting changed and the normal views and values of everyday life no longer apply. The women entered into a vulnerable state for which previous experience offered them little precedent. Separation occurred.

Transition

A journey through the sacred in a trance-like state where symbolic messages hold reverence was very apparent in the data. We found substantial evidence to suggest that the women experienced a phase of transition during their labour. They experienced physical sensations which put their normal reasoning powers, and in many cases personality traits, on hold. In this vulnerable condition they clung onto the cultural messages of the hospital setting. The reliability of the medical model became a source of comfort. The following examples show the type of things the women talked about:

> Sarah (NCT): They were intense my contractions. A very intense sensation… it was like a trance. Yes just like a trance, sort of drunk really. It distracted you from being able to sort of think of things that didn't actually seem pertinent to that actual moment in your labour. I didn't really care about the experience. I was just coping with the pain. I was soon screaming 'Pethidine, pethidine!' I thought I would be worried about the baby and things but I wasn't. I couldn't somehow think that far ahead.
>
> Alison (NCT): I think during the thing you are so involved with what's actually going on. Your mind never gets past the birth. All the things that are going on around you you don't care about. It's just a relief to know at least someone is in control here. Everything is just not important any more.
>
> Alex (NHS): I lost all track of time. I didn't know whether it was day or night. I remember John saying it was 2.30 and I had to ask him 'What 2.30 in the morning or the afternoon?' I didn't have a clue!

These examples show how the women experienced an altered state during their labours. They lost their sense of reality, experiencing a trance like state of consciousness indicative of the transitional stage of a rite of passage. Pain for these women frequently became overwhelming and they entered into another state of consciousness (Odent 1984, Kelpin 1992) where many previous beliefs and convictions become unimportant (Scarry 1987).

In this condition the women became very susceptible to the reassurances of the cultural props around them. The symbolic messages of the hospital setting gave them something to cling onto:

> Chris (NCT): It was such a relief to know that all was OK. I guess it was a kind of fix and in that way I felt that I really needed it (fetal monitoring). It was reassurance really.
>
> Kaz (NCT): I really think I could have coped on the TENS machine but it was just the way she said it really. I don't know why I just felt I needed a little bit extra. I think I needed reassurance really. It gave me a positive plan of action. I couldn't cope all on my own. So when she suggested it (pethidine) I said 'Yes please!'
>
> Alison (NCT): I just had gas and air for fifteen minutes I managed with that. I wanted something else to concentrate on I think really. I think it was just getting beyond my coping mechanism. I don't remember asking for it. I mean I tended not to talk at all. But you're really not aware that you're talking because you are talking in your head.
>
> Rosie (NHS): The nurse that was on that night was actually really nice, she stuck her head in the door and said 'what's the matter, have we got a water fall?' I says 'Yeah, I think so.' She came down and she moved all the pillows around 'Don't move.' Then it was all action like. The trolley comes. They don't like you to walk, you can't even sit on the trolley. You're just laid there on the spot. And that was it really I just did like they told me after that. And they put all them monitors on me and stuff so I just lay there.
>
> Ang (NHS): Oh thank God they've got all the stuff there that they have. Say years ago if you had blood pressure or the baby's heart went down, well did they know? Would they just leave you? Would you be poorly? You just don't know these things do ya. I'm so glad things aren't like that now. Who knows what would have happened. It's frightening really.

These examples demonstrate the type of symbolic messages the women experienced during there hospital confinements. We have established that separation has occurred, the women were now in a dangerous position where the surrounding symbols were very powerful. The women, therefore, experienced a sense of dependency upon things such as the 'high tech' medical equipment, the procedures such as confinement to bed and the aids such as pethidine and 'Entonox'. These were the type of cultural props offered to them by the staff in this crisis setting and the women relied upon them heavily. The cultural metaphor of medicine carried them through this transitional stage. Tracy (NHS) sums it up when she says:

> I'm a firm believer that if people take the time to invent these pain-killers and all that then you

28 In analysis of qualitative data, 'saturation' means:

a) The researcher has exhausted all possible ideas
b) The point at which no new analytical categories emerge from the data analysis
c) The point at which the researcher has mapped all the themes to underpinning relevant theory

29 Do you feel that the researchers achieved saturation in this study?

a) Yes
b) No
c) Don't know

30 Are the data they present clearly linked to their fieldwork?

a) Yes
b) No
c) Don't know

should take them, like that doesn't bother me. Childbirth can be a dangerous thing.

Reintegration

The movement back into the profane (normal). For some this transition was difficult:

> Alison (NCT): The midwife she offered just the presence of somebody who obviously knew what they were doing. And that if there were anything that were arising she would know what to do, she would be in complete control... You rely on her and she is absolutely wonderful and you're shipped off really before you come out of your involvement in the birth and you're on the ward with new people. People who weren't there really. People you've not shared all that with. I was quite sad when she went. 'Come back! I haven't finished yet. I would rather you saw me through the next twenty four hours really.'

For others it was a relief:

> Alex (NHS): I've never been in hospital before. I was pleased to come out. I was ready to come home. It was all over, so there was not much point being stuck in there like was there. No point in staying longer than you had to.

It is clear that with the onset of labour the setting for all the women in our sample was changed. They moved away from their everyday lives, and in doing so frequently found themselves abandoning the cultural themes which they had used to negotiate and make sense of their pregnancies. They entered into an area of transition, a special place. A place where they could safely change from the person they were to the person they will become, a limbo land. In this place the women felt bewildered and it would seem the authority of the metaphor of science and medicine, and the need to pass over the boundary to the safety of the white coats and medication, became overwhelming. At this time of crisis the women were reassured by the symbolic messages of the medical staff and their equipment.

By incorporating the structuralists' theory of ritual into the analysis of our ethnographic findings, we have been able to explain the power of the medical metaphor at the time of delivery. Our findings suggest that even if research could completely challenge the necessity of any medical intervention in childbirth, women in our culture would probably still need its presence to reassure in what is perceived by the UK culture as the life threatening, crisis ridden event of delivery.

In our Western culture science is a powerful belief system. In medicine it has helped to make many changes in the way we expect to be able to live. Science has become a metaphor for making everything safe, but metaphors have this ability to dominate where they are applied (Fernandez 1986), especially where it may be in the interest of certain groups who have the power to define what remains legitimate (Foucault 1976). All the women in this study had been encultured into the medical culture of childbirth, some were able to maintain an opposing position during pregnancy, but with the stress of childbirth their energy to maintain this position slipped. Ritual theory provided us with the tools necessary to analyse this slip, it is through using this analytical approach that we can clarify exactly how the dominant medical culture of childbirth remains authoritative even in a post *Changing Childbirth* (Department of Health 1993) environment, where it is hoped more choices might be available to women.

DISCUSSION

The evidence from our ethnography presented us with two problems. Firstly, we began to question whether the thrust for informed choice was universally appropriate. The pragmatic and utilitarian approach of working class women to childbirth has been well documented (Porter et al 1984, Mcintosh 1986), and our findings confirmed this trend. What is distinct about our research, however, is that it was carried out post *Changing Childbirth* (Department of Health 1993). Our findings, therefore, can be seen as a representation of the cultural bedrock onto which 'informed choice' will fall. This has serious implications for the implementation of the recommendations of this report, since it suggests that such a policy may serve to alienate the women most in need of support, advice and information because of its cultural inappropriateness (Prince & Adams 1978).

There is no point in assuming that one clear message will be effective when we are working in a society as rich and diverse as our own. The issues of empowerment and 'informed choice' may not always be relevant, and to advocate them without sensitivity may only serve to alienate the advocators from their client. We must give all women the opportunity to perceive childbirth outside the current dominant hegemony, be that the legacy of *Changing Childbirth* (Department of Health 1993) or the medical model. What we are suggesting is that health care providers should recognise that women will have existing cultural expectations and needs, which will provide what we might think of as the bedrock onto which any new ideas will fall. If the informed choice is going to gain further mileage it has to be sensitive to this existing bedrock.

The second problem, similarly, holds implications for the *Changing Childbirth* report. In the end both groups of women shared similar birth experiences. While the NHS women had anticipated a hospitalised childbirth experience with a sense of inevitability, the majority of the NCT women found their medicalised experience of childbirth rather shocking. For the NHS women the birth was a means to an end, once the end result was achieved, they had their baby, the birth tended to pale into

31 Are the links between the data and the conclusions clear? (Can you follow their decision trail?)

a) Yes, very clear

b) Reasonably clear

c) Not at all clear

32 Looking back at the whole paper, do you consider that the researchers were 'cultural strangers'?

a) Yes

b) No

c) Don't know

33 The researchers were anthropologists and not maternity care health professionals? Do you think, on balance, that this is:

a) A good thing because they can give a fresh 'outsider's' view of childbirth?

b) A good thing because they would not be caught up in a 'role conflict' - needing to work if the labour ward was short-staffed, for example?

c) A bad thing because they cannot understand all the complexities and real experiences of midwifery and childbirth?

d) A bad thing because they were 'outsiders' and therefore women would not tell them the truth?

34 Does the study have credibility? How do you feel about their findings? Do they 'ring true'? Does it tally with your own labour ward experience?

35 Is the study contributory? Has reading this paper increased your understanding of what happens to women on the labour ward?

84 *Midwifery*

insignificance. On the other hand the NCT women saw the birth as an end in itself and tended to be more traumatised by their experiences.

The NCT women had not expected to be so overwhelmed by the change in setting indicative of labour. They were surprised to find that their usual ideological props of control and autonomy were not strong enough to hold them in this altered crisis state. They turned to the dominant cultural props offered to them at the time, and these came under the umbrella of the medical model. We were able to explain this phenomena using ritual theory in our analysis. What this pattern tells us is that the medical metaphor continues to dominate the ethos of the intrapartum care. Women in labour are vulnerable; they are often not capable of choice, they are reassured by the safe boundaries set by medicalisation and are more susceptible to the symbolic messages of that environment. All the women in our research relied upon the medical model of childbirth during their labour because that was the cultural tool offered to them at the time by their attendants. Because birth is a ritualistic practice even the most determined anti-interventionist women may be easily swayed by the assuredness of obstetricians and midwives who may have the powerful metaphor of the safety of science on their side .

REFERENCES

Arms S 1975 Immaculate deception. Houghton Mifflin Co, Boston.

Brackbill Y 1984 Birth Trap. Mosby, St Louis

Campbell R, Macfarlane A 1990 Recent debate on the place of birth. In: Garcia J, Kilpatrick R, Richards M eds. The politics of maternity care. Clarendon Press, Oxford

Carrithers M 1992 Why humans have cultures. Oxford University Press, Oxford

Cartwright A 1979 Dignity of labour. Tavistock, London.

Chard T, Richards M eds 1977 Benefits and hazards of the new obstetrics. Spastics International, London

Clifford J, Marcus A 1986 Writing culture. University of California Press, Berkley, California

Davis-Floyd R E 1990 Ritual in the hospital: giving birth the American way. In: Whitton P, Hunter D, eds. Anthropology: contemporary perspectives. Scott Foresman, London

Douglas M 1980 Purity and danger. Routledge and Kegan Paul, London

Department of Health 1993 Changing childbirth, report of the expert maternity group. HMSO, London

Fernandez JW 1986 Persuasions and performances: the play of tropes in culture. Indiana University Press, Bloomington, Indiana

Foucault M 1976 Power as knowledge. In: Lemert C, ed. Social Theory. West View Press, Oxford

Geertz C 1973 Interpretation of other cultures. Hutchinson, London

Graham H, Oakley A 1991 Competing ideologies of reproduction. In: Currier C, Stacey M, eds. Concepts of Health illness and disease. Berg Press, Oxford

Hancock A 1994 How effective is antenatal education?' Modern Midwife 4 (5): 13–15

House of Commons Health Committee 1992 Report on the maternity services (Chairperson N Winterton). HMSO, London

Haire RA 1976 The cultural warping of childbirth. International Childbirth Association, London

Kelpin V 1992 Birthing pain. In: Morse J, ed. Qualitative health research. Sage, London

Kitzinger S 1978 The experience of childbirth. Penguin, London

Inch S 1984 Birthrights. Pantheon Books, New York

Leach E 1961 Rethinking anthropology. Athlone Press, London

Lomas P 1978 An interpretation of modern obstetrics. In: Kitzinger S, Davis J A, eds. Place of birth. Oxford University Press, Oxford

Lumley J, Brown S 1993 Attenders and non-attenders at childbirth education classes in Australia. Birth 20 (3): 123–130

Lupton D 1995 Medicine as culture: illness disease and the body in western societies. Sage, London

Machin D, Scamell A forthcoming Changing childbirth: ethnographic research suggests why 'informed choice' might not have the effect hoped for.

Malinowski B 1966 Argonauts of the West Pacific. Routledge and Kegan Paul, London.

Mcintosh J 1989 Models of childbirth and social class. In: Robinson S, Thomson A M, eds. Midwives, research and childbirth. Chapman and Hall, London, vol. 1

Morse J 1992 Qualitative research. Sage Publications, London

Nelson M 1983 Working class women middles class women and childbirth. Social Problems 30 (3): 284–297

Newson J, Newson E 1963 Infant Care in our Urban Community. Allen & Urwin, London

Nolan ML 1995 A comparison of attenders at antenatal classes in the voluntary sectors… Midwifery 11: 138–145

Oakely J, Callaway H 1992 Anthropology and autobiography Routledge, London.

Odent M 1984 How to help women in labour. In: Zander L, Chamberlain G, eds. Pregnancy care for the 1980s. The Royal Society of Medicine and Macmillan Press Ltd, London

Porter M, Macintyre S 1984 What is must be best: a research note on conservative or deferential responses to antenatal care provision. Social Science and Medicine 19 (11): 1197–1200

Prince J, Adams M 1978 Minds mothers and midwives. Churchill Livingstone, Edinburgh

Rabinow P 1977 Reflections on fieldwork in Morocco. University of California Press, Berkley, California

Reid M 1983 A feminist sociological imagination? Reading Ann Oakley. Sociology of Health and Illness 5 (1): 83–94

Scarry E 1987 The body in pain. The making and unmaking of the world. Oxford University Press, Oxford

Tew M 1990 Safer childbirth: a critical history of maternity care. Chapman and Hall, London

Topliss E 1970 Selection procedures for hospital domiciliary confinement' In McLachan G, Shegog R, eds. In: the beginning: studies of maternity services. Oxford Press, Oxford

van Gennep A 1960 The rites of passage. University of Chicago Press, Chicago

Zander L, Chamberlain G 1984 Pregnancy care for the 1980s. The Royal Society of Medicine and Macmillan Press Ltd, London

ANSWERS

Q1. b) No, the objectives are not clearly stated. The paragraph entitled 'Objective' in the abstract is not grammatically correct and therefore not understandable. Within the text it is explained that this paper is an analysis of data from an ethnographic study of women's experiences of pregnancy and childbirth in 1994–95, which aimed to investigate the way in which women assemble their understanding of pregnancy and birth. This, however, differs from and is not clearly linked with the objective outlined in the abstract

Q2. c) We are not given any information about the researchers, their personal/professional background, their reasons for being interested in this area or their motivations for conducting the study. Thus it is hard to assess for degrees of any possible bias

Q3. a) Yes, it is. The researchers are trying to understand the contemporary culture of pregnancy and birth from the perspective of women, in the time period following the implementation of *Changing childbirth*. Their aim is to study the 'whole' and not any one particular aspect of pregnancy or birth and therefore ethnography is a very suitable method

Q4. b) Critical ethnography. Descriptive ethnography simply describes what is observed, (through analysis of themes, patterns, etc.); critical ethnography aims to unravel larger sociopolitical agendas within a culture such as power and control to change/improve things. This study explicitly looks at the 'rhetoric versus reality' argument surrounding informed choice within maternity services following the publication of *Changing childbirth*; thus it is inherently 'critical'

Q5. True; it *could* be. We are not given any information about the Richard Stapely Trust – it could be a Engineering Trust for the Development of Birth Monitors or a Feminist Trust for the Advancement of Women. Who knows?! However, any reader who was considering using the findings and wanted to pursue this could look up the Richard Stapely Trust to find out more about the Trust's aims and objectives. It is enough, then, that the researchers acknowledged their funding source

Q6. a) and c). However, the researchers did not justify this satisfactorily. Why were all the women who chose not to attend NHS antenatal classes all from social classes four and five? Was this by intention or accident? The authors make quite a few stereotypical assumptions about 'NCT types' being 'naturally in accord with informed choice' and 'espousing the natural birth ideology'. Why did they choose attendance at classes or not as their focal point for these groups? What other factors could they have considered when defining the groups to study?

Q7. c) The focal culture of their study is that of childbearing women, during pregnancy, birth and the immediate postnatal period. It is not a study of the culture of the labour ward *per se* – this is more what Sheila Hunt did in her well-known ethnographic study of labour ward culture

Q8. a) The sample was primarily a homogenous one: a group of pregnant women all expecting their first baby within the North East of England. A homogenous sample consists of people who belong to the same subculture or have similar characteristics. However, they were also heterogenous with respect to one variable, in that the researchers chose to study two groups of pregnant women, one group who attended National Childbirth Trust (NCT) classes and one who did not attend any classes at all

Q9. a) This is a purposive sample of pregnant primigravid women, taken from two specific groups; those who had attended NCT antenatal classes and those who did not attend any classes

Q10. a) Yes. Qualitative research commonly uses small sample sizes (typically anything between 4 and 40 people), with the intention of obtaining in-depth, rich data from a small number of participants. However, there are no rigid rules for sample size within qualitative research. With the aim of ethnography being to study a 'culture' it is important that the number of participants is sufficient to reflect the culture being studied; 40 women (20 in each group) seems a reasonable size - small enough to be practical, yet large enough to reflect cultural norms and behaviours

Q11. a) Childbearing women. The researchers did not interview or 'hang out' with midwives or obstetricians

Q12. Primigravid women come to the culture of pregnancy and birth for the first time, and thus their interaction with it is relatively uncontaminated. Multigravid women obviously are hugely influenced by their previous birth experiences, good or bad, and have 'learnt how to behave' in the maternity culture; studying their understandings of pregnancy and birth is likely to have produced equally valid but very different results

Q13. c) The study proposal got ethical approval; that is, the ethics committee approved what the researchers said they were going to do. However, the ethics committee does not take any responsibility for the actualisation of the research proposal. This paper gives very little detail of how the women were recruited, consented, given the opportunity to choose not to take part or to withdraw at any stage and so on. We do not know how many women from the initial list refused to take part. However, it is reassuring that the researchers engaged in monthly progress peer review meetings with two departments at their university

Q14. d) We don't know. No details are given. It is often hard to gain truly informed consent for a qualitative, ethnographic study, as the aims may be quite open-ended at the beginning of the study. However, all research participants should be given written information about the study, time to read and consider it without feeling under pressure before deciding to take part, and a non-judgemental, comfortable way in which to decline should they decide to do so. Given the potentially intrusive nature of this study (the researchers accompanied the women to antenatal clinics and the labour and postnatal wards and several months into the postnatal period), it would have been reassuring to have more details of the recruitment and consent procedure

Q15. c). We don't know. The researchers do not state how many women, if any, that they approached declined to take part in the study. This is of concern from an ethical point of view, especially given the in-depth ethnographic nature of the study, particularly as the researchers worked from lists of women provided by NHS midwives and NCT antenatal class enrolment. As the women were going to be followed in antenatal clinics, labour and postnatal wards, it is likely that at least some would have declined. With the NHS group in particular, who were chosen specifically because of their lack of interest in NHS antenatal classes, one wonders how these women were consented to take part in this study, and whether they gave genuine informed consent. From the research report it is impossible to say

Q16. c) We don't know. This is very vague in the report. The researchers say that they accompanied the women into all the settings associated with their pregnancy, including the labour ward. Are we to assume that they were on call for the women and went with them to the labour ward at the onset of labour? Are we to assume that they were present at some or all of the births? Or are we to assume the researchers attended the labour ward as observers when some of the study women happened to be in labour? We simply can't tell from reading the research report. Given the nature of the analysis (that the division in views about birth between the two groups of women disappeared during labour), it would have been helpful to know this. Did they base this analysis primarily on data from the antenatal and postnatal interviews with the women? They do not quote from or even mention any field notes from the labour ward (or from anywhere else, for that matter) in the research report. One would expect in an ethnographic study to see reference made to the field notes taken whilst observing, and how they had been incorporated into the analysis process

Q17. a) and d)

Q18. c) Don't know. The researchers do not give any details about the content of the two semi-structured interviews which they undertook with each woman. This is of concern, as one would expect to see at least some indication of how they were structured and what topics were covered, particularly as the first antenatal interviews occurred before they had undertaken any period of observation. Typically, semi-structured interviews work from a loose schedule of topic areas to be covered

Q19. b), c) and d). Complete participant observation is when the researchers take a full 'insider' role, participating in all discussions and interactions as if one of the group. It can include 'covert' (secret) observation. Group members may gradually forget (or in some controversial studies, never even know) that they are the subject of observation and research, and perhaps reveal more than they intend. The researcher may become so much a part of the group that they lose the ability to be critically analytical

Q20. a), b) and c). All are true

Q21. d). In the labour ward and GP antenatal clinic setting it is most likely they were there as complete observers, not participating in any direct interactions. In women's homes and with groups of women they are most likely to have joined in discussions as participants

Q22. b) Although this is hard to assess. The researchers give little detail about their process of analysis. However, they do say that monthly meetings were held with two university departments in which the ongoing analysis was discussed. This is reassuring in there were some 'outsider' checks on the analysis process, as they trawled through their data looking for recurring patterns and themes. However, they did not perform 'member' checks: that is to say, they did not take their findings back to the women for them to check their validity, which would have enhanced the confirmability of the findings

Q23. b) The emic perspective is the viewpoint/perceptions of the insider; the etic perspective is the perceptions of the outsider/researcher. This paper presents a well-balanced combination of both emic and etic perspectives: that is, we see the women's perspectives and hear their voices, but also hear the researcher's analysis

Q24. They use ritual theory, which was well justified, plausible and illuminates the findings in an interesting and useful way

Q25. c)

Q26. Yes, I think so. The researchers have used ritual theory as a framework to analyse their data which provides an interesting and convincing interpretation of the data

Q27. d) We don't know. The researchers do not provide these details. It would have been helpful if they could have assigned each quotation to its source (e.g. field note in antenatal clinic; postnatal interview). This would have enabled us to assess the analysis process more thoroughly, especially given their analysis of how some women changed their viewpoints in the labour ward

Q28. b)

Q29. c) From the data given in the report, it is impossible to say

Q30. c) It is impossible to say. The researchers do not present a clear 'decision trail' at all. It is not clear whether the quotations they use come from the semi-structured interviews or fieldwork, whether they are from the antenatal or postnatal periods, or from observation on the labour ward. We are given no insight into their fieldwork in antenatal clinics or on the labour and postnatal wards, what approach to field note taking they used – in fact, we are given little detail about the data collection and analysis process, making this a hard study to evaluate thoroughly

Q31. c) This paper does not make explicit the links between all the data (the observation, the field notes and the semi-structured interviews) and the conclusions concerning the three themes of separation, transition and reintegration. They collected a large amount of data to which they never refer in the text (e.g. observation in antenatal clinics, the labour and postnatal ward and several months postnatally); thus it is hard to validate their decision trail. It is also hard to assess how recurrent the patterns/themes were

Q32. c) Don't know. A cultural stranger is someone who has no prior experience or knowledge of the culture being studied. Although we are told that the two researchers are anthropologists, we are not told whether the female researcher had children herself or whether the male researcher is a father with personal experience of the maternity services, and thus would have 'insider' knowledge and possibly corresponding biases. In this type of qualitative research where the researcher herself is the prime research tool, this is a valid question to ask

Q33. a) followed by b). There are both pros and cons of having non-maternity care professionals research childbirth but, on balance, I think that having other professionals study maternity care can bring a really fresh, 'out-of-the-box' perspective. Those of us who are in the middle of it, day in, day out, can sometimes struggle to see things afresh. Anthropology, in particular, can be a useful lens through which to view childbirth

Q34. They certainly 'ring true' with my own clinical experience of the labour ward, thus the findings have credibility for me

Q35. Yes, I personally feel it has. I found that the use of ritual theory helped me understand why women in labour are so vulnerable and suggestible, and why they seek certainty through clinging to the cultural icons with which they are surrounded

DISCUSSION

This process reveals how difficult it can be to evaluate ethnographic research reports. Given the word limit required by most professional journal articles (typically 1500–2000 words), it is common in published papers to include only a small amount of information about the methodology, analytical processes and ethical issues – just as we have found in this paper by Machin and Scamell. Most papers focus, quite understandably, on the more interesting results and discussion, which after all is what most readers want to read!

Let us go back to our four key principles. Is this study:

- *contributory* in advancing wider knowledge or research?
- *defensible in design* by providing a research strategy which can address the evaluation questions posed?
- *rigorous in conduct* through the systematic and transparent collection, analysis and interpretation of data?
- *credible in claim* through offering well-founded and plausible arguments about the significance of the data generated? (Cabinet Office 2003).

From answering the questions, we can confirm that it is certainly contributory in that it adds to our insight about women's behaviour on the labour ward, and credible in claim as it explains a phenomenon in a way that appears to reflect the real life of the participants. It is also defensible in design, in so much as ethnography is an appropriate method for this study. However, from the limited data included within the paper, it is not possible to say with confidence that it was rigorous in conduct. That is *not* to say that it was badly conducted, but simply that we are not given sufficient information to make that judgement. So should we dismiss this paper? I think not – remember that all the researchers are proposing is a 'theory' of what happens to women in labour. As with much qualitative research, the reader is invited to 'try on the theory for size', to see if it 'fits' and to see what insight it might provide.

This is a useful paper because it provides a theoretical explanation for a phenomenon that is commonly seen on the labour ward: a woman who has access to all the information, attended antenatal classes, and is articulate and educated, who starts off in labour planning for a natural birth yet ends up turning to the medical model. What the researchers don't do is consider any alternative or competing explanations for this phenomenon. For example, are these women simply naïve, with ill-informed expectations of the level of labour pain? Are they persuaded or coerced by health professionals into accepting medical interventions? Is the level of human support given to them inadequate, forcing them to rely on other, more technological things?

The application of ritual theory, taken from cultural anthropology, provides a useful tool for understanding the vulnerability of the labouring woman, who is in a potentially dangerous state of 'separation' of mind from body and who is likely to clutch at whatever she is offered to provide a sense of security and certainty. In a conventional labour ward setting that is likely to be a monitor, a clock or a doctor; in a different setting it could equally be a soft cushion, calming massage or the eyes of the husband or a trusted midwife. This paper helps us understand that the environment of birth is crucial to its outcome.

This paper raises two interesting dilemmas: one about the notion of informed choice for women and the other about the power of the midwife. If a woman is planning to give birth in a medical environment, such as a consultant-led labour ward, this research study tells us that she needs to know that she will find it very hard to resist the medical services on offer: analgesia, continuous fetal monitoring, artificial time limits, augmentation and so on. We know that midwives themselves also find these things extremely hard to shake off in face of the dominant medical hierarchy. As the authors state in their conclusion, 'the medical metaphor continues to dominate the ethos of intrapartum care'. Perhaps, as we continue to work to challenge this domination, antenatal preparation needs to be a lot more honest with women about the impact that simply being on a consultant labour ward will have on the way their labour is managed and the way they are likely to respond. The easy availability of pain relief when a woman is in pain, for example, is likely to be irresistible to her (Leap & Anderson 2004). Only then will women be able to make a more informed choice about where they want to have their babies.

If we accept the ritual theory of separation, it provides us with a stern reminder that midwives, although they don't perhaps always want to be, are very powerful when a woman is in labour. In our care we have women in a vulnerable state of 'separation', who are reaching out for anything that will provide safety and certainty, and likely to agree to pretty much anything we suggest. It's worth reflecting on how we use that power; do we use it to help women get the best long-term outcome for themselves and their babies or do we abuse it to get the best outcome for ourselves and the busy labour ward?

References

Cabinet Office 2003 Quality in qualitative evaluation: a framework for assessing research evidence. Strategy Unit, Cabinet Office, London

Leap N, Anderson T 2004 The role of pain in normal birth and the empowerment of women. In: Downe S ed Normal birth: evidence and debate. Churchill Livingstone, Edinburgh

Wagner M 2001 Fish can't see water: the need to humanise birth. International Journal of Gynaecology and Obstetrics 75(suppl 1):S25–S37

Resources

A QUICK GUIDE TO TABLES

I think it is important to acknowledge that it can be a bit scary to move from the relatively simple and straightforward ideas and tools in Section 1 to reading research itself, which can appear much more complex in reality. It is my experience that, for many people, the problem arises more in quantitative research with the tables and statistics, which can seem very mysterious and complicated. For this reason, there follows a quick guide to understanding the tables in research studies, using a couple of examples of common tables and then a list of tips. Hopefully, this will help the tables themselves be a bit less scary!

Usually, the first couple of tables or diagrams presented in quantitative research (and, of course, all studies vary, so this won't be the case all the time) show you how many people were in the study and whether the groups of people who were compared are actually similar. If you look at Section 6, Figure 1, you will see that this is a flow chart showing who was in a study at what time.

When you encounter the kind of diagram in Figure 1, you need to do two key things.

1. Follow the chart from beginning to end and see if the numbers add up. In the top box, we can see that the research starts with 1500 women, so we need to see that 1500 women are accounted for in the next row. 750 + 750 = 1500, so this is OK. If women are missing, perhaps because of lost forms or loss to follow-up

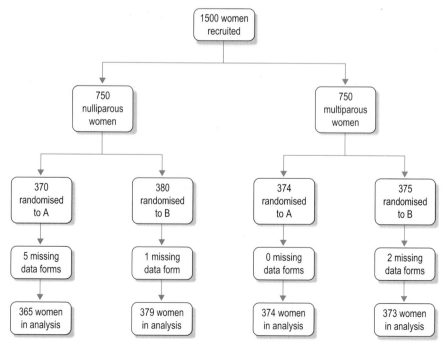

Section 6, Figure 1

(e.g. where the women moved house or were otherwise uncontactable by the researchers) we need to ensure that the researchers have told us why. Do the numbers add up in my chart, or can you spot any mistakes? (Answers at the end of this guide.)

2. Make sure that you understand what the chart is telling you – it will help you a great deal later on if you spend 5 minutes working out what it says. This kind of diagram often shows – much better than people can write in the text, and with fewer words – how the women were randomised into two or more groups, and what happened to any women who dropped out.

You'll see another example of a relatively simple flow chart in Figure 1 in the Hundley et al (2000) article in Chapter 3 and a more complex example of this kind of diagram in Figure 1 in the Smith et al (2002) article in Chapter 6.

The kind of table shown in Section 6, Table 1 is also quite common. This kind of table is included to demonstrate that randomisation was effective. For instance, if we began with 1000 women and randomised them into two groups, we can then go on to compile a table like this one to see whether the two groups we ended up with had relatively similar characteristics to each other. The note under the title of the table tells us that, unless noted otherwise in the individual row, each of the raw figures is given first (i.e. the actual number of women), followed by the percentage of women from that group that fell into this category. The exceptions to this are where standard deviation has been used: we'll talk about that in a bit so, at this point, it matters less whether you understand standard deviation than that you are able to compare two numbers! By the way, the 'n' at the top is simply an abbreviation for 'number' and tells us how many women were in each of the groups.

When you encounter this kind of table, all you need to do is to read across the information and compare the two (or more) groups with each other. You wouldn't expect to see that the two groups were exactly the same but you would hope that they were fairly similar in each of the areas. You might also want to check whether the numbers add up in other ways; for instance, do the numbers of nulliparous and multiparous women add up to 500 in each group? Don't forget, though, that while the whole numbers should add up, the percentages might not add up to 100 if the researchers have 'rounded up' the figures. If you do spot a problem, you need to have

Section 6, Table 1 Characteristics of participants in jelly baby and control groups*

	Jelly baby group (n = 500)	Control group (n = 500)
Mean {SD} age in years	38.5 {10.8}	38.9 {11.2}
Employed prior to course	335 (67)	355 (71)
Self-employed prior to course	80 (16)	75 (15)
Parity Nulliparous	314 (62.8)	307 (61.4)
Multiparous	186 (37.2)	193 (38.6)
Year of course First	180 (36)	188 (37.6)
Second	178 (35.6)	175 (35)
Third	142 (28.4)	136 (27.2)

* Figures are numbers (percentages) unless otherwise stated

a look through the text and see if the researchers have also highlighted and discussed this. If they haven't, you might decide that this is an error or a potential source of bias in the study.

Would you say that the two groups in my example (Section 6, Table 1) are similar, or is there cause for concern in one or more areas?

You can see another example of this kind of table in Chapter 6 (Table 1 in the Smith et al article). You can compare these tables with Table 1 in the Hundley et al article in Chapter 3, which simply describes the characteristics of the women in that study but does not compare them with another group of women.

You will also see lots of other kinds of tables presenting the results of studies, although, as there is a guide to statistics after this section, we'll not look at those tables here. The principles of understanding a table are the same no matter what kind it is.

- Begin by carefully reading the title of the table to make sure you understand what it is planning to tell you.
- Next, look at the titles for the rows and columns, to make sure you understand what they are comparing with what. If it makes you feel better, cover up the data in the middle of the table with a piece of paper until you understand the headings and are ready to face the rest!
- Keep your piece of paper handy and use it to cover parts of the table so that you are only looking at one row or column of data at a time. It is a good idea to do this with both the rows and the columns, as you will often be able to see different things in each.
- If at any point you get really stuck, read the text of the relevant section (e.g. results) to see if that can help you. I would suggest, if you are one of those people who just naturally dislikes tables, that you always read the text first and then come back to the tables when you understand what the text is saying.
- It is always good to work out whether they are talking about raw data (e.g. 15 women), the rate or percentage of something (e.g. 15% of primiparous women) or the average (e.g. the average score was 15). Sometimes researchers use two or more of these in the same table (as in Section 6, Table 1, where I used the average to express the age of the women, but raw numbers and percentages for each of the other factors). Sometimes, like in my table, they will use different kinds of brackets or parentheses to differentiate – like where I used {SD} and (per cent) – but this is not universal, so beware!

Answers

Section 6, Figure 1: Somehow I lost a woman in the multiparous group! If you look at the box saying that there were 750 multiparous women and then compare that to the numbers in the next row down, you will see that, if you add together 374 and 375, I have one woman who is not accounted for! She continues not to be accounted for all the way down the rest of the diagram. We can't tell from this table where I made the mistake (although you might be able to follow this through by seeing if the text says something different, or explains it), so it is enough to note that I have made a mistake that might affect the analysis.

Section 6, Table 1: These groups are probably similar enough to be comparable. You might notice that third-year students are underrepresented in the study, perhaps because they are busy writing their dissertations, although those that have entered are spread evenly amongst both groups. You might have (rightly) wondered why parity was relevant to my study – the answer is that it probably isn't (although you never know for sure until you explore these things!), but I wanted to show you an example using parity because this comes up so often in birth-related research. If you were really eagle-eyed, you might also have spotted that, in the control group, the numbers of students in each year added up to 499 rather than 500 and the percentages to

99.8 rather than 100! Somehow I have lost a student midwife without explaining how or why!

UNDERSTANDING STATISTICS

Facts are stubborn, but statistics are pliable.
MARK TWAIN

One of my favourite number-related quotations is attributed to Benjamin Disraeli, who talked about, 'lies, damned lies, and statistics'! By using this to begin this section, I don't mean to suggest that all statistics are lies. However, they are an attempt to get to the truth rather than actual, concrete truth in themselves, so they can be critiqued like any other aspect of the research process. There is always a possibility that the results of research are wrong and, indeed, one of the key functions of statistical tests is to help us see how likely it is that the results are right or wrong. This guide is designed to be a user-friendly way to take you through some of the statistical ideas and tests which are commonly used in birth-related research.

What are statistics all about?

In simple terms, the term statistics refers to the body of knowledge which is concerned with the collection, organisation, analysis, interpretation and presentation of numerical data. To break it down even further:

1. Researchers need to find ways of collecting data which will make the data easy to deal with later on, and they need to make sure they collect enough of the right kinds of data in the most accurate way possible. A knowledge of statistics can help them ensure these things.
2. They then need to organise those data in ways which will make them easy to handle and work with during the rest of their research.
3. Once the data are collected and organised, they will analyse them using specific statistical tests, which help to determine what the results of their research are, and how likely it is that they are significant.
4. It is then important to look at the results in relation to the wider picture, and interpret what they have found – again, a knowledge of statistics is vital to this step.
5. Finally, they will use one or more different ways to present their data and findings so that you, the reader, can see how they have reached their conclusions and decide whether you agree with them.

Because of all of this, it is handy to know a bit about how statistics are used, so that when you critique a piece of research that uses statistics, you will have at least a basic idea of what they have done, how they have done it, and whether it could have been done differently.

The research paper in Chapter 3 is an example of a piece of quantitative research which actually uses very few statistical tests. If you haven't read it already, have a flick through the tables, and you'll see that most of them use simple raw numbers and percentages, with only a couple of averages and their standard deviations added in.

Levels of measurement

Often, though, quantitative research uses more complex statistics, so it's helpful to have a grasp of the basics of those too. But before we get there, we need to talk a bit about four different terms that are used to describe the measurement of data. Although you don't need to be an expert in this to critique a research study, an understanding of levels of measurement will help you understand why a particular test has been used, and this knowledge also underpins much of what I will say about statistics in the remainder of this guide. These four categories begin with the one that is least useful from a statistical perspective, and move up the scale to the one which is the most useful.

If the level of measurement is *nominal*, this means that, although the data might be described with the use of numbers, these numbers don't actually mean anything – and you would certainly never do a test of significance on the numbers. For example, football players have different numbers on their backs, which helps people know who's who when they are all running around, and the numbers tend to define the order in which the team is listed in the match programme or on the TV screen. But no-one would suggest that the footballer wearing the number 7 shirt is seven times better than the goalkeeper wearing number 1. (Or perhaps they might, but it would have nothing to do with the numbers on their backs!) Other kinds of data that are measured nominally include gender, marital status and ethnicity.

Ordinal measurement is used when the different attributes can be put in order of rank but when the distances between different attributes don't have any meaning. For instance, you could give a value to each of a group of midwives depending on whether they were 1 = a first-year student, 2 = a second-year student, 3 = a third-year student, 4 = a qualified midwife with a degree, 5 = a qualified midwife teacher with a degree and a teaching qualification, 6 = a qualified midwife with a degree, a teaching qualification and a higher degree. People who have a higher number have more of the attribute (which, in this case, is education related to midwifery) but the distance between 1 and 2 cannot be said to be the same as the distance between 5 and 6, so we cannot use the interval between each number in drawing any conclusions. Other examples of ordinal data measurement include hotel star ratings, movie ratings in TV guides and the results of questions where you ask people to list things in order of preference or importance.

With *interval* measurement, the distances between the attributes do have meaning. Examples of data that can be measured in this way include the Fahrenheit temperature scale, where the difference between 94 and 96 degrees Fahrenheit is statistically the same as the difference between 96 and 98 degrees Fahrenheit. It might be useful to note at this point that it is important to differentiate whether something is *statistically* or *clinically* important: whereas there is no statistical difference between a person whose temperature drops from 98 to 96 degrees and a person whose temperature drops from 96 to 94 degrees, clinically, there is a big difference! (For those of you who work in Celsius, 95 degrees Fahrenheit is the temperature at which hypothermia is said to occur!) Although interval measurement is much more useful than the first two kinds of measurement, one problem it carries is that, even though 96 is two times 48, we cannot say that 96 degrees is twice as hot as 48 degrees, so it tells us nothing about the ratio of one value to another, which is why scientists measure temperature in kelvins and statisticians distinguish interval measurement from the final kind of measurement.

Ratio measurement describes the kind of measurement that carries all of the advantages of interval data but has one big addition – an absolute zero, which means that you can meaningfully describe fractions, or ratios. Attributes like height or weight are ratio variables, because we can say that someone who weighs 200 pounds is twice as heavy as someone who weighs 100 pounds. A lot of variables that 'count' things in birth-related research are ratio variables, because we can say things like 'twice as many babies were admitted to Special Care in January 2006 as in July 2005'.

So, you might wonder, what's the point of knowing all of this, then? Well, you can't make decisions about what kind of statistical test to use until you have thought about the attributes of the data you have, i.e. which one of the four categories (levels of measurement) they fall into. Some tests, for instance, are designed only for one level of measurement and if you used them with the wrong kind of data, your results won't be accurate. You wouldn't, for instance, do a *t*-test on nominal data because the numbers don't actually mean a lot and you would end up with complete nonsense!

Parametric and non-parametric data

There are a couple more terms that are useful to know before we carry on, and these are *parametric* and *non-parametric*. The word *parametric* basically describes data that meet certain parameters in relation to the way the data are distributed in the population as a whole. Interval and ratio data are said to be parametric and, if you think about the kinds of things they measure (height, weight, temperature), you'll be able to understand why this is the case. These kinds of things are normally distributed among the population (i.e. if we plot something like the height of lots of people on a bar chart and then join the tops of the bars together, we will get a curve that looks like a bell) and the numbers can be added, subtracted, multiplied, divided and thus analysed by parametric statistics.

You can probably work out yourself, then, that *non-parametric* data, which include ordinal and nominal data, are data that do not meet the same criteria around things like distribution and which cannot be added, subtracted, multiplied and divided (as in the numbers on the footballers' backs!). Non-parametric data require non-parametric statistical tests, which are considered to be less reliable than parametric statistics. However, if you want to research something that happens to be non-parametric in nature, you can hardly make it become parametric just because this is considered a more reliable kind of data! Having said that, parametric tests are sometimes used on non-parametric data, as explained further in the box.

FINDING THE AVERAGE

Most people will already be familiar with the concept of the average – or, to give it its mathematical name, central tendency (or, if you'd rather be more informal, what's in the middle) – and will know that it is possible to measure this in one of three ways.

The *mean* is what you get if you add up all of the values in a group and divide them by the number of values. So if we were to add up the heights of 10 jelly babies and the divide the number by 10, we would have the mean average height of the jelly babies in our group. The mean is used with interval or ratio data.

The *median* is what you get if you line up all of the values from the lowest to the highest (imagine asking a group of jelly babies to arrange themselves into a line with the shortest on the left and the tallest on the right!) and then take the height of the jelly baby in the middle as the average (Section 6, Figure 2). If you have an even number of jelly babies, you simply add together the heights of the two jelly babies in the middle and divide the result by two. The median is used with ordinal, interval or ratio data.

This can also be a more useful test of the average if you have one or more values that differ widely from the others. Imagine if we had nine jelly babies that were 2 inches tall and then a tenth giant jelly baby who was 22 inches tall joined the line (Section 6, Figure 3); if we used the mean, the average height would be 4 inches because the giant jelly baby would skew the results. In this case, it might be better to do the median; we would find out that the median height was 2 inches and the giant jelly baby that skewed the data wouldn't give us a misleading average.

The *mode* is simply the most commonly occurring value. It is possible to use the mode with ordinal, interval or ratio data, but this doesn't often happen. In fact, it is not generally used for numerical data unless these data are nominal; however, it would be the only way we could measure something like the most common jelly baby colour. As long as they haven't got bored yet, we could shake out a few packets of jelly babies

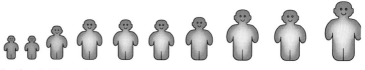

Section 6, Figure 2

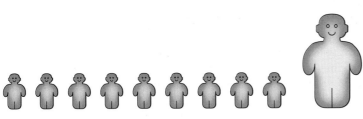

Section 6, Figure 3

and ask them to arrange themselves in groups, according to colour. We would then be able to count the numbers of jelly babies in each group and could see which colour occurred most often. (Personally, I think it is green, but I might be biased because that's my least favourite colour!)

So you can see from all of this that each of the measures of central tendency is used for different levels of measurement. As a general rule of thumb:

If you have nominal data → Use the mode
If you have ordinal data → Use the median
If you have interval data → Use the mean if the data are symmetrical
→ Use the median if the data are 'skewed'
If you have ratio data → Use the mean if the data are symmetrical
→ Use the median if the data are 'skewed'

When looking critically at the question of how researchers calculated the average, you simply need to know about whether the method they have used was the one best suited to the kind of data they were looking at. Sometimes researchers will present more than one kind of average to answer the same question; this might be to show you that there was little difference between the mean and mode average, thus reducing the risk of potential bias. If there was a difference between the mean and the median, you should check out if and how they justified which one they used in the rest of their analysis. It is very easy to fool people with measures of central tendency, as the example of the giant jelly baby shows, which is why we'll talk about dispersion next.

DISPERSION

As I've just mentioned, the average can sometimes be misleading unless you know other things about the data. Let's go back to the group of jelly babies that included the giant jelly baby. Here are the things we already know about measuring the average height of the jelly babies in that group.

- If we use the mean, the average height would be falsely high because the giant jelly baby would skew the data.
- If we use the median, the average height would be a more accurate representation of the data as a whole, because the giant jelly baby would not skew the median in the same way it would skew the mean.
- *But* if we simply reported the median average height of the group (2 inches) without any other information, we would have no idea whether the group of jelly babies we were looking at were:
  - 10 jelly babies who were 2 inches tall
  - nine jelly babies who were 2 inches tall and one who was 10 inches tall
  - eight jelly babies who were 2 inches tall, one who was 1½ inches tall (perhaps because she had got a bit squashed in the packet) and one whose head and upper body had been eaten and was only ½ inch tall.

I could go on; if you think about it, there are lots of ways that the data set could be skewed enough for us to have chosen the median but contain anomalous jelly babies on one or other end of the line, but I'll stop now in the hope that you've got the picture!

In the example I have used on the right, where the median is 2 and the range is 8, I said that we could deduce from this that we have at least one really tall jelly baby, because no jelly babies can have a height of less than zero. If you can get into the habit of looking for things like this when you are reading the data given in research papers, you can weave these into your responses to papers and thus demonstrate that you really understand what you are talking about. You might even be able to spot something that someone else hasn't! Some of the best ways of doing this are to think about the people 'behind' the statistics, and/or to think about how you would have answered a question, and/or to think about your own experience of the world and of practice and see how the statistics given relate to this. If the numbers given in a research paper disagree with your own experience it doesn't make either you or them wrong, but it might highlight something interesting which you can discuss.

So this is why we need to also talk about *dispersion*, or *spread* or *variability*, all of which mean essentially the same thing and describe the ways in which the data are arranged around the average. The tools that calculate things under the umbrella term of dispersion can give us a clearer picture of the other jelly babies in the line or, indeed, with a line where we would use the mean average but still want to know more about the variation. There are a number of different ways of calculating and talking about different aspects of dispersion, which are described below.

The *range* shows us the extent of our data set: the difference between the minimum and maximum values in the group. In the group that included the 10-inch jelly baby and its nine 2-inch friends, the median average height was 2 inches, with the lowest height being 2 inches and the highest height being 10 inches. The range is calculated by subtracting the lowest value from the highest, so in this case the range would be $10 - 2 = 8$.

If the range is a low number, you know that all of the data in the group are quite similar, whereas if the range is a high number, you know that you have a wider range of data. If we have a median jelly baby height of 2 and a range of 0, we know that all of the jelly babies in the group are 2 inches tall.

The range doesn't always tell us which way the data are skewed; if the median of a data set of jelly baby tummy circumferences was 30 mm and the range was 20 mm, we know that we either have some fat or thin jelly babies, but we don't know which. With our example where the median is 2 and the range is 8, we can deduce that we have at least one fairly tall jelly baby because no jelly baby could have a height of less than zero!

Although the range can be used with both the median and the mean, it still doesn't tell us all that much and other measures can give us a further sense of how the data are spread around the average without us having to look at every single value. Sometimes, the easiest way of doing this is to plot a chart or graph which shows the spread (i.e. the curves and bar graphs which sometimes show distribution of data pictorially), but there are also numerical ways of showing this which take up less space in an article.

The *interquartile range*, which is used with the median, builds upon this idea and tells us about the range of the scores in the middle half of a distribution. To calculate it, you first need to find the numbers that describe the 25th quartile and the 75th quartile. Statisticians have a number of different ways of defining quartiles, but we are certainly not going to worry about that here! For our purposes we will define them as follows.

- The 25th quartile is the point below which a quarter of the data lies.
- The 75th quartile is the point below which three-quarters of the data lie (so one-quarter of the data lies above it).
- The 50th quartile, by the way, is the median, which you already know about.

Another way of thinking of it is like this.

- The 25th quartile is the median point of the data between the lowest value and the median value.
- The 75th quartile is the median point of the data between the median and the highest value.

The interquartile range (IQR), then, is the difference between the 25th and 75th quartiles. To calculate it, you subtract the 25th quartile from the 75th quartile and the result is the IQR. Like the range, it is expressed as one number. Let's have another quick look at our group of jelly babies that includes the giant.

We already know that the median value of this group is 2 and the range is 8. The IQR is 0 ($2 - 2$). Although I am showing you the picture of the data set so that you can see how these calculations are made and how they relate to the data (Section 6, Figure 4), if you weren't able to see the picture you could now be more certain from the statistics alone that most of the values are very close to the median value.

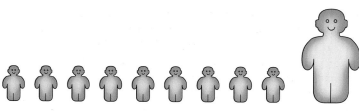

Section 6, Figure 4

Additionally, the combination of the median, the range and the IQR also gives us a fair idea that there might be one or two extreme values which are skewing the data set.

Variance and *standard deviation* (SD) are also used when we are looking to add information to a mean average, as they can tell us about how close the scores in the distribution are to the average and give us more of an idea of how the data are dispersed around the average.

By this point, many statistical textbooks will have piled into the equations that help you calculate things like standard deviation. Although I've described the simple calculations like the range, I'm not going to describe these more complex equations; partly because if you want to know this stuff, you can find it in any statistics book; partly because that's the point where the statistics books usually lose the attention of anybody who doesn't find maths easy; and partly because, at the level of being able to understand and critique research for practice, you don't actually need to know how they are worked out; you just need a basic idea of what they represent and a few key points. So, instead of the equations, here are the key points.

- Both variance and standard deviation involve looking at how each of the individual values deviates from the average value. In other words, it can tell you whether the values in the data set are closely arranged around the average or whether they are widely spread out.
- Variance involves squaring the deviation of each number from the average, so, if you are looking at a study that gives the average height of jelly babies in mm, you can expect the variation to be expressed in mm^2.
- Standard deviation involves squaring values and then finding the square root (don't worry, we're not going to get into how you do that!) so it is expressed in the same terms as the average. So, if the average height is expressed in mm, the standard deviation will also be expressed in mm.
- Just as the mean can be affected when there are outliers, or extreme values, in the data (like the 10-inch jelly baby), the standard deviation can also be affected. If the standard deviation is high, then this might be because there are outliers in the data.
- The standard deviation can be very useful when you are comparing two data sets with each other, as in the example in 'A quick guide to tables' (see p 143), where we talked about the kind of table researchers use to show that, after randomisation, the two groups were similar. If the averages of two data sets are similar but one of the data sets has a larger standard deviation than the other, we know that the data set with the larger standard deviation has a wider spread of data around the mean and may include more people with very low or very high values. Ideally, if we are looking at two groups of people who are entering an RCT, we want to see that both the mean average and the standard deviation (or the IQR in cases where the median is used) for each variable are similar in both groups.
- In other words, a value from a data set that has a low standard deviation is closer to the mean average than a value from the data set that has a higher standard deviation.
- Standard deviation is never expressed as a negative value.
- As we discussed with the IQR, if all the values in one data set are exactly the same (e.g. 10 jelly babies who are all 2 inches tall), then the standard deviation will be 0.

A brief digression on centiles

Even though you are less likely to see centiles than quartiles in birth-related research, we do encounter centiles in practice, so here's a little bit of information about those, in case you've always wondered…

Centiles, or percentiles, are a bit like quartiles, except that whereas quartiles divide the data into four equal parts, percentiles divide it into 100 equal parts. They are quite handy for telling us about how an aspect of an individual relates to the same aspect in the population as a whole, which is why you commonly see them on baby growth charts. A baby whose height (or weight, or head circumference, whatever you are looking at) is on the 50th centile is exactly in the middle of the population in relation to that variable, whereas a baby whose growth is on the 3rd centile is smaller than 97% of other babies.

As with other ways in which we use numbers in practice, this tool has advantages and disadvantages. It can be useful to note that an individual baby's weight was on the 75th centile but, 2 weeks later, is now on the 13th centile, as this can highlight issues in relation to her growth. On the other hand, it can be dangerous to automatically assume that a baby who is on the 1st or 99th centile is intrinsically abnormal – by definition, some babies have to be on the 1st and 99th centile, otherwise the graph itself wouldn't be an accurate representation of the population!

LOOKING FOR CORRELATIONS

Because quantitative research related to childbearing in the Western world is so focused on interventions and outcomes, one of the key areas of statistical theory used in data analysis is called *relational statistics*. You may have already noticed that the words *relational* and *correlation* are very similar – in fact, they relate (no pun intended!) to the same thing, which is whether two or more things that have been measured in a research study can be shown to have a relationship to each other. In other words, if we want to find out whether there is a correlation between the amount of jelly babies someone eats and their level of happiness, or perhaps their weight, then we need to use relational statistics. Again, we can only use some of these if we have the right kind of data – you can't generally use these tests with nominal data – but the focus in this section is to enable you to understand the basics of what the tests mean when you see them in research papers.

Before we go on, there are a couple more things to note here.

1. Just because something can be shown to correlate (*co-relate*) to something else with statistics does not mean that there is a causal relationship between the two. Don't forget that statistics are an attempt to get to the truth, they are not absolute truth in themselves! This was shown very well in a study by Hofer et al (2004), who managed to show a correlation between an increase in the stork population in one part of Germany and an increase in the home birth rate in the same area! However, the statistical association between the two things was, according to them, entirely coincidental.

2. Even if a correlation can be shown to exist between two things, statistics can only show us that a relationship appears to exist, not *why* it exists or *what* it means. To explore these questions, we need to use other ways of knowing.

The analysis of relationships can be *univariate*, *bivariate* or *multivariate*.

Univariate analysis is actually very simple and you already know about most of the tools used to summarise the individual variables in a data set, because we have just looked at them! Univariate analysis uses tools like the mean (or median or mode), the range and the standard deviation (or variance or IQR) to describe the data. It might also end up on the page as a pictorial representation in the form of a bar graph, pie chart or line graph (among other possibilities).

Bivariate analysis measures the strength of the relationship between two variables. This does not, by the way, mean that we are interested in whether the marriage of two given jelly babies is likely to last; instead, it means we are interested in things like whether the mood of a group of jelly babies is linked with the time of the year, or whether there is a link between the weight of the baby at birth and the weight of the sweets or chocolates given to her or his midwife! (This, by the way, was a real study, conducted by Nordin in 1993!)

The main statistical test used to see if there is a relationship between two variables is called *correlation*, and correlations are represented by *correlation coefficients*, which include tests with long and complicated names like Pearson's product moment correlation coefficient (for parametric data) or Spearman's rank correlation coefficient (for non-parametric data), but we won't worry about these equations either because these are the things you need to know about correlation coefficients.

- They can be positive or negative: a positive correlation coefficient means that, as one thing increases (e.g. average number of jelly babies eaten in a day), something else increases at the same time (e.g. happiness or weight). A negative correlation coefficient means that as one thing increases (e.g. the amount of bursary that a student midwife gets), something else (perhaps the stress level of the student midwife) decreases.

- Positive correlation coefficients are expressed in values that fall between 0 and 1, so they involve figures like 0.35, 0.76 and 0.2.

- Negative correlation coefficients are expressed in values that fall between 0 and −1, so they involve figures like −0.5, −0.83 and −0.2.
- The higher the number, the stronger the correlation between the two things is. So a correlation coefficient of 0.68 implies a stronger correlation than a correlation coefficient of 0.54.
- It is generally perceived that a correlation coefficient of:
  - 0.8 to 1.0 is very strong
  - 0.6 to 0.8 is strong
  - 0.4 to 0.6 is moderate
  - 0.2 to 0.4 is weak
  - 0 to 0.2 is very weak.

There are other aspects to this, and other statistical tests that can help explore different kinds of relationships between variables, because not all relationship are linear – some are curved, or S-shaped, or logarithmic, but relatively simple linear correlations are the kind you are most likely to see in birth-related research.

If researchers find that a strong correlation appears in their data, they might then go on to do something called *regression*. Regression comes under the heading of *inferential statistics*, because it can help us see whether *inferences* can be made about a population from the data collected about the sample. Regression, then, is simply about trying to plot a line on a graph to link the two things that seem to correlate, so that you can make predictions about other values from the graph. For instance, if you find that there is a strong correlation between the height of a jelly baby and how good that jelly baby is at basketball, you might decide to use regression to see if you could make predictions about how a jelly baby who was not in the study might fare at basketball. Or, to use a practice-related example, if you found a correlation between the height of mothers and the weight of their babies, you could use regression analysis to try to predict how heavy the baby of any particular mother might be. In reality, relationships are not always simple and linear, and this is one of the main problems with using quantitative research and statistics when we are trying to learn more about childbearing.

Multivariate analysis is about looking at whether more than one thing correlates with others. Unfortunately for us, the term can be used to mean more than one thing and a large number of techniques fall under this umbrella (and some, like regression, fall into the category of inferential statistics). Some examples are given in Section 6, Table 2, although this is only so that you can identify what they are; as I have said before, you do not need to understand how they all work to be able to critique research! We will have a look at one of the most common tests used in birth-related research: multiple regression analysis.

Although it is much simpler and 'cleaner' to look at just two values in relation to each other, the world we live in is very complex and there are often lots of factors that need to be taken into account. After conducting my 'jelly baby study' for a number of years with different groups of midwives and students, I have never found that jelly babies make a significant difference to midwives' or students' happiness. When I change the focus of my study around completely and run a qualitative focus group asking student midwives what makes them happy, they talk about things like their family situation, their assessment workload and the financial pressures of being a student midwife. From my qualitative study I then have a number of factors that could contribute to students' happiness. (There's a bit more about this idea on the next page.)

For my next piece of quantitative research, I might choose to ask lots of students to complete a questionnaire that asks them questions about different areas of their life and about things like their happiness. I might also decide to include their academic grades to see if any of these factors can be correlated with how well they are doing. I would then need to use a test like multiple regression analysis to compare their responses in each of these areas to see if I could find any relationships between the different things.

Logarithmic! What does that mean?

For anybody who has noticed the words 'logarithm' or 'logarithmic' and doesn't know what they mean, logarithms are a kind of number that is used as a substitute for other numbers. A well-known example of a logarithmic scale is the Richter scale, which measures earthquakes. Because the magnitude of earthquakes can vary by an enormous amount, there would be a lot of zeros if we used simple numbers to measure them by. Instead, each of the logarithmic numbers – or steps – on the Richter scale denotes that the earthquake released 10 times as much energy as the number representing the previous step. So an earthquake measuring 7.0 releases 10 times as much energy as an earthquake measuring 6.0.

So, if you use the logarithms of a series of numbers, you can sometimes work more easily than if you use the numbers themselves. In statistics, if you would need to perform complex multiplications with the original numbers, you can sometimes use the logarithms of the numbers instead and then use addition instead of multiplication. There are different kinds of logarithms, but all you really need to know is that they are a way of substituting where you might have to multiply the original numbers, and can be a way of representing things that might vary widely and might otherwise be difficult to show on a graph.

Section 6, Table 2 Types of multivariate analysis

Multiple regression analysis	Logistic regression
Multivariate analysis of variance	Cross-classification analysis
Multidimensional scaling (MDS)	Cluster analysis

The circle of research

The example I have discussed of the quantitative and qualitative jelly baby studies is a good example of how different kinds of research can be used to generate knowledge in a cyclical way. The discussions in Chapters 1 and 2 of this book look at how, if you employ both quantitative and qualitative elements in a study on a particular area, you can often learn different but complementary things from each. The example of the jelly baby study further shows how different kinds of research can help us move in circles of knowing (Section 6, Figure 5).

This circle links *inductive* kinds of research, which enable us to generate knowledge and hypotheses without necessarily having had a fixed agenda about what those hypotheses might have been beforehand, and *deductive* kinds of research, which enable us to test very specific questions or hypotheses.

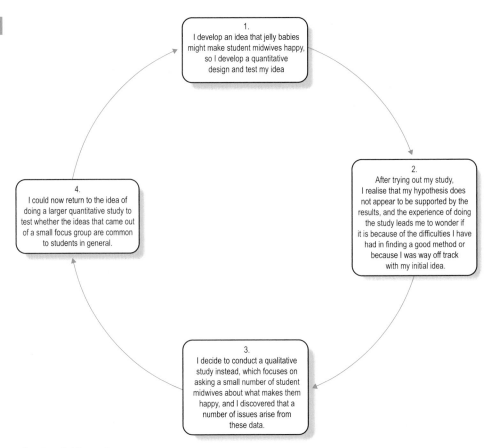

1.
I develop an idea that jelly babies might make student midwives happy, so I develop a quantitative design and test my idea

2.
After trying out my study, I realise that my hypothesis does not appear to be supported by the results, and the experience of doing the study leads me to wonder if it is because of the difficulties I have had in finding a good method or because I was way off track with my initial idea.

3.
I decide to conduct a qualitative study instead, which focuses on asking a small number of student midwives about what makes them happy, and I discovered that a number of issues arise from these data.

4.
I could now return to the idea of doing a larger quantitative study to test whether the ideas that came out of a small focus group are common to students in general.

Section 6, Figure 5

(Before I go on, I want to point out that some of the kinds of data I have suggested gathering for this study are exactly those kinds that I have already said might not be OK with certain statistical tests, i.e. ordinal data, but, just for now, I am hoping we can just pretend that this is not the case so that we can stay with the simple examples that I've been using throughout this section!)

Multiple regression, then, would allow me to look at all of the factors on which I have gathered data in relation to each other. I could look at the effect of any number of factors on a certain outcome at the same time. I could also look at how a number of different factors explain differences in outcomes between different people, or I could look at the effect of one specific factor while taking into account other factors which might have influenced the outcome. This last example is seen relatively often in birth-related research, and a related statistical test called logistic regression is used in the research in Chapter 5.

As before, this is just one example of inferential statistics, which are used to see if inferences can be made about a population from the data collected about the sample. One of the other most important aspects of inferential statistics in birth-related research occurs where they are used to calculate whether a finding or result is statistically significant.

TESTING YOUR HYPOTHESIS

Let's say that we are going to do a very simple RCT to compare whether a group of people who each eat 20 jelly babies in 5 minutes have a higher blood sugar than a control group of people who don't eat anything. We have recruited enough people who have fasted for a few hours before the study, randomised them into groups and used descriptive statistics to ensure that the two groups are similar enough to continue. We have recorded the blood sugar of everyone in the groups and given the intervention group their jelly babies, following whatever research protocol and data collection method we agreed on previously. We now have a lot of data, perhaps a sheet of A4 for each person, which might summarise some of their demographic and other details but also, most importantly of all for the purposes of the next paragraph, records their blood sugar before and after the experiment.

If the data we have are normally distributed, we could use the *t*-test (which, by the way, was developed to measure the similarity of different batches of Guinness!). It comes in two forms.

- We could do a one-sample *t*-test and compare the blood sugars of the people who had the jelly babies to the blood sugar of the population as a whole (assuming we know this). To do this, we would compare the mean score in our sample with the mean average blood sugar level in the population at large. The test takes into account the size of the sample and the standard deviation, and churns out a *t*-number. The *t*-number and the number of people in the sample can then be put together to work out the *p* value (which is explained further below), which tells us if our result is statistically significant.
- We could also do a two-sample *t*-test, where we compare the blood sugars of the people who had the jelly babies to the blood sugars of the people who didn't have the jelly babies but who were similar to them in every other regard. In this case, the mean score of the people in the intervention group is compared with the mean score of the people in the control group. All of the numbers are sent into the equation and out comes a *t*-number which, again, can be used to calculate the *p* value.

Given that we have done an RCT, it would seem silly not to do the two-sample *t*-test, and this is a very common statistical test in birth-related research, but you need to know about the one-sample *t*-test as there is not always a handy control group available! One of the big advantages of the *t*-test is that you can use it even if you only have a small number of people. If your data are not normally distributed, you would have to use something like the Mann–Whitney U-test, which is defined below.

Section 6, Box 1 But what's a *p* value?

I think I might have mentioned before that statistics are not absolute truth; one of the reasons for this is that there is always a possibility that we got some results that look significant but which actually came about by chance.

Imagine that I asked 100 student midwives to toss 10 coins and record how many heads and how many tails they got. You might expect that most of them will get five heads and five tails, or four and six, and you probably wouldn't be surprised if quite a few got three of one and seven of the other. But would you be surprised if somebody got 10 heads? What about if they were asked to toss 20 coins and someone got 20 tails?

Although we tend to expect that most experimental results will fall around the average, it is important to acknowledge that, sometimes, unlikely things do happen by chance alone. The more student midwives you ask to participate in the coin-tossing experiment, the more likely it is that someone will get 10 heads or 10 tails. If they are all in the same room when it happens, the person who got 10 of something won't be that surprised, because they will be able to see that they have the 'anomalous' result and that most people have the kind of results you'd expect to see.

The same thing is true with research statistics. If you conduct enough studies, some of them will get results that appear to be significant simply by chance. That is, the results will look as if they are significant, but they actually won't be; the difference in the results of the two groups (or the one group when compared to the population as a whole) will have come about simply by chance. They will be the research equivalent of getting 10 heads. However, we are no more able to predict which studies will get anomalous results than we can predict which student will get 10 coins landing heads up. We also have an additional problem with research statistics – we can't even tell in retrospect which studies' results came about merely by chance, although this might be one of the reasons why you sometimes see 10 studies which find one thing and the eleventh study on the same topic saying something completely different.

Continued

Tips to impress your tutor: 4

When you are looking at quantitative research studies, have a look at the tables and statistics and see what p value the researchers considered to be statistically significant and how they talk about the significance of their results in the text of their paper. Sometimes, you will see results that are significant (but not highly significant) and which appear to be given more weight in the text of the article than this might merit. Sometimes, the opposite happens, and one result comes out to be much more statistically significant than other results, yet this is not picked up in the discussion. Although this might be because it was not the main aim, or may be due to a lack of wordage, it might also be indicative of bias, and a useful point for your discussion of the paper.

Section 6, Box 1 But what's a p value?

Here's one important thing to remember:

You can never completely rule out the possibility that the results came about by chance, in any study. It doesn't matter how well the study is designed!

So this is where our friend the p value comes in. It can be helpful to think about the p standing for 'the possibility that we got our results by chance alone'. And this is what the p value tells us. Remember, there is *always* a chance that they came about by chance...

p values are represented on a scale from 0 to 1, where 0 would represent no chance of the results having come about by chance (which doesn't actually happen, because, as I have just said, there is always a chance that they came about by chance!) and 1 would mean they definitely came about by chance (which also doesn't happen because we can't be certain about that either!).

Once you get the hang of it, it is simple to translate p values into terms that are generally easier for non-mathematicians to understand. If the p value is 0.1, this means that there is a 1 in 10 chance that the results came about by chance. If the p value is 0.5, there is a 1 in 2 chance that the results came about by chance. You need to translate the decimal into a fraction, and then you know how likely it is that the results came about by chance. However, if you've just switched off at the idea of having to turn a decimal into a fraction, there is an even simpler way, which I'll come back to in a minute, but you will have to brace yourself to learn a couple of other things instead!

It is generally accepted that if the p value is 0.05 or less, then the results of a study are considered statistically significant. There is still a 1 in 20 chance that the results turned out the way they did by chance alone (which means that if you line up 20 study results with a p value of 0.05, odds are that one of them is an interloper!) but this is the generally accepted point at which results are said to be significant. If the p value is 0.005 or lower, then there is only a 1 in 200 chance that the results came about by chance alone, and this is considered to be highly statistically significant. It's still not 'truth' but it's a better result than, say, a p value of 0.08.

Even if all you can do is to remember that 0.05 is significant and 0.005 is highly significant, you are halfway there! The other thing you have to get your head around is that, when it comes to numbers after the decimal point, numbers that appear bigger mean lower significance! So a p value of 0.8 is less significant than a p value of 0.1, although neither of these would be considered statistically significant. Finally, the more zeros that come straight after the decimal point, the more statistically significant the result is said to be.

PUTTING A FEW MORE NAMES TO FACES...

One issue that cannot easily be avoided when we discuss statistics is that many of the more complex tests and ideas you will see in birth-related research can be used for more than one thing, which makes it difficult to categorise them easily. Now that we have come this far and, hopefully, you have a better understanding of some of the key concepts, I'll use this last section to help you put a few more names to faces as far as statistical tests are concerned, and give you a little bit of information about how they are used.

ANOVA stands for *AN*alysis *O*f *VA*riance, and this is one of the tests that can be used for a number of things, but is basically designed to determine whether there are significant differences between the mean averages of different groups or variables. You can see an example of ANOVA in use in Table 2 of the study in Chapter 6 (see p 102).

Chi-square is used to evaluate hypotheses. It enables researchers to see whether relationships between two variables in a sample are either statistically significant or due to chance alone. The test is relatively simple and compares what you would expect to see if there was no relationship between the variables with what you actually observe in your sample. Julie Frohlich has a bit more to say about chi-square in Chapter 5.

F-tests are used a bit like *t*-tests but they are far more powerful (and also much more complex!). You might see them in birth-related research in conjunction with regression and ANOVA.

The *Kruskal–Wallis test* is another kind of analysis of variance, which is used for non-parametric data. It enables researchers to rank the values of different sample groups so that they can see whether one or more of the groups are significantly different from the other(s).

The *Mann–Whitney U-test* (and the *Wilcoxon signed-rank sum test*) can be used with ordinal as well as interval and ratio data, and it enables comparison of the data from two independent samples to determine whether any differences are statistically significant.

Z-tests are used for a number of things, including to test whether correlation coefficients are statistically significant and to compare samples to populations.

Section 6, Box 2 Confidence intervals

By now, we've talked several times about how statistical tests can't give us the exact, spot-on, precise truth that our brains might yearn for but that many people's hearts know doesn't really exist. Instead of claiming that they have the exact answer, researchers usually have to say things like, 'well, we think the answer is around about y, and we are pretty sure that the answer lies somewhere between x and z, but we can't be certain at all, so we have to acknowledge there is a small chance that it is totally outside even this wider range.' In research papers, though, there generally isn't room to say all of that, so, instead, you see something like this:

Section 6, Figure 6

Of course, the lines and dots are pretty meaningless without numbers, so you will either see numbers written next to each of the ends and the dot, or the little 'bar and dot' pictures might instead be placed on a graph so that you can read the numbers from the axis of the graph. In the text, they read something like (relative risk 6; 95% CI 4–8), which means, our results show that the relative risk is 6 and that, given that this might not be exactly accurate, there is a 95% chance that the relative risk lies somewhere between 4 and 8.

The *confidence interval* (CI), then, is not the main finding, it is a way of expressing a range *around* the main finding, which tells us how precise the main finding is and therefore how much attention we should pay to it. If the proposed answer is y, then the confidence interval in the case above is x–z.

By the way, confidence intervals do not always use 95% as the level of significance; you might also see confidence intervals that use 90% or 99%. With a 95% level of significance, you have a 5% chance of being wrong (and, like with a p value of 0.05, that's 1 in 20), with a 90% confidence interval you have a 10% (1 in 10) chance of being wrong, and with a 99% confidence interval you have a 1% (1 in 100) chance of being wrong.

Sometimes you will see several results and confidence intervals plotted on the same graph so you can compare the results of several studies on the same topic: the meta-analyses carried out by the Cochrane Collaboration are a good example of this. Confidence intervals can tell you a number of things, and there are different things to look at with them, especially when you are able to compare several together.

- A narrow confidence interval is more significant than a wide one.
- A symmetrical confidence interval (where the line is about the same length either side of the dot) is generally preferable to a non-symmetrical one (which has a longer line on one side of the dot than the other).
- With something like an RCT, if the graph containing the confidence interval is split into two sides, where one side means that *A* works better and the other side means that *B* works better, we can be more confident about the confidence intervals that do not cross the central line. If a confidence interval crosses the line, this means that, even though the dot itself might be on one side of the graph, the results are less trustworthy than if the entire confidence interval was on one side of the graph than the other.

A FINAL REMINDER

Don't forget: whether you are looking at confidence intervals, *p* values or any other kind of number, your statistics are only as good as the data you collected, which in turn are only as good as the methods you used to collect them! One of my statistics lecturers used to say, 'If you put garbage in, you'll get nothing but garbage out!'. Even if someone has managed to get the most significant result in the world after they've performed the 'perfect' statistical analysis, this could be because their data collection tool was biased because they didn't adequately randomise participants or because of any number of other flaws in the design of their study. Although it is important to be able to look at the separate parts of the study in depth, it is also important to think about the whole, and about whether potential bias in one part of the study could lead to more potential bias later on. It's a bit like working in the garden really – you have to dig around the different parts of the research in order to weed out the problems, but you also have to step back sometimes and take a wider view of what's going on to make sure you're digging in the right place. And, often, it's only at the end of the day – when you get to relax in a comfy chair and admire your work – that you decide it was worth it, after all!

References

Hofer T, Przyrembel H, Verleger S 2004 New evidence for the Theory of the Stork. Paediatric and Perinatal Epidemiology 18(1):88–92

Nordin AJ 1993 A prospective study of postpartum candy gift net weight: correlation with birth weight. Obstetrics and Gynecology 82(1):156–158

DRAWING IT ALL TOGETHER

Here, I am simply outlining a few tips for recording your thoughts about different studies and drawing them together when you are asked to present a critical review of several studies, for instance in a dissertation or literature review.

The index card approach

This is a way of recording and prioritising your thoughts about studies, rather than just reading or appraising them, but some people have found it useful as an approach. You can use it in conjunction with any of the approaches to critiquing discussed in Section 1 (or, indeed, any other approach that is not mentioned here). As you read a study, you note down up to five key points about the design of the study (e.g. that it only included women having their first baby, that it set out to look at the difference between two methods of suturing, and that it was an RCT). You can then note down up to five key points that arise from the study, which you will focus on in your critique. If you already have five points and find another, you will need to decide whether the latest point is more important than one of those that you already have, thus limiting yourself to a few key points rather than lots of points of differing importance.

This method is not much use if you are being asked to write a 4000-word critique of one paper, as you will need to look at lots more than five key points, but it can be helpful if you are writing something like a dissertation and need to summarise or précis a lot of studies on the same subject and pull the salient points out of each. It can also help you think about what the really significant issues from each study are, as you will have to decide whether, for instance, the fact that a study excluded women under 18 was more or less important than the fact that one of the main outcome measures could have been interpreted differently by different midwives. I sometimes use this kind of approach if I am writing a short critique for a journal or digest like MIDIRS, where you only have around 500 words and have to get to the key issues really quickly.

Pulling it all together

Finally, if you are writing an overview of several studies, such as in a dissertation, the following information might be useful, although please don't take my word for it if you are undertaking a course and your lecturer wants something different from this!

Generally, the students who gain the most marks are those who integrate their discussion of several studies rather than writing about each one separately, and one after the other. One way in which you can do this is to draw a table with different headings so you can put your notes from each study in a separate row and then pull out points. Here is a very simple example, which considers four imaginary studies that looked at the question of whether jelly babies make student midwives happy. (These include the kinds of study that were discussed in Chapter 1.) Because this is such a simple example, you might well find you need to add more columns to cover all of the issues in the area you are looking at.

Section 6, Table 3 Integrating and comparing research

Author	Study design	Participants	Number of participants	Main results	Key points
A	RCT	Student midwives	150	No difference detected between jelly baby and no jelly baby	No blinding
B	RCT	Student and qualified midwives	200	Students who had a jelly baby were not significantly happier than students who did not, but authors noted a statistically significant reduction in the happiness of the control group	No blinding. Difficult to see what was going on for individuals because of quantitative design
C	Prospective case control	Student midwives	1500	Students who were continually given jelly babies over a period of time were significantly happier than the control group, but researchers note that it was impossible to separate out whether this was due to the effect of the jelly baby or to the extra attention students received from the lecturer running the study	Problems with possible confounding variables (as researcher notes)
D	Grounded theory	Student midwives	25	When asked what made them happy, students didn't mention jelly babies at all, but discussed issues concerning finance (or lack thereof), different teaching and learning methods and whether lecturers were perceived as being interested in and responsive to their needs	Difficult to generalise because of qualitative design Specific questions re jelly babies were not asked

With this example, you might note some of the following points.

- Two RCTs and one case control study looked at the question at hand; there was also one qualitative study that did not look at the exact same question but which might throw additional light on the topic.
- Both of the RCTs were small and no blinding was used, which has implications that you can discuss further...
- The results of both RCTs showed no positive effect of having a jelly baby, although the case control study did (but, as the researchers themselves noted, this may have been affected by confounding factors, which you might want to expand on a bit as well...)
- One RCT showed that students who did not get jelly babies were unhappier as a result, which might have been an unexpected finding, and has more implications that you can discuss...
- The qualitative study, although not specifically designed to look at jelly babies, might throw additional light onto the issue of what makes student midwives happy. This could be explored in relation to the results of the case control study,

where students receiving jelly babies might also have been exposed to different teaching methods. However, when we also add in the results of the RCTs, it begins to look as though jelly babies *per se* are not the issue...

- With this example, it is entirely possible to come to one of a number of conclusions, including that:
  - There is no real evidence to support the idea that jelly babies make student midwives happy (with this conclusion we are rejecting the results of the case control study because it contradicts all of the others and because of the possibility of confounding), and there is no point in exploring this any further...
  - Although there is not much evidence to support the idea that jelly babies make student midwives happy, the case control study, although methodologically flawed, did show some difference and therefore we should think about attempting a larger RCT which attempts to find a placebo and a method of blinding...
  - Although there is little evidence to support the idea that jelly babies make student midwives happy, the results of both the case control and the qualitative study seem to suggest that there may be a case for exploring the use of creative teaching methods (with or without jelly babies) further...

CERRIDWYN AND THE PIXIES: A HOLIDAY FAIRYTALE

This article was first published in *The Practising Midwife* in December 2004, and has been included here by kind permission of *The Practising Midwife*. It sets out to illustrate, in story form, some of the points discussed throughout the book about the current dominance of the RCT in relation to other forms of research.

Once upon a time, four research pixies, Reggie RCT, Patti Phenomenology, Connie Cohort and Clive Case-Control, went for a walk in the woods. On the way, they collected their friends, Edward Ethnography, Gillie Grounded Theory and Leonard Longitudinal. They decided to explore a part of the woods they hadn't been to before, and walked through the trees, talking about the different perspectives they brought to generating knowledge. Each had always thought that their own perspective was the best, and they had long debates about which was the most useful way to find things out.

'Of course phenomenology is best,' Patti said. 'I get much deeper than some of you, who only look at numbers. I can see way beyond the numbers to find out what people really think and feel.'

'Which is all very well,' snorted Reggie, 'if you want to know how a few people think, but what about when you need to see if something you think is true really is true for whole populations? Then you need an RCT!'

'Or a cohort study,' shouted Connie, 'especially if it's not fair to force people to take the option that you choose for them, Reggie.'

And so they continued, bickering about who was best, as they had done every day for all the years they had known each other.

Soon, they came upon a clearing. In the middle of a clearing there was a circle of happy fairies, and in the middle of the circle sat the most beautiful woman they had ever seen. They stopped in their tracks, awed by the sight. The woman beckoned them into the circle, explaining that she was Cerridwyn, the knowledge fairy, and wanted to tell them that their approaches were all of great value. As she spoke, the pixies looked at each other: as if by magic, each pixie intuitively realised that their perspective to research brought advantages and challenges, and that the ideal way forward was to work together.

The pixies talked with the knowledge fairy until dusk began to fall. Reluctantly, they left the lovely fairy and carried on through the woods, trying to find a short cut home so they could talk about their new-found friend and her words of wisdom.

As they walked, the woods became very dark and, suddenly, they saw two yellow eyes peering out of the trees. Scared, the pixies huddled together, as a man stepped out of the trees, holding several banners in his hands.

The man laughed. 'I haven't seen you here before. Have you been to see Cerridwyn?'

Some of the braver pixies nodded.

The man laughed again. 'I suppose she's told you that you're all valuable, in different ways?'

The pixies nodded again and the man laughed a third time, longer and louder than before.

'Well that would be lovely if it were true, but those nice humans have been getting together and they have made their own decisions about which of you is the more valuable, and sent me with a standard for each of you to carry, so you'll know where you stand.'

Some of the pixies shrunk back, as the man silently handed out the flags: pink for Gillie, Patti and Edward and varying shades of green for Connie, Clive and Leonard. The biggest and most beautiful flag of all he handed to Reggie, who looked in awe at its golden colour. The pixies were so busy looking around at the flags that they didn't realise the man had disappeared.

'Well I guess that answers it,' said Reggie haughtily. 'RCTs are the best. I said so all along, and now my flag proves it. I shan't be needing to hang out with you losers any more.' And, so saying, he walked off, his head held high and his flag flying behind him.

The other pixies looked rather dejected, but did not want to stay in the dark woods any longer, and began trudging home, in silence. They were too tired and sad even to argue. They had enjoyed their debates, and each had always secretly thought that they were all equal.

All of a sudden, Connie looked thoughtful. She looked at her flag, then at the others, then back in the direction from which they had come.

'You know,' she said. 'I don't think there is anything extra-special about Reggie RCT at all. He didn't get the gold standard because his way of knowing is any better than ours. His ability to test interventions is great, but so is my way of comparing groups, and Edward's way of finding out what really happens in people's lives.'

'You're right,' replied Edward, the truth suddenly dawning on him too. 'He got the gold standard because those humans who want research to help them know things value interventions more than anything else. And that's what his way tests.'

The six pixies got up again and walked in silence for a while. Then Gillie, who was lagging behind, suddenly stopped.

'I just realised something else,' she said. 'One day, the nice people will realise we all have something to offer, and maybe we can work together to find things out!'

That made the other pixies very happy. They joined hands, and began skipping back home through the woods, dreaming about what they would have for their supper and knowing – in each of their different ways – that they would all live happily ever after. Even Reggie RCT.

Index